The Ultimate Guide to Point-of-Care Ultrasound-Guided Procedures

Srikar Adhikari • Michael Blaivas
Editors

The Ultimate Guide to Point-of-Care Ultrasound-Guided Procedures

Springer

Editors
Srikar Adhikari
Department of Emergency Medicine
University of Arizona
Tucson, AZ
USA

Michael Blaivas
Department of Medicine
University of South Carolina
Columbia, SC
USA

ISBN 978-3-030-28265-3 ISBN 978-3-030-28267-7 (eBook)
https://doi.org/10.1007/978-3-030-28267-7

This Springer imprint is published by the registered company Springer Nature Switzerland AG
The registered company address is: Gewerbestrasse 11, 6330 Cham, Switzerland

Preface

One of the things I recall most distressingly from medical school and internship is struggling with procedures. Those were days when central and arterial lines were daily occurrences, every cardiac arrest got a pericardiocentesis, and thoracentesis and paracentesis were done frequently and all blindly. My many failures are still vivid in my mind, including the feeling of procedural incompetence compared to my fellow residents. Many clinicians have had the frustration of wanting to learn a new procedure or simply become more successful at ones they have tried before. Unlike those experts who act as procedure wizards and scoff at our attempts to cannulate a vein or artery, drain, or inject something or even float a temporary transvenous pacemaker, many of us would benefit from a method to significantly improve and become as good as these experts tell us they are. This is not a feeling for open discussion in the halls of academia but one which spills out in the trenches of clinical practice. How can we get a leg up and become accurate, precise, and expert-like in our procedure outcomes? It is no accident that this magical method is real, and it turns out to be ultrasound guidance.

Erasmus of Rotterdam said: "In the land of the blind, the one-eyed man is king." Ultrasound is that one eye which not only levels our playing field with the experts using blind techniques but elevates us far beyond their sightless capabilities. Is it somehow cheating to visualize a needle approaching a nerve, the location of which I had forgotten immediately after the gross anatomy test? Maybe it is, but not to our patients. They benefit from precision and ultrasound-created expertise at the bedside, not far away in a procedure room or another facility. The ability to perform procedures not previously possible or to perform old procedures with a new level of accuracy benefits patient and clinician alike. I have seen many tired senior colleagues get a second wind upon discovering ultrasound guidance for procedures.

This text is for those who are interested in improving their procedural skills or expanding their procedure toolkit and may not be diagnostic ultrasound gurus. Many clinicians just want to use ultrasound for procedure guidance and are reluctant to attend days-long courses or read massive textbooks which focus on diagnostic ultrasound use and contain occasional hidden procedural gems. If you are interested in applying ultrasound to procedure guidance, this book is for you and your patients. We both hope it improves your practice, your patients' experiences, and their access to expert procedure delivery like it has for us. We sincerely hope this text will help increase patient safety and contribute to universal adoption of ultrasound guidance for procedures.

Tucson, AZ, USA Srikar Adhikari
Columbia, SC, USA Michael Blaivas

Acknowledgments

To my wife for her love, patience, and tolerance, my daughters for constantly reminding me of the priorities in life, and my sisters and parents for their unconditional love and support.

Srikar Adhikari

To my family, I owe them everything. My incredible wife and daughters.

Michael Blaivas

Contents

Contributors

Josie Acuña, MD Department of Emergency Medicine, Banner University Medical Center-Tucson, Tucson, AZ, USA

Srikar Adhikari, MD, MS Department of Emergency Medicine, University of Arizona, Tucson, AZ, USA

Richard Amini, MD University of Arizona, Department of Emergency Medicine, Tucson, AZ, USA

Hina Arif-Tiwari, MD Department of Medical Imaging, University of Arizona, Tucson, AZ, USA

Adam Ash, DO Department of Emergency Medicine, North Shore University Hospital, Manhasset, NY, USA

Arthur Au, MD Department of Emergency Medicine, Thomas Jefferson University Hospital, Philadelphia, PA, USA

Tanya Bajaj, DO Department of Emergency Medicine, North Shore University Hospital, Manhasset, NY, USA

Michael Blaivas, MD, MBA Department of Medicine, University of South Carolina, Columbia, SC, USA

Andrew R. Bodenham, MBBS, FRCA Department of Anesthesia, Leeds General Infirmary, Leeds, UK

Brian Burke, MD Department of Radiology, North Shore University Hospital, Manhasset, NY, USA

Samita S. Das, MD, MBA Department of Anesthesiology & Critical Care Medicine, Ochsner Health System, New Orleans, LA, USA

Paola Devis, MD Medical Imaging and Gastroenterology, University of Arizona College of Medicine, Staff Interventional Radiologist, Southern Arizona Veterans Affairs Health care System, Tucson, AZ, USA

Eitan Dickman, MD, MMM, FACEP, FAIUM Department of Emergency Medicine, Maimonides Medical Center, Brooklyn, NY, USA

Robert Ellspermann, MD Department of Emergency Medicine, North Shore University Hospital, Manhasset, NY, USA

Timothy Faust, MD Department of Emergency Medicine, Thomas Jefferson University Hospital, Philadelphia, PA, USA

J. Matthew Fields, MD Department of Emergency Medicine, Thomas Jefferson University Hospital, Philadelphia, PA, USA

Maged A. Guirguis, MD Department of Interventional Pain Management, Ochsner Health System, New Orleans, LA, USA

Joshua Guttman, MD Department of Emergency Medicine, Emory University Hospital, Atlanta, GA, USA

Parisa Javedani, MD Colorado Permanente Medical Group, Denver, CO, USA

Brian Johnson, MD University of Washington – Valley Medical Center, Emergency Department, Renton, WA, USA

Dimitrios Karakitsos, MD Department of Internal Medicine, University of South Carolina, School of Medicine, Columbia, SC, USA

Pete Keenan, MD Lakewood Regional Medical Center, Lakewood, CA, USA

Los Alamitos Medical Center, Los Alamitos, CA, USA

Nat Kittisarapong, DO Department of Emergency Medicine, North Shore University Hospital, Manhasset, NY, USA

Samuel Blake Kluger, MD Ultrasound Faculty, Emergency Care Specialists, Grand Rapids, MI, USA

Ahmed Labib, FRCA Medical Intensive Care Unit, Hamad General Hospital, Doha, Qatar

Emily Lovallo, MD Department of Emergency Medicine, University of Pittsburgh School of Medicine, Pittsburgh, PA, USA

UPMC Mercy and Magee Hospitals, Pittsburgh, PA, USA

Sean Maley, MD Northwest Medical Center, Tucson, AZ, USA

Veena Modayil, MD Department of Emergency Medicine, North Shore University Hospital, Manhasset, NY, USA

Arun Nagdev, MD Highland General Hospital, Alameda Health System, Oakland, CA, USA

Bret Nelson, MD Department of Emergency Medicine, Mount Sinai Hospital, New York, NY, USA

Mathew Nelson, DO Department of Emergency Medicine, North Shore University Hospital, Manhasset, NY, USA

Kay Odashima, MD Department of Emergency Medicine, Maimonides Medical Center, Brooklyn, NY, USA

Matthew E. Patterson, MD Department of Anesthesiology & Critical Care Medicine, Ochsner Health System, New Orleans, LA, USA

Ashley Shilling, MD Department of Anesthesiology, University of Virginia, Charlottesville, VA, USA

Elaine Situ-LaCasse, MD Department of Emergency Medicine, Banner University Medical Center-Tucson, Tucson, AZ, USA

David Spinner, DO Department of Rehabiliation Medicine, Mount Sinai Hospital, New York, NY, USA

Lori Stolz, MD University of Cincinnati, Department of Emergency Medicine, Cincinnati, OH, USA

Azeem Tajani, MD Department of Emergency Medicine, Thomas Jefferson University Hospital, Philadelphia, PA, USA

Abdullah Sulieman Terkawi, MD Department of Anesthesiology, Perioperative, and Pain Medicine, Stanford University, Stanford, CA, USA

Department of Anesthesiology, King Fahad Medical City, Riyadh, Saudi Arabia

Syrian Expatriate Medical Association - US (SEMA US), Santa Clara, CA, USA

Alison Thurber, MD Emergency Medicine, SUNY Upstate University Hospital, Syracuse, NY, USA

William K. White, MD Department of Anesthesiology & Critical Care Medicine, Ochsner Health System, New Orleans, LA, USA

1 Introduction

Srikar Adhikari and Michael Blaivas

The widespread availability of portable ultrasound has increased bedside use of this technology in a variety of healthcare settings [1]. Ultrasound technology is relatively cheap and delivers no ionizing radiation to the patient or the provider. Concomitantly, the house of medicine is witnessing the largest expansion to point-of-care ultrasound in history as it moves beyond fields such as emergency medicine, critical care, and anesthesiology. With internal medicine, family medicine, and others quickly taking up point-of-care ultrasound and expanding its utilization, ultrasound may soon be at the bedside of most patients being treated in the developed and developing worlds. The use of point-of-care ultrasound for procedural guidance is rapidly increasing in clinical practice as providers realize that ultrasound allows guidance of almost any needle or device as long as an image can be obtained from the skin surface to the target organ or tissue [2]. Recent data suggests that nonradiologists are performing more ultrasound-guided procedures than radiologists and are responsible for a majority of growth in procedure volume [3].

S. Adhikari (✉)
Department of Emergency Medicine, University of Arizona, Tucson, AZ, USA
e-mail: sadhikari@aemrc.arizona.edu

M. Blaivas
Department of Medicine, University of South Carolina, Columbia, SC, USA

Performing invasive procedures safely is an important aspect of both medical education and clinical practice. Ultrasound guidance helps visualize the target precisely for directing a needle's path and avoiding adjacent structures. Ultrasound procedural guidance may involve use of a freehand technique or utilize some sort of guidance device such as a needle guide. Needle guides can take on varied shapes and sizes depending on the ultrasound transducer they will be attaching to and the type of procedure for which they will be used. Further, needle and other guides have matured significantly in the last two decades, becoming more streamlined, functional, and versatile [4].

The use of ultrasound as an adjunct to perform invasive procedures has been shown to enhance procedural success, decrease complications, improve satisfaction, and decrease time required to perform procedures. There is a robust body of evidence demonstrating that ultrasound guidance can significantly increase the safety and quality of patient care, while reducing complications and costs among patients undergoing invasive procedures [5]. The clinical efficacy of ultrasound guidance for performing procedures can be translated into significant cost savings in multiple fashions, including reduction of procedure-related complications and associated costs, decreased procedure times, reduced hospital length of stay, improved throughput, and more consistent success across a broader range of qualified healthcare providers [6].

S. Adhikari, M. Blaivas (eds.), *The Ultimate Guide to Point-of-Care Ultrasound-Guided Procedures*, https://doi.org/10.1007/978-3-030-28267-7_1

Ultrasound guidance has been shown to improve success for a simple procedure, such as peripheral intravenous catheter placement, to the most complex and technically challenging procedure, such as transvenous pacemaker placement. The use of real-time ultrasound guidance not only improves success rate but also reduces the number of attempts and the amount of anesthetic needed for certain procedures. Although less well studied, the introduction of ultrasound guidance can have a tremendous impact on provider satisfaction, feeling of competence, or mastery and even breathe new life into some clinician practices by allowing them to competently perform procedures which were once out of reach such as nerve blocks in emergency medicine, precise tendon injections in primary care, and many other examples. The use of ultrasound guidance for central venous access has become the standard of care after being recommended by multiple medical societies and supported by ample number of studies in the literature [7]. Although currently the highest quality evidence may be present for ultrasound-guided vascular access, the evidence for the use of ultrasound guidance for other procedures is rapidly increasing as well. Considerable evidence is building which demonstrates the benefits of real-time ultrasound guidance for procedures such as paracentesis, thoracentesis, arthrocentesis, and other procedures.

This technique can be broadly categorized into two groups: ultrasound assistance and real-time ultrasound guidance. Ultrasound-assisted procedures refer to evaluating patient anatomy and localization of procedure site (including target and surrounding structures) with ultrasound and do not involve real-time visualization of the needle and the target. This static method is less favored because of the potential for complications. Real-time ultrasound-guided procedures refer to the continuous visualization of the needle to direct needle placement while performing the procedure. This is the preferred technique since the location of the needle tip and target structure are continuously visualized.

Successful performance of ultrasound-guided procedures is dependent on training, experience, competence, and skills of the operator. Ultrasound-guided technique has been shown to increase operator confidence and is frequently replacing the anatomical landmark approach as the new standard for various invasive procedures. However, healthcare providers who perform ultrasound-guided procedures should be qualified to perform invasive procedures within their scope of practice. It is crucial to understand the principles of needle guidance to achieve success while using ultrasound for procedural guidance. They should receive training in the basic physical principles, ultrasound equipment, imaging modes, scanning planes, relevant sonographic anatomy needle guidance techniques, and limitations of ultrasound as they pertain to invasive procedures.

Despite growing evidence referenced above, the use of ultrasound-guided procedures is growing more slowly in nonacademic clinical settings [8]. Most of the research published to date has naturally occurred in academic settings, and more attention needs to be paid in community practice settings which represent the majority of patients seen worldwide. To have a larger and meaningful impact on patient care, it is imperative to integrate ultrasound guidance into clinical practice outside of academic centers. Providers in these settings may not even be aware of the potential available with ultrasound technology, its ever-lowering cost, and its ease of use as well as its capability. Technological advances such as beam steering software can potentially increase the ease of use and therefore adoption. In addition, artificial intelligence is rapidly making an impact on medical imaging, and multiple studies of deep learning applications in point-of-care ultrasound will soon be emerging as well and as commercially available artificial intelligence aps for real ultrasound machines.

In summary, adopting ultrasound guidance for procedural performance can increase safety, improve speed, simply comply with the new standard of care, improve patient satisfaction, and also radically improve the feeling of mastery and accomplishment by clinicians who gain access to procedures they were once unable to perform. Anecdotally, we have seen this in a variety of practice settings, and this repeatable finding is not limited to any provider age or experience group. It is likely that ultrasound guidance will one day be the standard of care for virtually every procedure in which ultrasound can visualize the intended target, but long before that, both providers and patients are increasingly benefiting from its increased utilization. We hope this book will move you forward in your discovery and mastery of ultrasound guidance in procedural performance.

References

1. American College of Emergency Physicians. Ultrasound guidelines: emergency, point-of-care and clinical ultrasound guidelines in medicine. Ann Emerg Med. 2017;69(5):e27–54.
2. Rippey J. Ultrasound guidance should be the standard of care for most invasive procedures performed by clinicians. Australas J Ultrasound Med. 2012; 15(4):116–20.
3. McGahan J, Pozniak M, Cronan J, et al. Handheld ultrasound: threat or opportunity? Appl Radiol. 2015; 44(3):20–5.
4. Ueshima H, Kitamura A. The use of a needle guide kit improves the stability of ultrasound-guided techniques. J Anesth. 2015;29(5):803–4.
5. Patel PA, Ernst FR, Gunnarsson CL. Evaluation of hospital complications and costs associated with using ultrasound guidance during abdominal paracentesis procedures. J Med Econ. 2012;15:1–7.
6. Nicolaou S, Talsky A, Khashoggi K, Venu V. Ultrasound guided interventional radiology in critical care. Crit Care Med. 2007;35:S186–97.
7. Adhikari S, Theodoro D, Raio C, Nelson M, Lyon M, Leech S, Akhtar S, Stolz U. Central venous catheterization: are we using ultrasound guidance? J Ultrasound Med. 2015;34(11):2065–70.
8. Amini R, Wyman MT, Hernandez NC, Guisto JA, Adhikari S. Use of emergency ultrasound in Arizona Community Emergency Departments. J Ultrasound Med. 2017;36(5):913–21.

Principles of Ultrasound Guidance

2

Elaine Situ-LaCasse and Josie Acuña

Introduction

Procedures guided by ultrasound have been proven to be far safer than the conventional landmark-based technique [1]. Central venous catheter placements are expected to be placed using ultrasound, and it is now considered the standard of care [2].

For those who are not trained in the use of bedside ultrasound, ultrasound-guided procedures may appear daunting. However, the principles and techniques are straightforward, and with some education and practice, any healthcare provider can safely perform procedures under the guidance of ultrasound, taking the guesswork out of the needle tip location. It is important to understand that the basic procedure remains the same and is not affected by the addition of ultrasound guidance per se. Thus, providers should not view adding ultrasound guidance as having to relearn how to perform a procedure. This chapter covers the basic principles of ultrasound and its use for procedural guidance, and once these principles are understood, they can be applied to the most commonly performed procedures.

E. Situ-LaCasse (✉) · J. Acuña
Department of Emergency Medicine,
Banner University Medical Center-Tucson,
Tucson, AZ, USA
e-mail: esitu@aemrc.arizona.edu

Basic Physics

Although one does not need to know ultrasound physics to operate the machine, understanding the basics will allow the user to improve image quality and better utilize the technology. Physics topics will be briefly reviewed in this chapter, and they can be directly applied to clinical ultrasound use.

Sound is energy transmitted through a medium, be it air, liquid, or solid. Ultrasound is beyond the audible range of humans, which means any sound frequency greater than 20,000 Hz. Ultrasound has been harnessed into imaging technology, and diagnostic ultrasound typically ranges between 2.5 MHz and 15 MHz. There are newer ultrasound transducers that emit higher frequencies for improved imaging of superficial structures [3]. Clinical indications for use of the various transducers will be discussed later in the chapter.

Ultrasound systems transmit electrical current through the cord of the ultrasound transducer, causing special piezoelectric crystals in the probe to vibrate. This energy from the vibrations is transmitted into the patient's body in the form of sound. As the sound travels through the body, it collides with various structures, and the sound waves bounce or reflect back toward the transducer. The transducer is constantly monitoring for returning sound waves while recording them. This information travels back to the machine,

S. Adhikari, M. Blaivas (eds.), *The Ultimate Guide to Point-of-Care Ultrasound-Guided Procedures*, https://doi.org/10.1007/978-3-030-28267-7_2

and the processed data becomes the ultrasound image on the monitor.

To understand diagnostic ultrasound, one must understand the interaction between the sound waves and the structures of the human body. *Impedance* is the resistance to the propagation of sound, and ultrasound uses sound waves to detect impedance mismatch to differentiate structures [4]. Different tissues have varying levels of impedance. For example, bone has higher impedance, which means it reflects most of the ultrasound signal back to the ultrasound transducer, yielding a brighter image. On the contrary, fluid has little to no impedance, so the ultrasound signal travels through the fluid with no reflection of the signal, yielding black image on the screen. Liver is a structure that has levels of impedance between bone and fluid, appearing as various shades of gray on the monitor (Fig. 2.1).

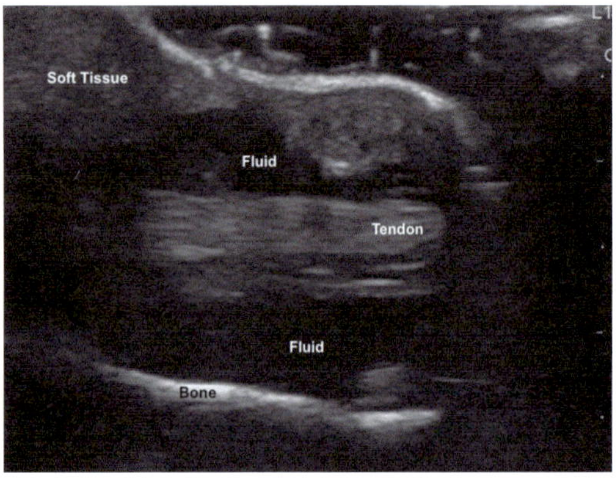

Fig. 2.1 This image shows tissues of various impedances. Note that the fluid is dark, having little to no impedance. The bone has high impedance, which is seen as bright on this image. The rest of the tissues have levels of impedance between the bone and fluid, appearing as various shades of gray

Attenuation is defined as the decrease in intensity, power, and amplitude of a sound wave as it passes through a medium. This can also be described as acoustic loss [5]. There are three components of attenuation: absorption, scattering, and reflection [6]. Air has the most attenuation, and that is why gel is used to remove air from the path of the sound beams when performing an ultrasound study. Bone attenuates less than air, absorbing some but reflecting more sound. Water attenuates the sound energy the least, transmitting almost all the sound beams and reflecting very little.

Learning about attenuation segues into learning echogenicity. *Echogenicity* is the brightness of an object on the ultrasound image. If a structure is *hyperechoic*, it is white or bright. If a tissue is *hypoechoic* or less bright, it is seen as shades of gray. An object that is *anechoic*, such as a fluid-filled structure, will appear black on the image (Fig. 2.2). The term isoechoic describes two adjacent structures or tissues that are the same echogenicity.

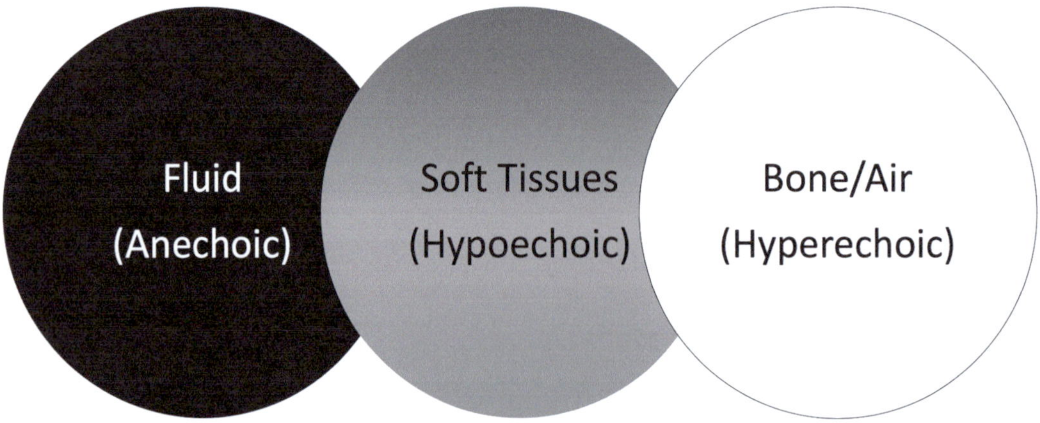

Fig. 2.2 Echogenicity refers to brightness of structures. Fluid is considered anechoic, tissues such as liver can be considered hypoechoic, and bone on ultrasound is hyperechoic

Knobology

Ultrasound machines and their control panels vary widely in design depending on manufacturers, but the functions are essentially the same (Fig. 2.3a, b). The understanding of the different knob functions, or knobology, is necessary to operate an ultrasound machine. The basic functions are gain, time gain compensation (TGC), depth, zoom, freeze, measurements, and calculations. Advanced knobology includes M-mode, Doppler, color Doppler, power Doppler, focus, harmonics, optimization, and presets [7]. Most of the listed functions above will be discussed in the coming sections of this chapter.

a

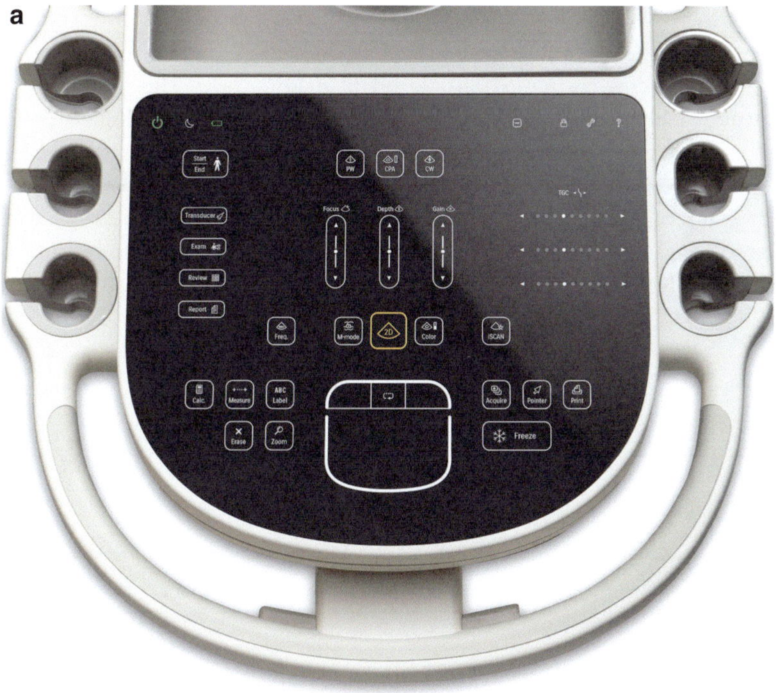

b

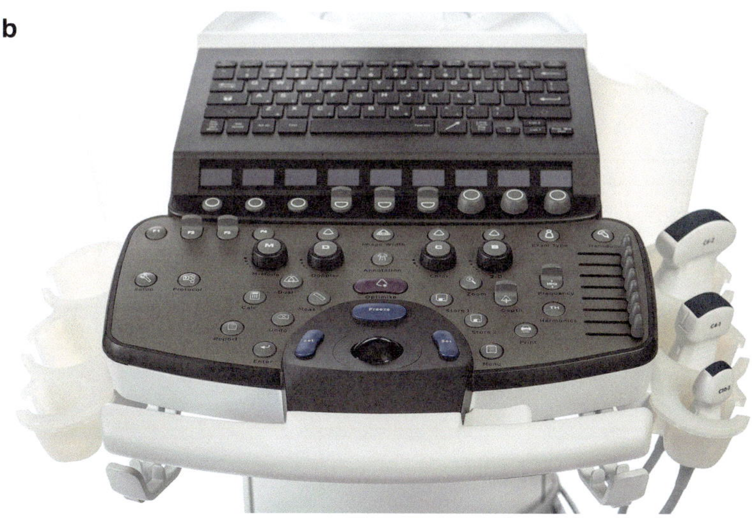

Fig. 2.3 (**a**, **b**) Examples of different control panels from different manufacturers. (**a**) Touch screen control panel from Philips. (**b**) Control panel with knobs from Zonare

Probes/Frequency

Ultrasound probes, or transducers, have a wide range of frequencies, and one should choose the correct frequency range or bandwidth, to best image the body region of interest [5]. The most common transducers are linear array, convex or curved array, and phased array (Fig. 2.4a, b).

Linear array probes produce higher frequencies, designed to image superficial structures. Some linear probes are designed to produce lower frequencies, which allow imaging of deeper structures. For linear array probes, groups of in-line crystal elements are turned on and off in increments, creating individual echo lines as each group of elements is activated, creating a rectangular image [5]. These probes generally have a flat scanning surface, and the section of tissue being imaged, or sector, is exactly the surface area of the probe footprint (Fig. 2.5a, b). The frequency of linear probes is generally considered to be 10–5 MHz. However, modern broadband transducers often range from 5 or 6 to as high as 14 or even 16 MHz. There are linear probes that operate at a much higher frequency, significantly improving image quality of superficial structures. Breast and musculoskeletal ultrasound imaging have transitioned to using higher-frequency linear array transducers [5].

Curved array probes have a curved footprint and produce lower frequencies, so the sound waves penetrate deeper into the body. These transducers are similar to the linear array, except the crystal elements are arranged on a curved surface. This is typically used for imaging of the thorax, abdomen, and pelvis. For patients with a larger body habitus, the curved array or curvilinear probe can be used to image the buttocks or thighs. The image sector is wider than the footprint of the probe itself (Fig. 2.6a, b), similar to a pie slice with a bite taken out of the top [5].

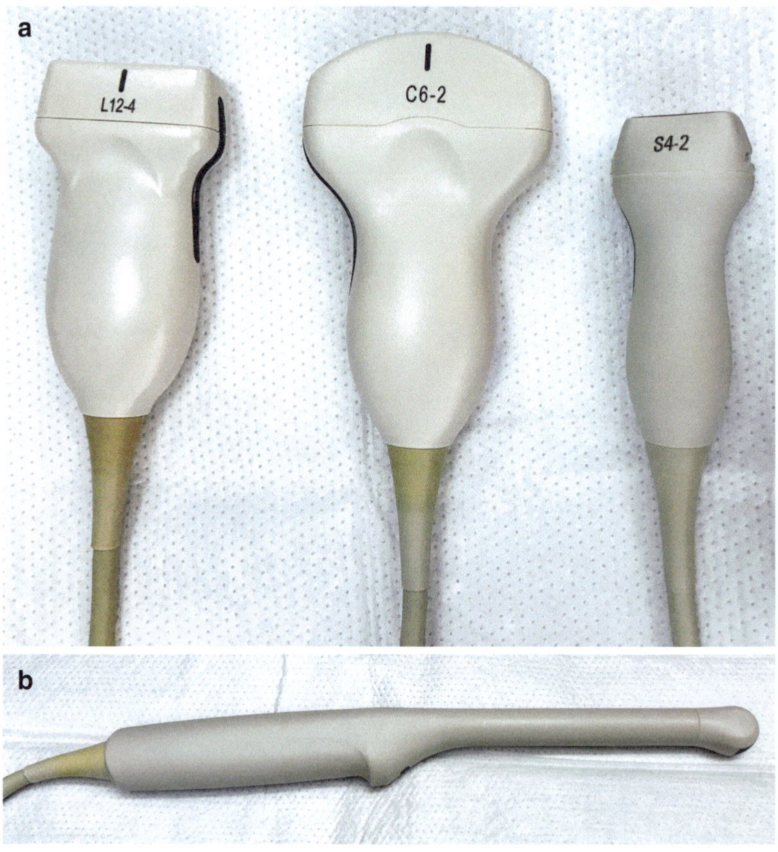

Fig. 2.4 (**a**, **b**) The most commonly used ultrasound transducers. (**a**) From left to right: linear array, convex array, and phased array. (**b**) Endocavitary transducer, which is another example of curved array probe

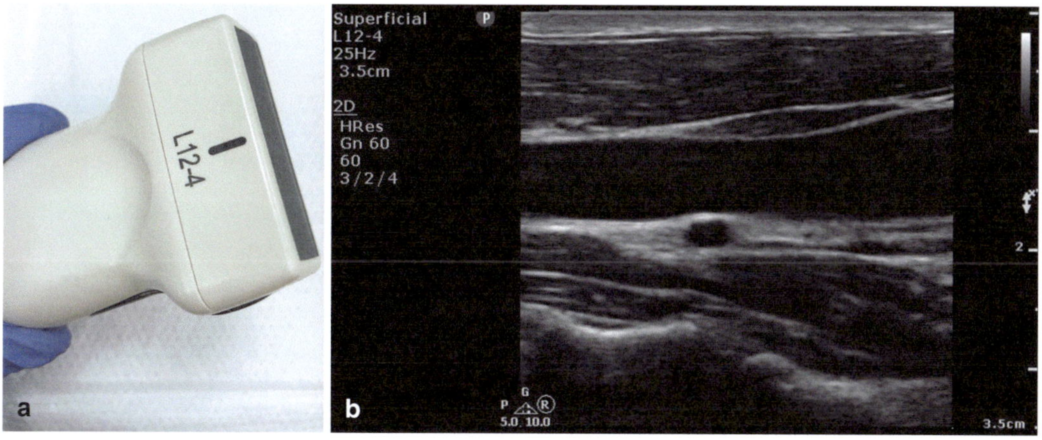

Fig. 2.5 (**a**) Rectangular, flat scanning surface of a linear transducer. (**b**) The image sector of a linear transducer is a rectangle, exactly the length of its footprint

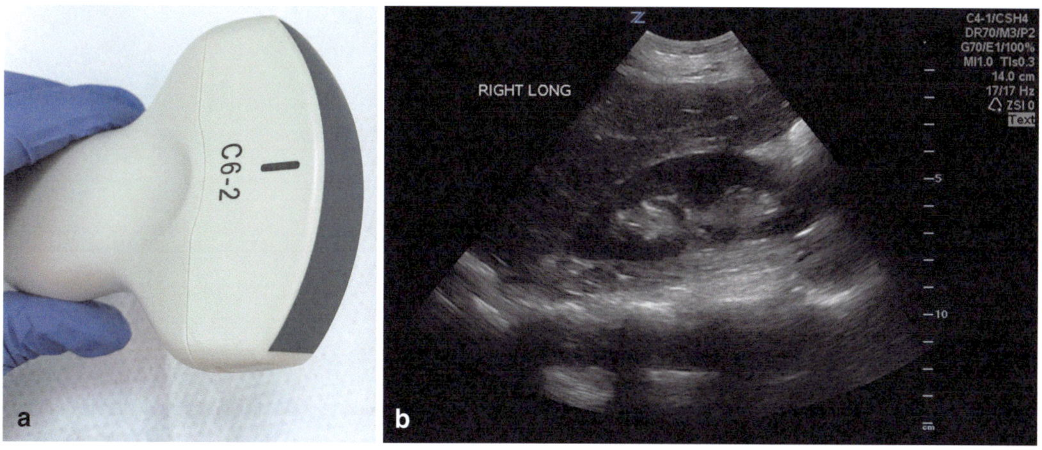

Fig. 2.6 (**a**) Convex array probe emits lower-frequency sound waves. (**b**) It creates a wedge-shaped image that fans out, exceeding the footprint of the scanning surface

Another curved array probe is the endocavitary probe. The crystals and scanning surface are at the end of a long handle. This is designed for intraoral, transvaginal, and transrectal imaging. The sector of imaging is quite wide, up to almost 180° (Fig. 2.7a, b). This probe sends out higher frequencies (13–8 MHz), producing high-resolution images of structures with little tissue between the probe and the structure of interest [7]. The endocavitary probe can be used intraorally to diagnose and drain peritonsillar abscesses. It can also be used transvaginally to better evaluate pelvic structures, such as evaluating for early pregnancy, ectopic pregnancy, torsion, tubo-ovarian abscesses, etc. Urologists use the endocavitary probe for prostate evaluation as well [5].

Phased array probes have a flat scanning surface. The crystals are grouped tightly, and each crystal element is activated with each ultrasound pulse [7]. The probe creates a wedge-shaped image. Phased array probes are mainly used for echocardiograms, but it can also be used for thoracic and intra-abdominal imaging. The small footprint fits well in between the ribs, increasing maneuverability (Fig. 2.8a, b).

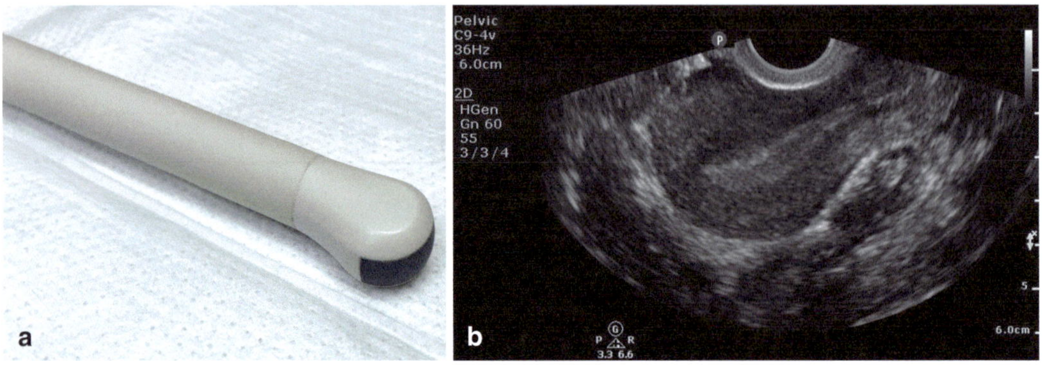

Fig. 2.7 (**a**) The scanning surface of an endocavitary probe is convex and small. (**b**) The generated image is wide, almost giving 180° view

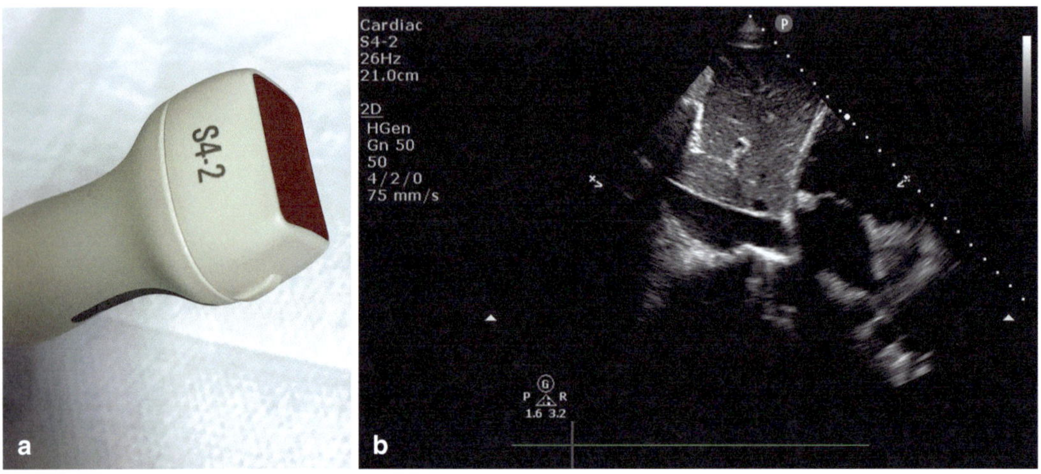

Fig. 2.8 (**a**) Phased array probe with small footprint, which fits between ribs well to image the heart. (**b**) The image generated is wedge-shaped

Presets

Ultrasound machines have various examination presets for different probes (Fig. 2.9). Acoustic power, gain, focal zones, lines per sector, sector size, and other settings are optimized to the ideal level for that particular exam [7]. For example, obstetric presets lower the power output to FDA-approved levels [7, 8]. Cardiac settings increase frame rate at the expense of image quality so it can keep up with the cardiac activity. There are also calculation packages that have preset formulas. An example is calculating cardiac stroke volume. The user needs to activate the calculation package and make a few measurements, and the calculation package will give you the results after using its preprogrammed formula (Fig. 2.10). Presets can also be customized, depending on the machine manufacturer.

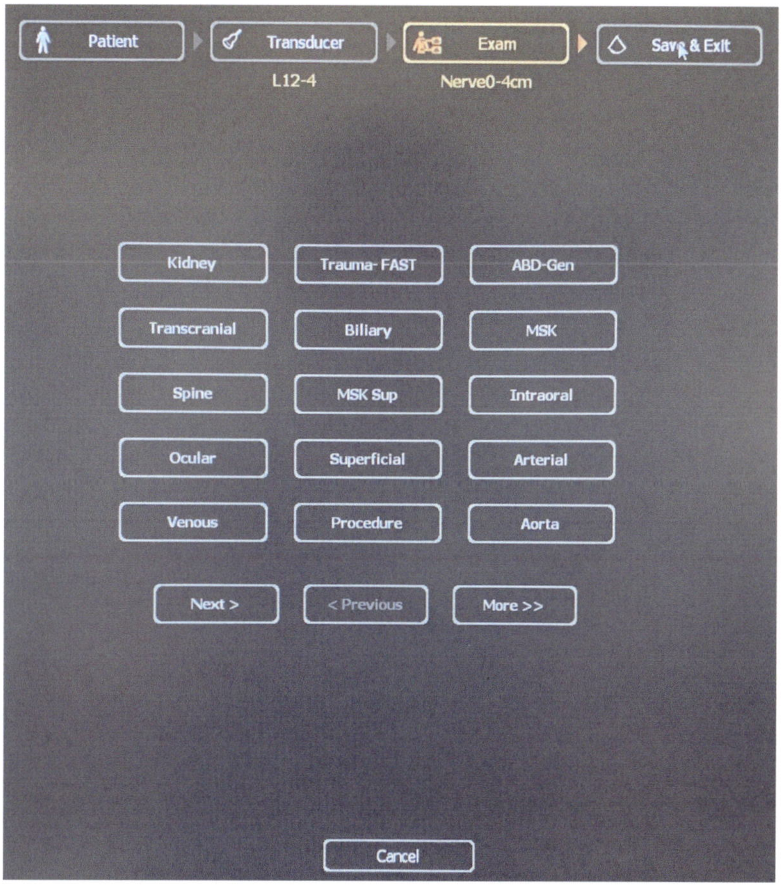

Fig. 2.9 Example of presets for linear probe

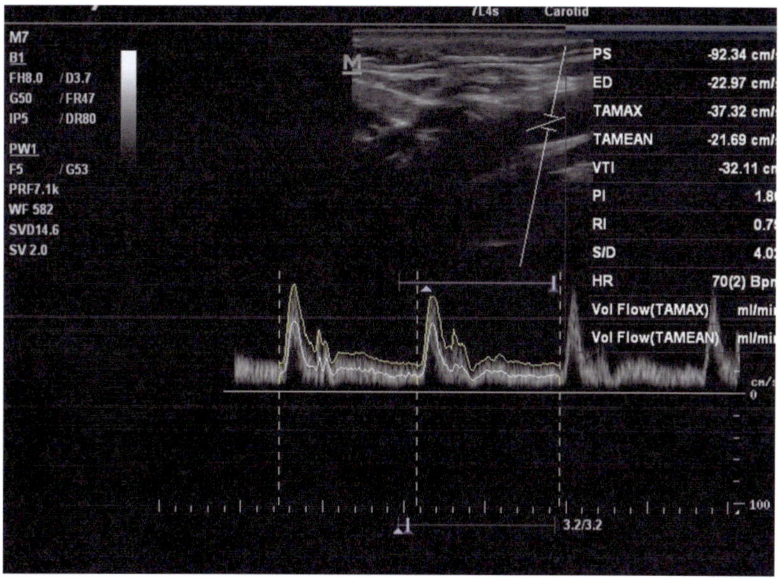

Fig. 2.10 Example of calculation package preset for carotid VTi for stroke volume calculation

Depth and Gain

There are buttons on the machine's control panel that allow you to adjust the displayed image field in one centimeter (or half centimeter) gradation increments. When increasing the *depth*, the structures in the image sector become smaller to accommodate imaging of the deeper structures and vice versa. It is important to remember to decrease the depth if you do not need deeper imaging, so the structures of interest are better visualized with higher resolution (Fig. 2.11a, b). The machine also monitors longer for reflected sound waves when the depth is increased, which reduces the frame rate, hence the temporal resolution. This means the stream of images will not be as smooth. This can be an issue with diagnostic accuracy and procedural guidance [7].

Another common adjustment to improve image quality is to increase *gain*. Increasing gain of an image means increasing the brightness of the image. The machine increases the amplitude of the signals after they have returned to the probe [9]. If the gain is increased above the optimum level, subtler findings may be obscured (Fig. 2.12a, b).

To adjust the gain of the various levels of an image, one can adjust the time gain compensation (TGC). Ultrasound beams are progressively

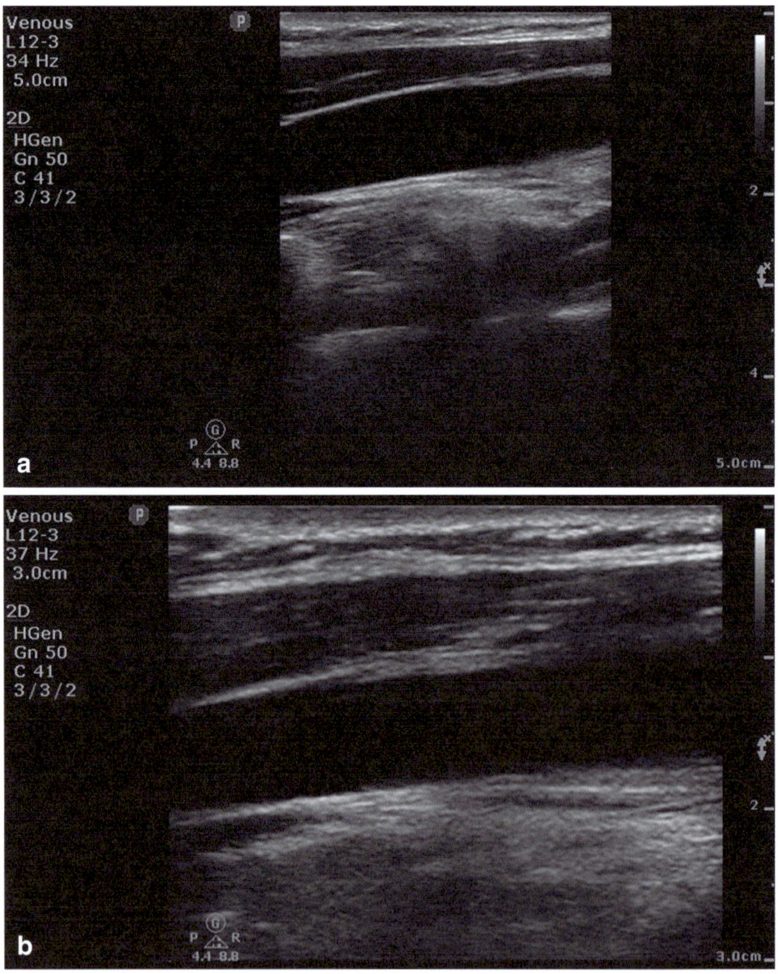

Fig. 2.11 (**a**) The structure of interest, the vein, is not in the center of the image. The imaging of deeper structures is not necessary, so the depth should be decreased to place the vein in the middle of the image. (**b**) Example of appropriately adjusted depth to visualize the vein

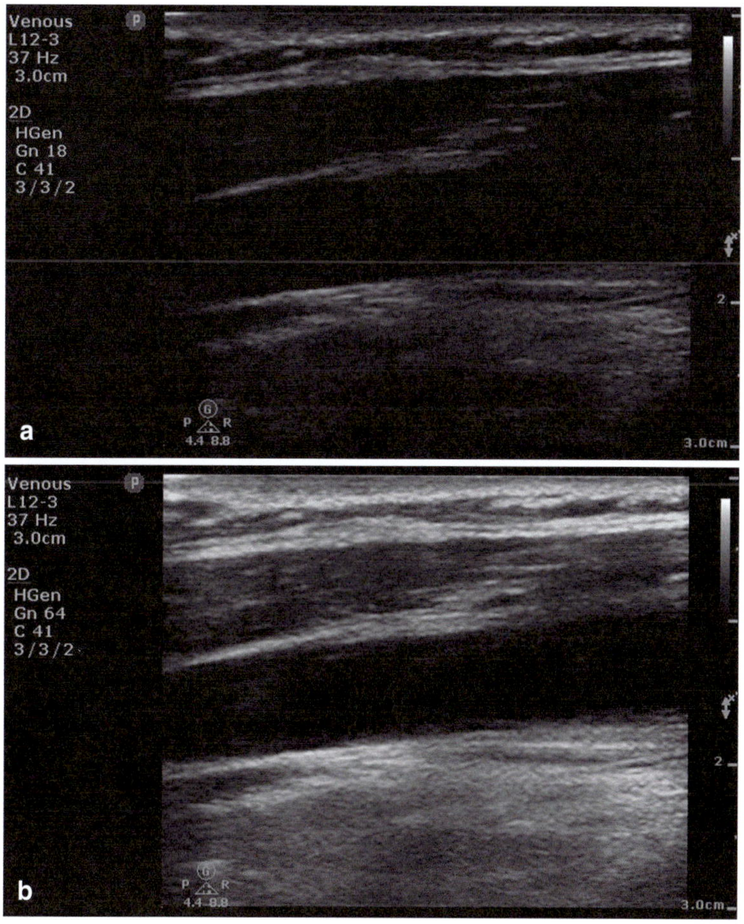

Fig. 2.12 (**a**) Example of a poorly gained image. This image is too dark, obscuring details of the structures. (**b**) Well-gained image after optimizing the gain settings on the ultrasound machine

attenuated as they travel through different tissues in the body. Therefore, strength of echoes returning from greater depths is weaker. TGC function allows to selectively amplify the signals returning from greater depths, so that equal reflectors at varying depths are displayed as structures of equal brightness on the screen [9]. At times, the machine may automatically overgain or undergain certain parts of the image depending on the type of tissue ultrasound beams go through, and the user can optimize the image manually by using TGC. Machines can vary on what type of buttons is used to adjust TGC. Some use knobs, allowing the user to turn the knobs to adjust the gain in the near field or far field. Other machines have sliders that correspond to different depths of the image, allowing the user to adjust the brightness of multiple levels more smoothly (Fig. 2.13a–d).

Focus

Ultrasound probes transmit sound waves in the shape of an hourglass, with the best resolution typically in the narrowest point (center) of the hourglass which is known as focal point [5]. The area just above and below where the ultrasound beam is still relatively narrow is the focal zone, and the sound waves converge to focal zone and then diverge from the focal zone. The broad converging beam above the focal zone near the footprint of the transducer is the near field, and the diverging broad beam beyond the focal zone is the far field. Machines allow the user to adjust the location of the focus or even add multiple foci to the region of interest (Fig. 2.14). However, although this may increase the lateral resolution, the temporal resolution will decrease, since the machine is taking more time to listen to returning signals.

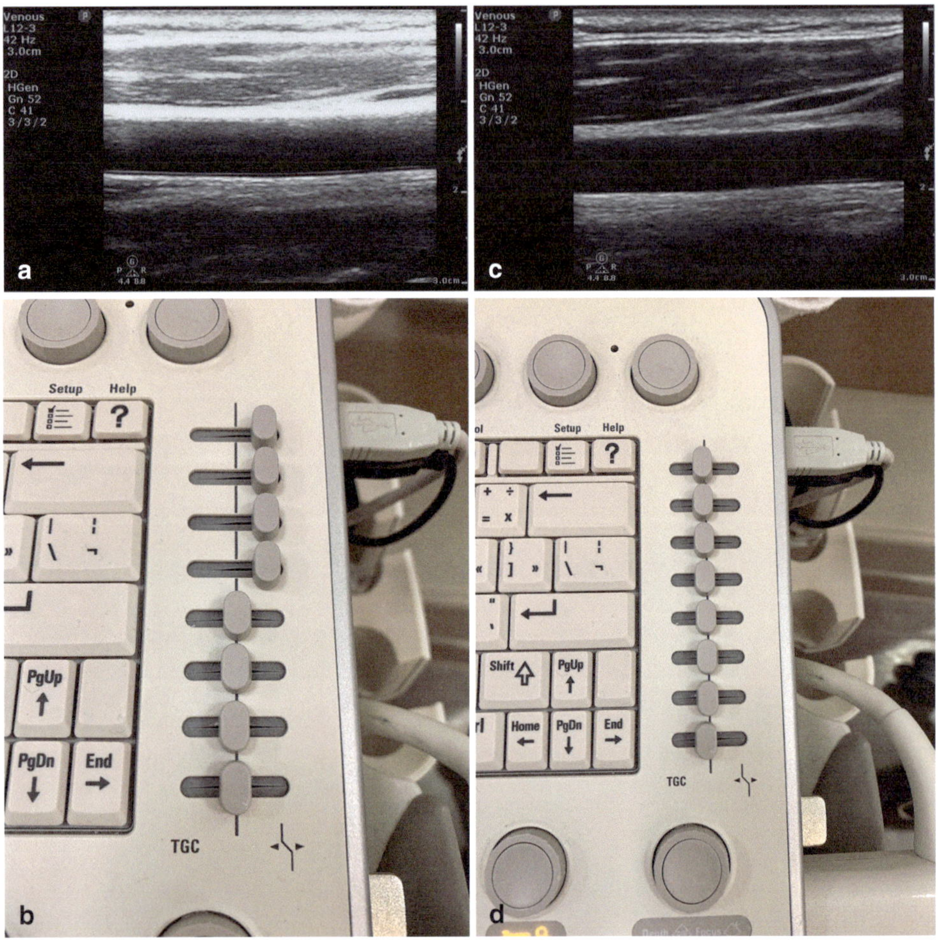

Fig. 2.13 (**a**–**d**) Examples of gain adjustments with TGC. (**a**) The image shows the near field being over-gained, causing the details to be unclear in the more superficial structures. (**b**) The TGC knobs with the over-gained near field. (**c**) The image's gain has been improved by adjusting the TGC knobs in the near field. (**d**) The TGC knobs after decreasing the near field gain to optimize the image

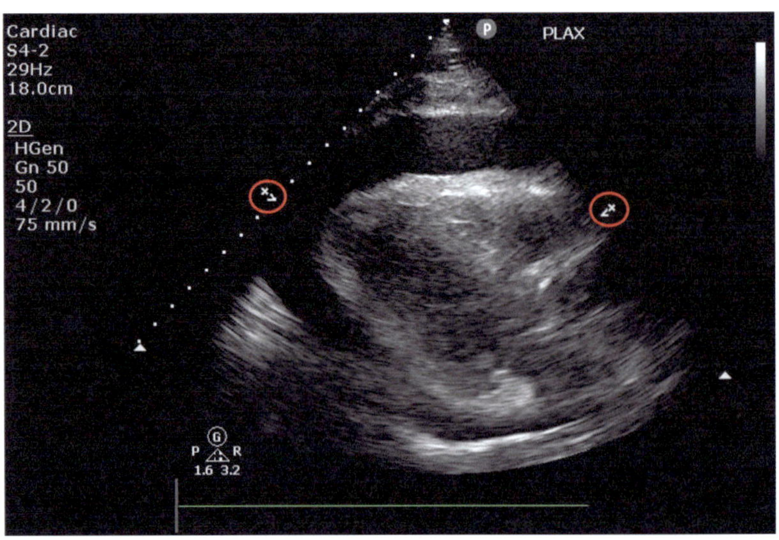

Fig. 2.14 The focal point of the image is denoted by a unique symbol on the ultrasound image. In this cardiac image, the circles highlight the location of the focus. This can be adjusted on the ultrasound machine

Optimization

Perhaps the most frequently used button on the control panel is the button that automatically optimizes the image by changing the acoustic power, gain, focus, and harmonics [7]. There are various names for this button, but the principle is the same. This is a good start to improving image quality, since it is simple and effective, but the user should also know how to change each of the above settings separately (Fig. 2.15a, b).

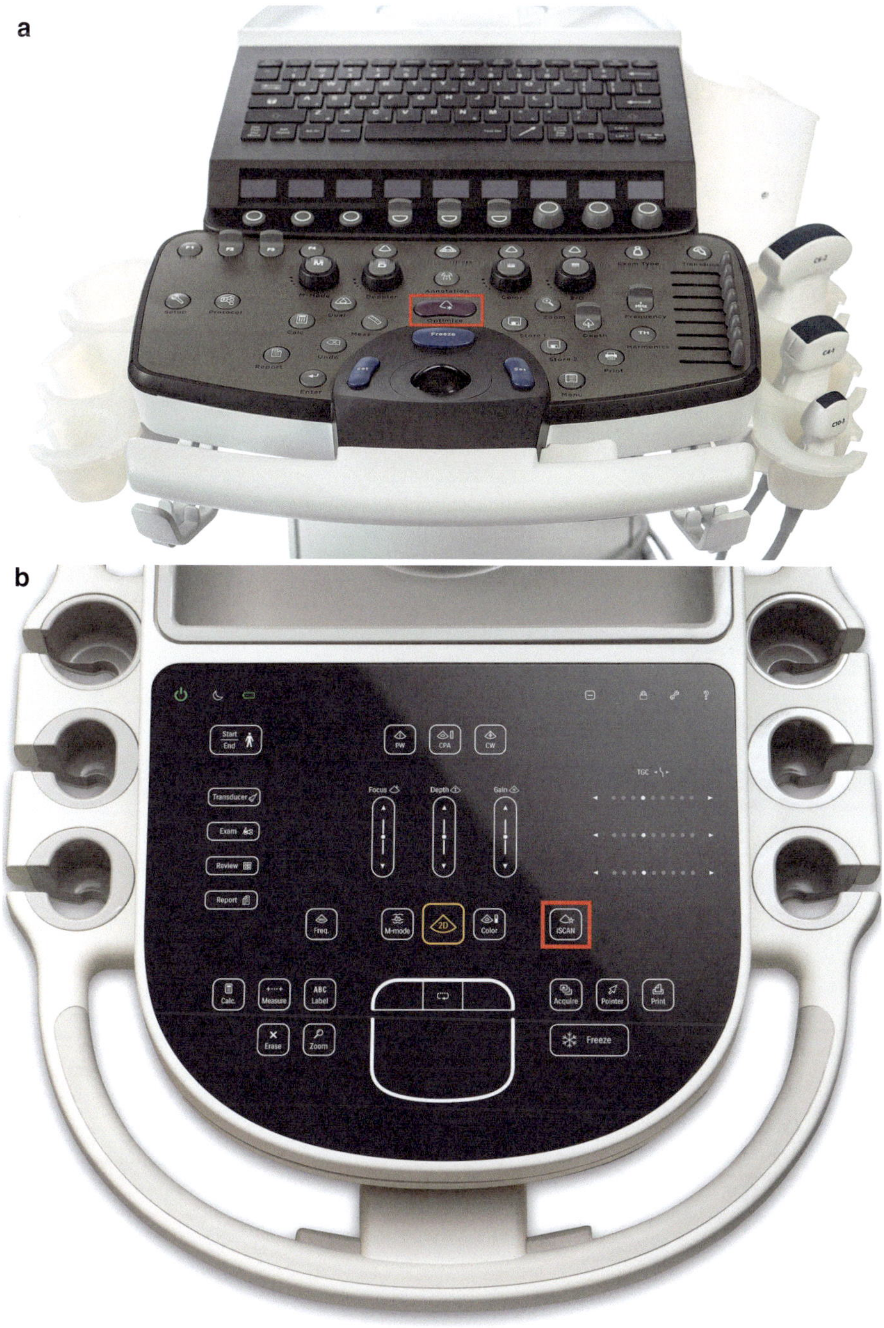

Fig. 2.15 (**a**, **b**) Optimization button automatically adjusts multiple settings to improve the image quality. Manufacturers can give the button a different name, but it will do the same thing. (**a**) Optimize button on Zonare control panel. (**b**) Another button design for the same function from Philips

Freeze and Image Saving

One of the key functions of the ultrasound machine is the ability to capture a still image with the "Freeze" button. Pressing the "Freeze" button will preserve a snapshot of whatever is on the screen. This still image will stay on the screen until you press the "Freeze" button a second time, and the image will be in real-time again. To save a frozen image to the machine or to an ultrasound image repository, the "Save" or "Clip" button should be pressed (Fig. 2.16). Typically, there is a button on the control panel that allows you to save the image. After pressing the "Freeze" button, the operator can also scroll through the previous frames on the internal memory of ultrasound machine hard drive to select the best image for saving. A benefit of ultrasound is the dynamic nature of image acquisition, so machines will also allow recording of a cine loop prospectively or retrospectively. The length of each clip can be adjusted as well.

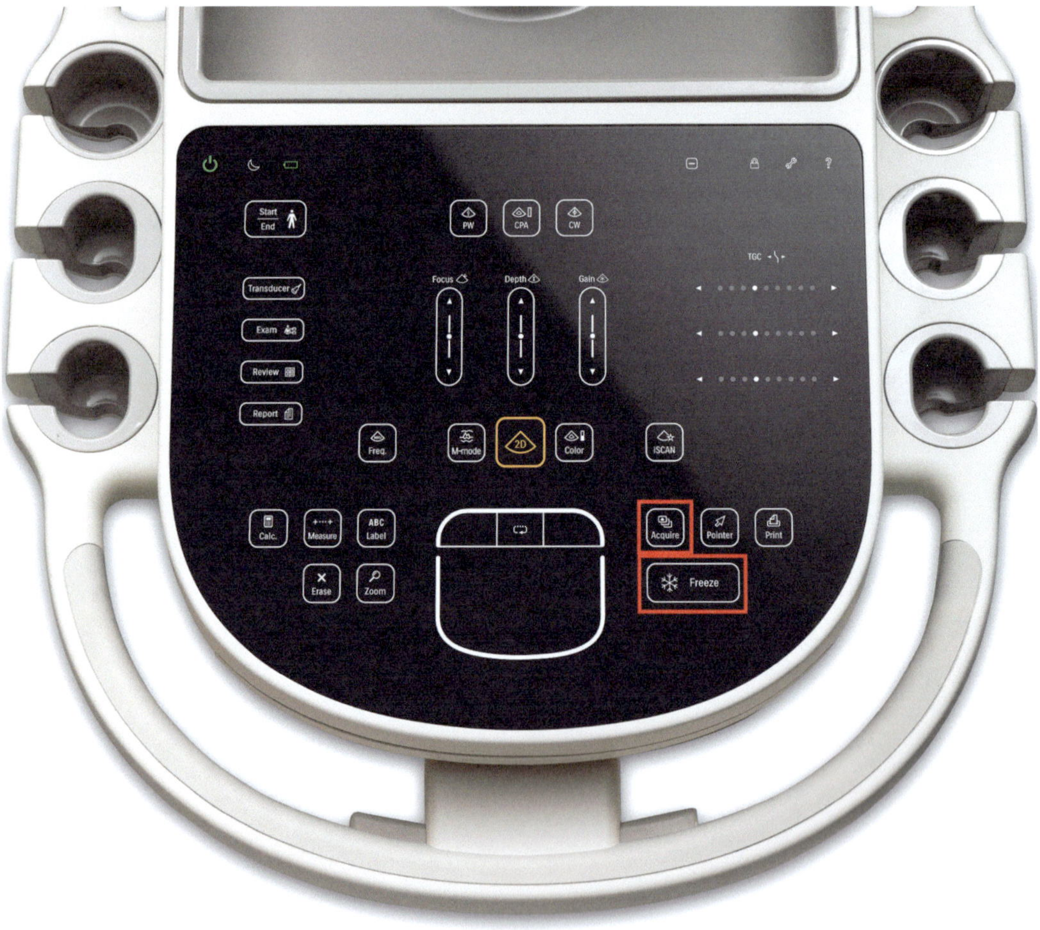

Fig. 2.16 The "Freeze" and "Acquire" (image saving) buttons on Philips machine

Color Doppler, Power Doppler, and Pulsed-Wave Doppler

In the mid-1950s, Japanese researchers took mathematician and physicist Christian Doppler's theories on the color differences between stars and used them to describe flow velocities in blood vessels. They determined that Doppler signals were being generated when sound waves were reflected by moving red blood cells, with frequency shifts determined by the speed of the flow and the output voltage determined by the number of particles [10, 11].

In the 1970s, Doppler was incorporated into clinical ultrasound [10, 11]. Doppler detects movement toward or away from the transducer, and *color Doppler* is typically represented by gradients of red and blue on the screen. The brightness of the color is proportional to the flow velocity, and turbulence is seen as small sections of yellow or green [10, 11]. The color key is located on the side of the screen. Typically, the color at the top of the color key means flow toward the probe, and the color at the bottom of the key means away from the probe. It is important to remember that the typical red-blue color scheme is unrelated to arterial or venous flow. There is a weaker Doppler signal if the probe is held at 90° to the flow. To improve the signal, angle the probe away from 90°. For low-flow states, consider using power Doppler.

Power Doppler detects and displays flow without taking into account the direction of the flow. Instead of two or more colors, power Doppler is usually various shades of one color (frequently orange) [7]. Power Doppler is more sensitive, so it picks up slower flow, but at the same time, it is more vulnerable to motion artifact (Fig. 2.17a, b). The angle of the probe is less important in power Doppler as compared to color Doppler.

Because the Doppler settings send more energy into the body creating heat, avoid using Doppler on sensitive structures, such as a fetus during an obstetric exam or the back of the eye during an ocular ultrasound [8].

Pulsed-wave Doppler (PW Doppler) is used to measure the velocity of blood flow at a single point or a small, user-determined window of area. The transducer sends out short, quick pulses of sound and waits for that pulsed signal to return, allowing the calculation of the flow at that single point. With the need to wait for the signal to return, there is a limit to how quickly and how accurately the machine measures the velocity. PW Doppler waveforms can be used to distinguish a normal arterial wave form which demonstrates pulsatility from a normal venous waveform which shows respiratory phasicity. This can assist in the placement of a needle or catheter into a vein while performing vascular access procedures using ultrasound guidance (Fig. 2.17c–e) [7].

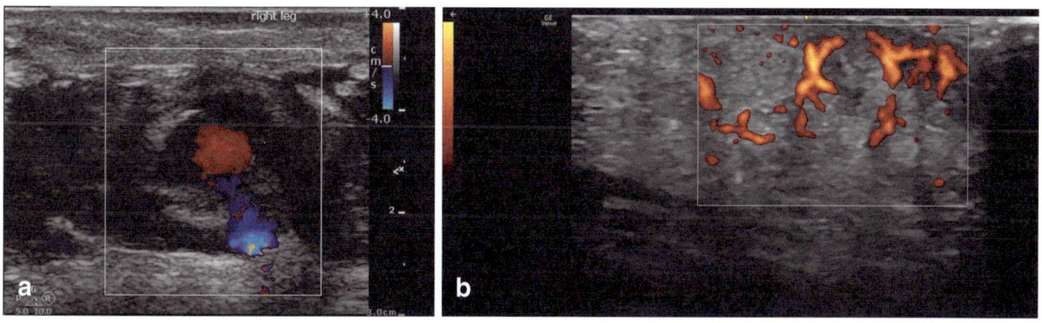

Fig. 2.17 (**a**) Color Doppler signal denoted by red and blue. Red for flow toward the probe and blue for flow away from the probe. (**b**) For low-flow states, power Doppler may be used. Power Doppler does not account for the direction of the flow. (**c**) Example of pulsed-wave Doppler arterial waveform demonstrating pulsatility. (**d**) Pulsed-wave Doppler venous waveform showing phasicity. (**e**) The buttons on the Mindray for color (C), power (P), and pulsed-wave (PW) Doppler settings

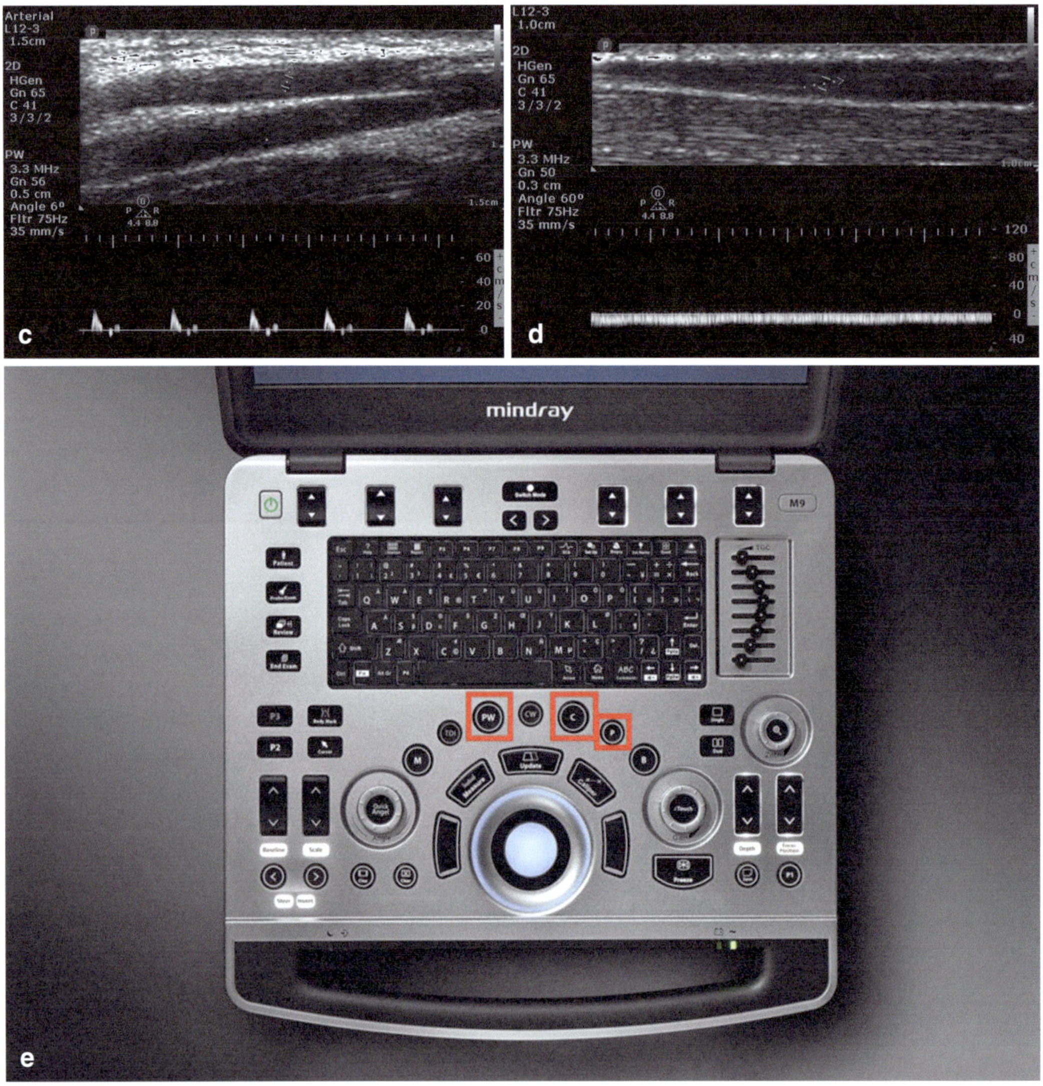

Fig. 2.17 (continued)

Compound Imaging

Compound imaging combines three or more images together to create an image with fewer artifacts and shadows (Fig. 2.18a, b) [12]. Echoes from the probe are sent from multiple angles to image the same tissue, increasing resolution and edge detail. Only linear and convex transducers are capable of compound imaging. Compound imaging can improve contrast resolution and tissue differentiation for imaging of peripheral blood vessels, breast tissue, and various musculoskeletal injuries [12]. Very superficial structures will not benefit from this technology, and it is less effective for imaging of deep structures.

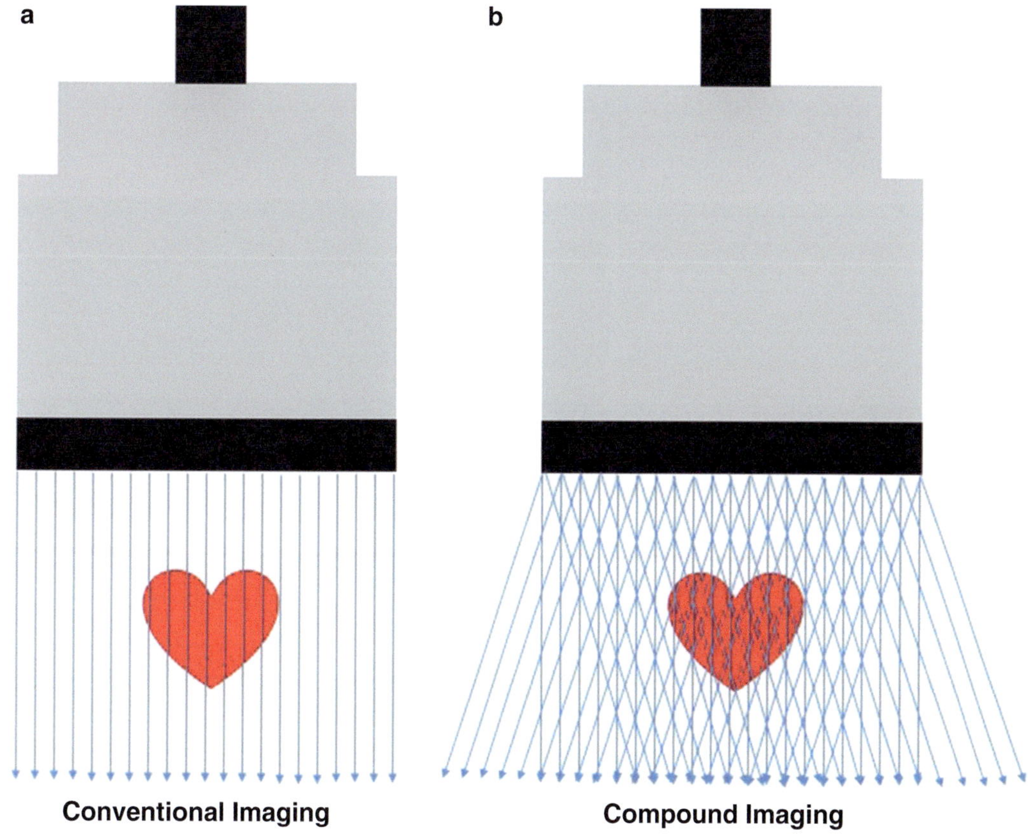

Fig. 2.18 (**a**) Conventional ultrasound imaging emits one set of sound waves. (**b**) Compound ultrasound imaging emits multiple sets of sound waves from different angles to better image a structure, decreasing artifacts and shadows

Tissue Harmonic Imaging

When ultrasound probes send out sound pulses and listen for the signal, those signals return at the primary frequency and harmonic frequencies (2×, 4×, 6×, 8×) of the original [7]. Harmonic frequencies produce less scatter and side-lobe artifacts (occurs when ultrasound beam strikes a highly reflective structure to the side of a hypoechoic structure), creating a crisper image [13]. This means that these harmonic frequencies can penetrate into deeper tissues and produce a higher-resolution image. *Tissue harmonic imaging* is a filtration setting that can be turned on and off. It filters the primary frequency signal and only uses the harmonic frequencies to generate the image [5]. This can be helpful in difficult-to-scan patients but can worsen image quality in others.

Improving Needle Visibility

One of the challenges of ultrasound-guided procedures is the ability to continuously visualize the needle tip for efficacy and safety. Irrespective of the skill of the operator in ultrasound-guided procedures, there is always the potential risk of the needle penetrating adjacent structures and thereby causing damage to surrounding structures such as arteries, nerve bundles, and pleura. Even if the target structure is clearly defined and recognizable, achieving optimal needle placement can still be an obstacle. There is a variety of advancements to enhance nee-

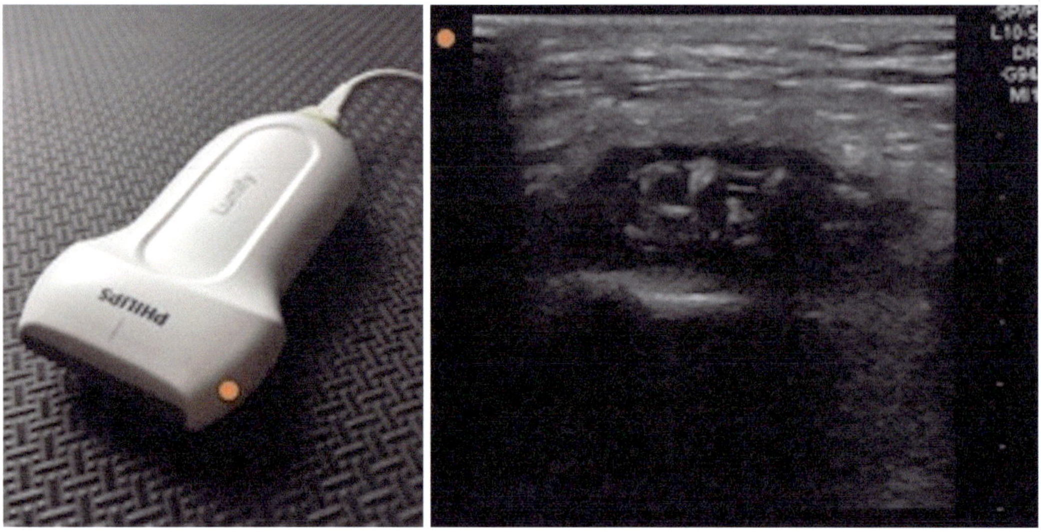

Fig. 2.19 There is a physical marker found on each ultrasound probe that corresponds to a side of the display screen

dle visibility such as improvements in transducer technology and echogenic needle design [14].

Ultrasound Probe Orientation

A true understanding of probe orientation is vital to performing a successful and safe ultrasound-guided procedure. Each transducer has an indicator marker. This marker corresponds to an indicator on the machine's display (Fig. 2.19).

To best explain ultrasound-guided procedures, ultrasound-guided intravenous (IV) access will be used as the main example, and the linear array probe is to be used. There are three main needle visualization approaches to all venous access: out-of-plane (short axis), in-plane (long axis), and oblique. In the out-of-plane (short-axis) needle visualization approach, the marker on the ultrasound probe and the marker on the ultrasound machine screen should correspond. If the needle moves to the right side of the ultrasound probe, the needle also moves to the right on the ultrasound machine display. This helps to accurately move the needle right to left while directing the needle toward the target structure. In the in-plane (long-axis) or oblique needle visualization approach, it is imperative to determine which way the probe marker is directed so the operator knows which side of the screen the needle will come into view (i.e., the right or left of the image). For each approach explained below, needle probe alignment, angle of approach, and skin insertion site and angle will be discussed.

Utilizing the Out-of-Plane (Short Axis) Approach

The out-of-plane (short-axis) needle visualization approach allows visualization of the target in cross section. This view is obtained by placing the ultrasound probe perpendicular to the long axis of the target (Fig. 2.20). Place sterile ultrasound gel on the skin above the vein and on the footprint of the sterile ultrasound probe. Grasp the ultrasound probe with the nondominant hand and the needle with the dominant hand. Reidentify the target structure and the optimal site of needle insertion. Adjust the ultrasound probe to center the target on the ultrasound machine display. The midpoint of the ultrasound probe now becomes the reference point for needle insertion.

Select the skin entry site to maximize the possibility of the tip of the needle puncturing the vein as well as intersecting the ultrasound probe scan plane. The geometry of the Pythagorean theorem ($a^2 + b^2 = c^2$) can be used to assess the distance to insert the needle into the skin and away from the ultrasound probe (Fig. 2.21). Measure the distance from the skin surface to the center of the target structure on the ultrasound

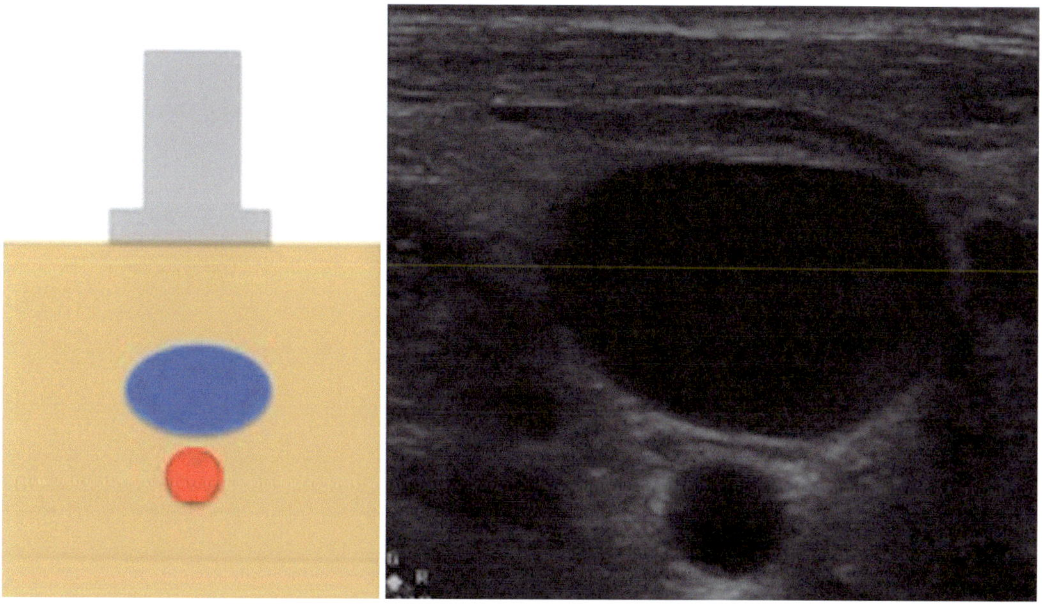

Fig. 2.20 This view is obtained by placing the probe perpendicular to the long axis of the target

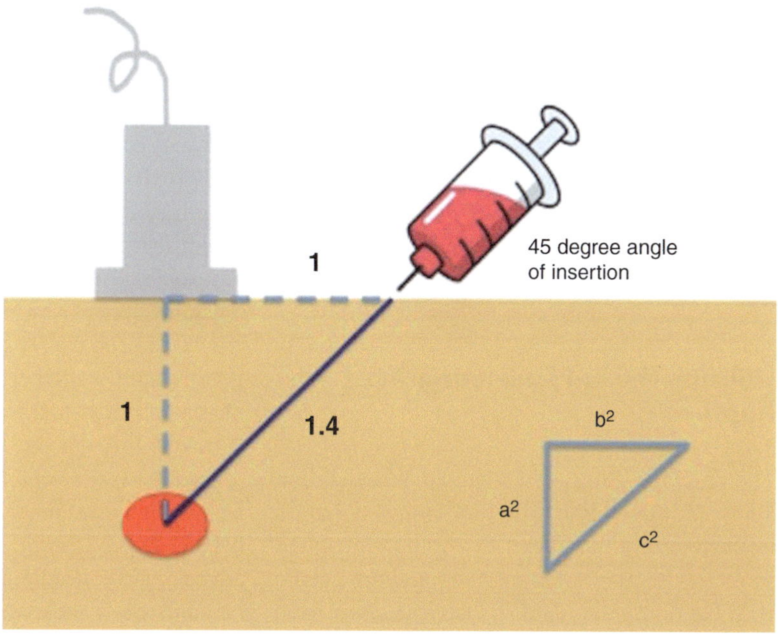

Fig. 2.21 Use of the Pythagorean theorem to determine the site of needle insertion

screen. This distance is equal to the distance from the probe to where the needle punctures the skin at a 45° angle. For example, if the distance from the skin surface to the center of a target vein is 1 cm, make the skin puncture 1 cm from the midpoint of the ultrasound probe along the trajectory of the target structure. Insert and advance the needle at a 45° angle. The vein will then be punctured after the needle is inserted 1.4 cm. It is very useful to assess the distances using this method before puncture to avoid complications. If the vein is not punctured within the expected inserted needle length, the needle trajectory may not be accurate and should be reassessed.

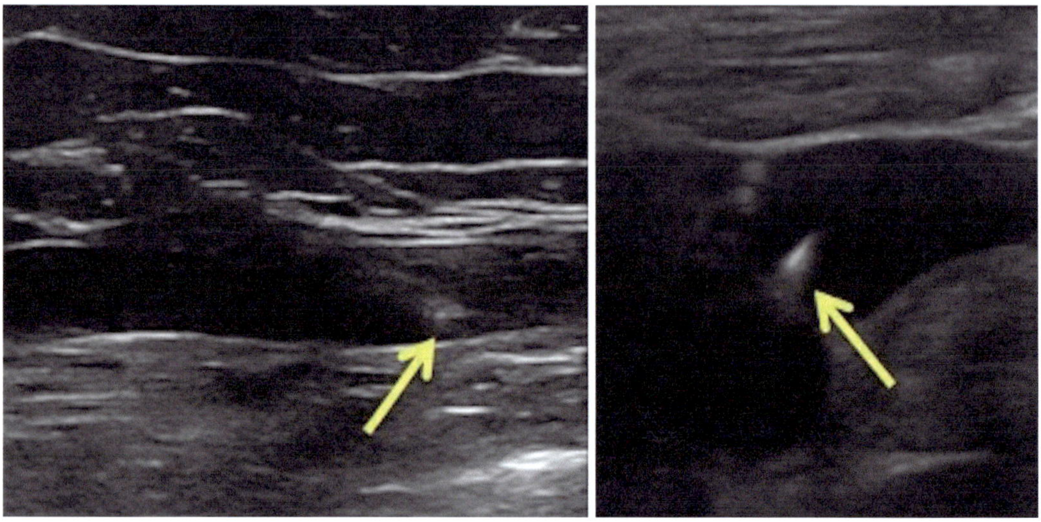

Fig. 2.22 Needle tip can be identified as a hyperechoic dot

It is important to understand that the ultrasound beam is very narrow and only 1–2 mm wide despite the ultrasound probe being approximately 1 cm wide. The needle will be visualized only when it is within this narrow beam width. The cross section of the needle in the out-of-plane (short-axis) approach will be seen only when it crosses the ultrasound scan plane that is oriented perpendicular to the needle. The needle tip or shaft will appear hyperechoic (Fig. 2.22).

Utilizing the In-Plane (Long-Axis) Approach

The in-plane (long-axis) needle visualization approach targets the structure along its length in the longitudinal plane. Grasp the ultrasound probe in the nondominant hand and the needle with the dominant hand. Locate the target vein using the short-axis approach. Slowly rotate the ultrasound probe to visualize the vein in the long axis. The ultrasound probe should be positioned so that the long axis of the probe is parallel to the long axis of the target structure (Fig. 2.23). The probe position can then be adjusted slightly to visualize the structure at its greatest anteroposterior diameter.

The needle should be inserted through the skin at approximately 30° angle adjacent to one end of the ultrasound probe. The needle should be in the plane, that is in line with the long axis of the ultrasound probe, and in the exact same plane as the ultrasound beam. With this approach, it is crucial to keep the probe steady and over the target structure. As the needle is advanced, the needle tip and shaft will be visualized in real time as it travels through the subcutaneous tissues and toward the target vein. If the needle is not visualized on the ultrasound display, then the planes of the needle and probe are not aligned. Prior to advancing the needle any farther, the probe can be adjusted or the needle may need to be withdrawn and redirected to align it with the ultrasound beam and the long axis of the target structure.

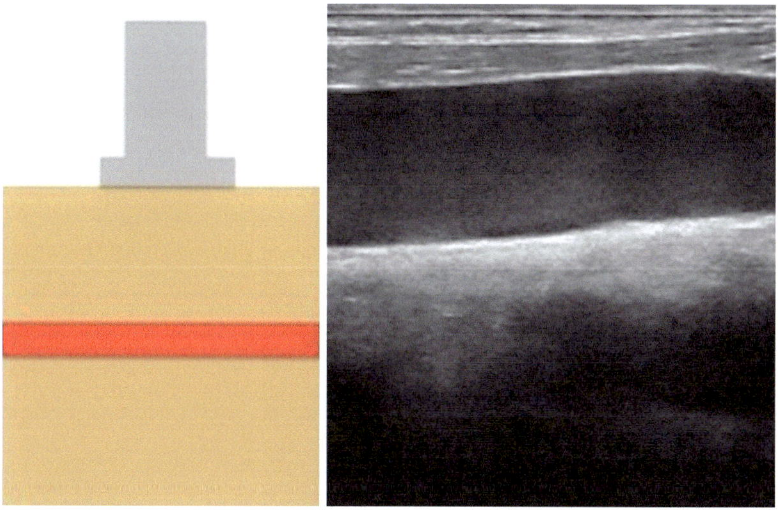

Fig. 2.23 The ultrasound probe should be positioned so that the long axis of the probe is parallel to the long axis of the target structure

Utilizing the Oblique Approach

The oblique approach is a hybrid between the short- and long-axis approaches. This approach allows for the visualization of the structures adjacent to the target vessel as well as full needle tip evaluation throughout the procedure. The advantage of this needle visualization approach is the ability to visualize structures adjacent to the target vein and observe the needle tip continuously throughout the procedure [14]. The oblique approach is not as commonly utilized as the short- and long-axis approach, which may be due to it being more difficult to learn.

To perform the oblique approach, the probe needs to be placed at an oblique angle to the target structure. This can be performed by first identifying the target structure in short axis then rotating the probe approximately 45° to almost midway between the short- and long-axis views. The needle is inserted into the skin on one end of the probe in plane with the ultrasound beam. The needle tip and needle shaft will be fully visible as it travels at an oblique angle toward the target. As in the long-axis (in-plane) approach, if the needle tip is not visualized, retract the needle and realign it with the ultrasound beam.

Software for Improving Needle Guidance and Ultrasound-Guided Procedures

Over the last two decades, ultrasound technology has advanced at a rapid pace. New imaging modes have been developed that may further assist the operator with needle guidance and ultrasound-guided procedures. These include compound imaging, tissue harmonic imaging, beam steering, and color Doppler imaging.

- *Compound Imaging:* As mentioned above, compound imaging involves acquiring multiple images of the same object and combining them into a single image. Spatial compound imaging is when the images may be acquired from different angles in the same plane. Spatial compound imaging is available on most of the newer portable ultrasound machines. When compared with conventional B-mode imaging, spatial compound imaging consistently improves needle visibility [15, 16]. Frequency compound imaging is when images are acquired at different frequencies. Frequency compound imaging does not appear to have a significant effect on needle

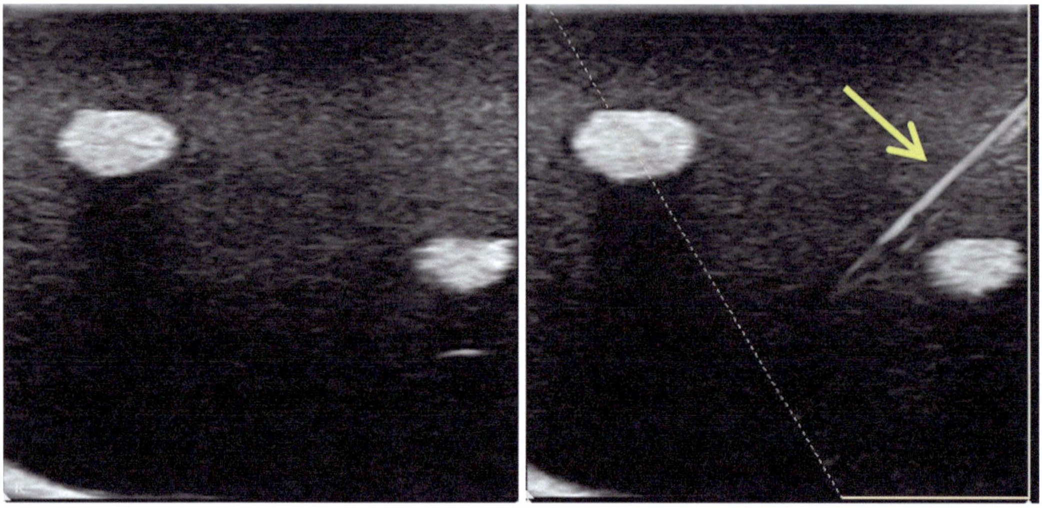

Fig. 2.24 This image with poor needle-tip visualization (left) is significantly enhanced after utilizing electronic beam steering technology (right)

visibility as compared to spatial compound imaging.

- *Tissue Harmonic Imaging:* Tissue harmonic imaging forms an image using echoes at twice the emitted frequency; this higher-frequency harmonic signal is spontaneously generated by propagation through tissues. When compared with conventional B-mode imaging, tissue harmonic does not seem to have a positive effect on needle visualization. However, harmonic imaging may improve the visibility of hypoechoic target structures [17, 18].
- *Electronic Beam Steering:* Electronic beam steering is a technology that allows the ultrasound beam to be tilted relative to the transducer, thus increasing the needle beam angle of incidence toward 90°. This has been shown to greatly improve needle tip and shaft visibility [19]. While this feature has not typically been standard on most machines, it is now becoming more widely available on newer devices (Fig. 2.24).
- *Color Doppler:* Color Doppler has shown to aid in the detection of the needle tip. Movement of an object within an ultrasound beam produces a Doppler shift in the frequency of the reflected echoes [20]. These frequency shifts are depicted by a color signal on the display. Today, the majority of newer ultrasound devices have this function. While clinically color Doppler is most commonly used to detect flow, it can also be used to localize a moving needle tip. Other devices exist to enhance this feature. For example, the ColorMark device (EchoCath Inc., Princeton, NJ) clips onto the needle shaft and induces tiny high-frequency, low-amplitude vibrations at the needle tip to improve visualization. These vibrations are able to generate a signal detected by color Doppler. Although manually induced needle motion has been described, there is currently no clear evidence to support the efficacy of this method in improving needle visualization.

Echogenic Needles

Full needle visualization can be extremely challenging with traditional needles. The needle tip can often be visualized even when the shaft cannot. This is because the cutting bevel at the needle tip has an irregular surface. The portion of the ultrasound beam that interacts with this surface is scattered in all directions. Therefore, only some of the beam will be reflected back to the transducer, even when the shaft of the needle is nearly parallel to the ultrasound beam [21]. This problem has been addressed by the development of echogenic needles. Many echogenic needles are now available, with a variety of textured needle surfaces designed to reflect the ultrasound waves back to the transducer. Most echogenic needle designs include a polymer coating that traps microbubbles and a dimpled distal shaft [22]. Echogenic needles have been shown to improve tip visibility during ultrasound-guided procedures in phantoms and cadavers, as well as in a number of clinical studies [23–25] (Fig. 2.25).

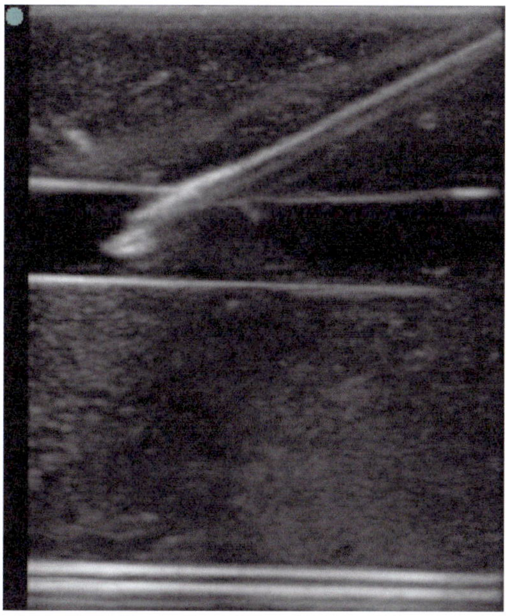

Fig. 2.25 An echogenic needle demonstrated on a phantom model

Imaging Artifact

Ultrasound machines rely on physical assumptions to assign the location and the intensity of each received echo and create an image on display screen. An imaging artifact is a term used to describe any part of the image that does not accurately represent the anatomy or physiology within the subject being imaged [26]. Imaging artifacts are commonly seen and can be useful in ultrasound-guided procedures. The operator's ability to recognize certain artifacts can help to more accurately determine needle localization. There are three major artifacts that are most commonly identified in ultrasound-guided procedures: reverberation, refraction, and acoustic shadowing.

Reverberation Artifact In reverberation artifact, the ultrasound wave bounces back and forth at the interface of two tissues with varying acoustic impedance, prolonging the beam time of flight and creating the imaging artifact [27]. It appears as multiple reflections that progressively weaken over time. A needle is highly reflective, and reverberation artifacts known as "ring-down artifacts" are frequently seen posterior to needles during ultrasound-guided venipuncture (Fig. 2.26).

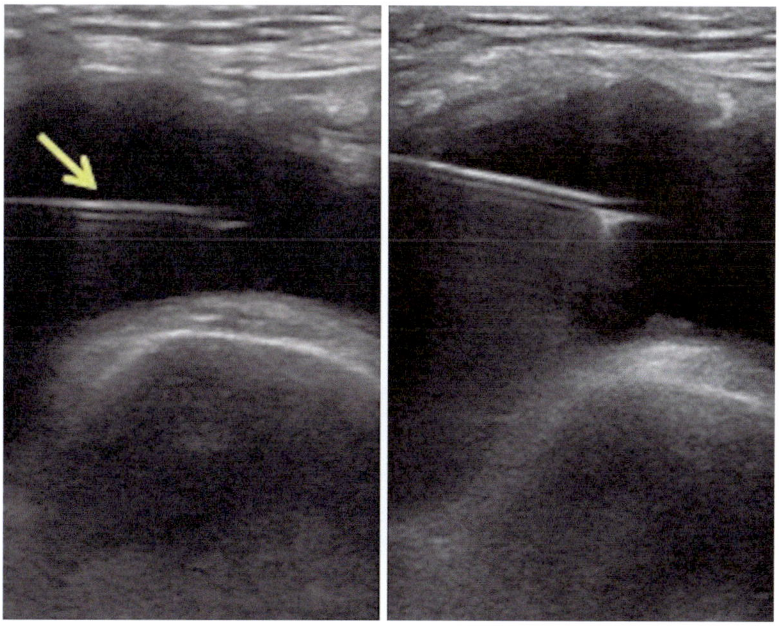

Fig. 2.26 Reverberation artifact from a needle

Refraction Artifact Refraction is a change in direction of the sound beam and is usually seen at the curve of a rounded object, such as a vessel when in short axis. This will appear as a deletion of information known as an "edge artifact" (Fig. 2.27).

Acoustic Shadowing An acoustic shadow is the result of a highly attenuating structure, such as the metal of a penetrating needle. Posterior to a structure, there will be a reduction in the amplitude of the sound beam (Fig. 2.28).

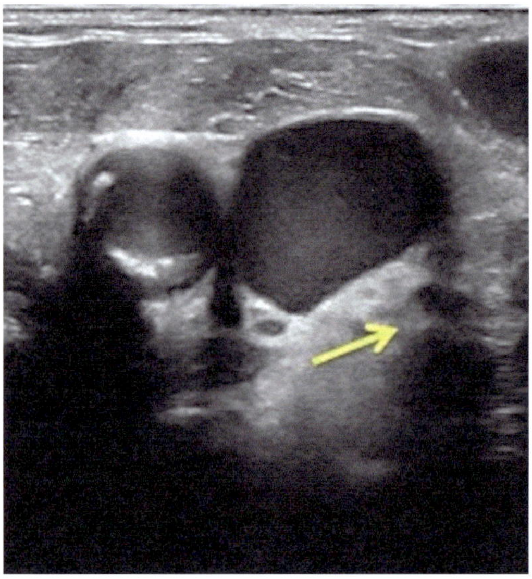

Fig. 2.27 Edge artifact seen as a vertical band on both sides of the vessel

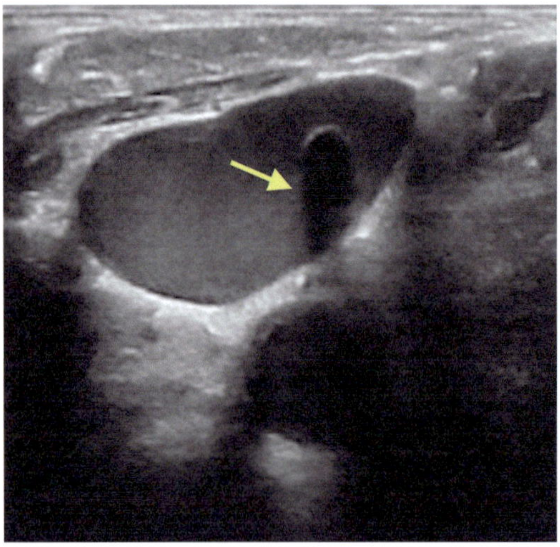

Fig. 2.28 Posterior shadowing from a highly attenuating structure

Needle Guides

The needle guide is designed to be directly applied onto the ultrasound probe. The guide aids the operator in restricting lateral movement of the needle and keeping the needle trajectory in line with the long axis of the probe. As demonstrated in a number of studies, needle guides can provide significant improvement in needle tip visibility [28–30]. In a clinical study, in addition to increasing needle visibility, the use of a needle guide also led to shorter procedural time and greater operator satisfaction when compared to the traditional freehand technique in an ultrasound-guided procedure [31]. However, other studies argue that while needle guides may minimize challenges with obtaining alignment in the in-plane approach, they bring about another obstacle restricting needle redirection [32]. Needle guides are not routinely used by point-of-care ultrasound users to perform ultrasound-guided procedures.

References

1. Brass P, Hellmich M, Kolodziej L, Schick G, Smith AF. Ultrasound guidance versus anatomical landmarks for internal jugular vein catheterization. Cochrane Database Syst Rev. 2015;(1):CD006962.
2. Feller-Kopman D. Ultrasound-guided central venous catheter placement: the new standard of care? Crit Care Med. 2005;33:1875–7.
3. Bodor M, Fullerton B. Ultrasonography of the hand, wrist, and elbow. Phys Med Rehabil Clin N Am. 2010;21:509–31.
4. Moy WJ, Su E, Chen JJ, Oh C, Jing JC, Qu Y, He Y, Chen Z, Wong BJF. Association of Electrochemical Therapy with optical, mechanical, and acoustic impedance properties of porcine skin. JAMA Facial Plast Surg. 2017;19:502–9. https://doi.org/10.1001/jamafacial.2017.0341.
5. Szabo TL, Lewin PA. Ultrasound transducer selection in clinical imaging practice. J Ultrasound Med. 2017. https://doi.org/10.1002/jum.14351.
6. Edelman SK. Ultrasound physics and instrumentation. Woodlands: ESP, Inc.; 2016. Print.
7. Ma OJ, Mateer JR, Reardon RF, Joing SA. Ma and Mateer's emergency ultrasound. New York: McGraw-Hill Education; 2014. Print.
8. Barnett SB. Intracranial temperature elevation from diagnostic ultrasound. Ultrasound Med Biol. 2001;27:883–8.
9. Mari J, Hibbs K, Stride E, Eckersley R, Tang M. An approximate nonlinear model for time gain compensation of amplitude modulated images of ultra-

sound contrast agent perfusion. IEEE Trans Ultrason Ferroelectr Freq Control. 2010;57:818–29.
10. Richards JR, Awrey JM, Medeiros SE, McGahan JP. Color and power Doppler sonography for pneumothorax detection. J Ultrasound Med. 2017;36:2143–7. https://doi.org/10.1002/jum.14243.
11. Coman IM. Christian Andreas Doppler: the man and his legacy. Eur J Echocardiogr. 2005;6:7–10.
12. Entrekin RR, Porter BA, Sillesen HH, Wong AD, Cooperberg PL, Fix CH. Real-time spatial compound imaging: application to breast, vascular, and musculoskeletal ultrasound. Semin Ultrasound CT MR. 2001;22:50–64.
13. Socransky S, Wiss R. Point-of-care ultrasound for emergency physicians: "The EDE Book". Canada: The EDE 2 Course Inc; 2013. Print.
14. Dillane D, Tsui BC. From basic concepts to emerging technologies in regional anesthesia. Curr Opin Anaesthesiol. 2010;23:643–9.
15. Cohnen M, Saleh A, Lüthen R, Bode J, Mödder U. Improvement of sonographic needle visibility in cirrhotic livers during transjugular intrahepatic portosystemic stent-shunt procedures with use of real-time compound imaging. J Vasc Interv Radiol. 2003;14:103–6.
16. Saleh A, Ernst S, Grust A, Fürst G, Dall P, Mödder U. Real-time compound imaging: improved visibility of puncture needles and localization wires as compared to single-line ultrasonography. Rofo. 2001;173:368–72.
17. Mesurolle B, Bining HJ, El Khoury M, Barhdadi A, Kao E. Contribution of tissue harmonic imaging and frequency compound imaging in interventional breast sonography. J Ultrasound Med. 2006;25:845–55.
18. Karstrup S, Brøns J, Morsel L, Juul N, von der Recke P. Optimal set-up for ultrasound guided punctures using new scanner applications: an in-vitro study. Eur J Ultrasound. 2002;15:77–84.
19. Baker JA, Soo MS, Mengoni P. Sonographically guided percutaneous interventions of the breast using a steerable ultrasound beam. AJR Am J Roentgenol. 1999;172:157–9.
20. Taylor KJ, Holland S. Doppler US. Part I. Basic principles, instrumentation, and pitfalls. Radiology. 1990;174:297–307.
21. Chapman GA, Johnson D, Bodenham AR. Visualisation of needle position using ultrasonography. Anaesthesia. 2006;61:148Y158.
22. Chin KJ, Perlas A, Chan VW, Brull R. Needle visualization in ultrasound-guided regional anesthesia: challenges and solutions. Reg Anesth Pain Med. 2008;33:532–44.
23. Hebard S, Hocking G. Echogenic technology can improve needle visibility during ultrasound-guided regional anesthesia. Reg Anesth Pain Med. 2011;36:185–9.
24. Deam RK, Kluger R, Barrington MJ, McCutcheon CA. Investigation of a new echogenic needle for use with ultrasound peripheral nerve block. Anaesth Intensive Care. 2007;35:582–6.
25. Miura M, Takeyama K, Suzuki T. Visibility of ultrasound-guided echogenic needle and its potential in clinical delivery of regional anesthesia. Tokai J Exp Clin Med. 2014;39:80–6.
26. Kremkau FW. Diagnostic ultrasound principles and instruments. 5th ed. Philadelphia: Saunders; 1998: 147Y157, 377Y436.
27. Prabhu SJ, Kanal K, Bhargava P, Vaidya S, Dighe MK. Ultrasound artifacts: classification, applied physics with illustrations, and imaging appearances. Ultrasound Q. 2014;30:145–57.
28. van Geffen GJ, Mulder J, Gielen M, van Egmond J, Scheffer GJ, et al. A needle guidance device compared to free hand technique in an ultrasound guided interventional task using a phantom. Anaesthesia. 2008;63:986–90.
29. Whittaker S, Lethbridge G, Kim C, Keon Cohen Z, Ng I. An ultrasound needle insertion guide in a porcine phantom model. Anaesthesia. 2013;68:826–9.
30. Ball RD, Scouras NE, Orebaugh S, Wilde J, Sakai T. Randomized, prospective, observational simulation study comparing residents' needle guided vs free-hand ultrasound techniques for central venous catheter access. Br J Anaesth. 2012;108:72–9.
31. Kim C, Ratnayake M, Lethbridge G, Ng I. Comparing the use of a needle guidance device vs. free-hand technique in performing ultrasound-guided TAP blocks: a prospective randomised trial. J Anesth Clin Res. 2014;5:429.
32. Matalon TA, Silver B. US guidance of interventional procedures. Radiology. 1990;174:43–7.

Disinfection and Sterile Techniques

3

Sean Maley and Alison Thurber

Definitions

Cleaning the removal of visible soil (i.e., organic and inorganic) from an object

Disinfection a process that eliminates many or all pathogenic microorganisms, except bacterial spores, from an inanimate object

Sterilization a process that eliminates all living microorganisms, including bacterial spores

Probe Contamination Risks and Multidrug-Resistant Organisms

As drug-resistant organisms become more prevalent in the community and healthcare facilities, clinicians must be aware of possible baseline microbial probe contamination [1–4]. Two studies have shown baseline bacterial probe contamination rates of 17.5% and 22.6% [5, 6]. With the prevalence of methicillin-resistant *Staphylococcus aureus* (MRSA) as high as 36%, MRSA has become one of the leading causes of skin and soft-tissue infections in patients throughout various clinical settings [7, 8]. Outbreaks have been associated with bacterial colonization of ultrasound probes secondary to inadequate cleaning of a transesophageal probe and ultrasound-guided needle guides [9, 10]. An outbreak of methicillin-susceptible *Staphylococcus aureus* (MSSA) causing pyodermas in neonates was reportedly due to contaminated ultrasound gel [11].

S. Maley (✉)
Northwest Medical Center, Tucson, AZ, USA

A. Thurber
Emergency Medicine, SUNY Upstate University Hospital, Syracuse, NY, USA

Transducer Cleaning and Decontamination

While there are no universally established guidelines for transducer cleaning and decontamination, the Center for Disease Control and many manufacturers of ultrasound equipment have adopted the Spaulding Classification scheme to determine the level of recommended decontamination for transducers [1]. The American Institute of Ultrasound in Medicine approved guidelines for transducer cleaning and handling as well as use of ultrasound gel in 2018 [12]. These guidelines, available on their website, are comprehensive, but they are radiology practice driven and poorly disseminated into the point-of-care ultrasound world. In addition, universal precautions should be taken on every patient. This means that appropriate cleaning and disinfection should be performed between every patient ultrasound

S. Adhikari, M. Blaivas (eds.), *The Ultimate Guide to Point-of-Care Ultrasound-Guided Procedures*, https://doi.org/10.1007/978-3-030-28267-7_3

examination, a deviation from some common practices in the early years of point-of-care ultrasound.

Prior to disinfection, proper cleaning techniques should be applied. Cleaning should result in the removal of any debris, ultrasound gel, or body fluid that is visible on the transducer. This can be done with paper towels or using soap/detergent with water. This is a necessary prerequisite to disinfection and sterilization. Failure to adequately clean can result in the decreased effectiveness of a disinfectant as the foreign material works as a barrier between microorganisms and the disinfectant (Fig. 3.1).

The Spaulding Classification scheme categorizes medical equipment decontamination based on the risk of infection that is posed to a patient. The categories of medical instruments are classified as critical, semi-critical, and noncritical, as described below:

Critical	device exposed to or enters normally sterile tissue
Semi-critical	transducer exposed to mucous membranes or non-intact skin
Noncritical	transducer in contact with only intact skin [13]

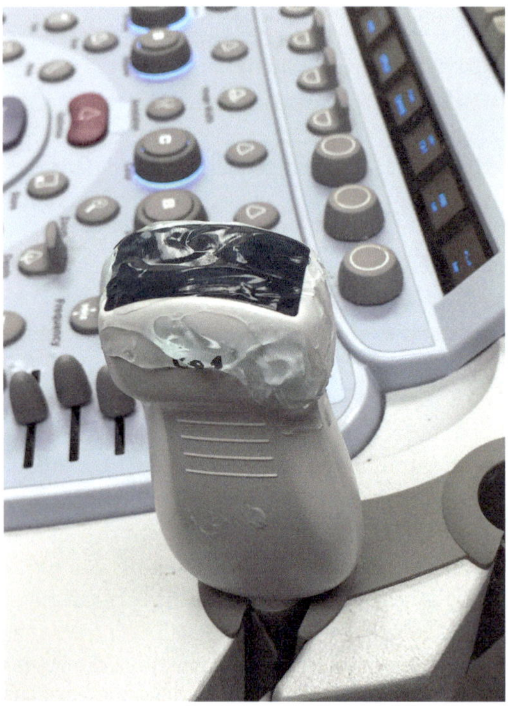

Fig. 3.1 Cleaning of all visible soil and contaminant should be done before any disinfection

Critical items are associated with the highest risk of infection and require sterilization. This is usually reserved for intraoperative ultrasound use and does not generally apply to the use of point-of-care ultrasound. In situations where an ultrasound probe is needed, a sterile sheath should be used, and the probe should be sterilized between each patient. If sterilization of the ultrasound probe is not possible, then high-level disinfection should be performed along with the use of a sterile probe cover [1].

A semi-critical exam results in the exposure of the transducer to mucous membranes, body fluids, or non-intact tissue. This necessitates that the transducer undergoes high-level disinfection (HLD). HLD is a disinfecting process that will eliminate all microorganisms with the exception of microbial spores. It is also recommended that the probe be covered with either a sterile sheath or appropriate nonsterile barrier during semi-critical exams. For example, a commercial sterile ultrasound transducer sheath should be used for procedures such as central venous line insertions, while a properly disinfected endocavitary transducer would be covered with a commercial nonsterile condom-like cover for a diagnostic scan in the absence of a sterile field. One study on decontamination practices of transvaginal ultrasound probes found that 0 of 68 hospitals performed high-level disinfection following their use, although all facilities used some type of probe cover [14]. The use of a probe cover has been interpreted by some as changing the Spaulding device Classification, but in general, the examination type and risks involved should determine the level of decontamination. Little is known about potential liability from contaminated ultrasound transducers in point-of-care settings. However, the fact that great variability exists among point-of-care ultrasound providers in disinfection standards adherence coupled with persistence of pathogens on probe surfaces in studies even after intermediate disinfection measures

Table 3.1 Spaulding classification in point-of-care ultrasound

Device classification	Risks involved	POCUS examples	Level of decontamination
Critical	Invasive sterile tissue/vascular system	Intraoperative liver biopsy	Sterilization
Semi-critical	Contact with mucous membranes, body fluids, or non-intact tissue	Transesophageal echocardiography, transvaginal ultrasound, intraoral ultrasound	High-level disinfection
Noncritical	Transfer of microorganisms on intact skin	Transabdominal/transthoracic ultrasound	Low-level disinfection

suggests risk potential [15, 16]. Experience in other areas such as endoscopy and transesophageal echocardiography (TEE) laboratories suggests that large-scale infective agent exposure is possible in some cases and carries considerable liability both civilly and in terms of public relations for an institution. All of these factors should lead providers to adhere to hospital and published standards for all ultrasound examinations. One of the few point-of-care medical societies to release guidelines to date, American College of Emergency Physicians, has released guidelines covering the breadth of current point-of-care ultrasound practice and relevant transducer care and decontamination [17].

If a transducer only comes into contact with intact skin, then only cleaning and low-level disinfection are needed. Intact skin will serve as a barrier against microorganism transmission which decreases the risk of transmission. Low-level disinfection means that most bacteria, some viruses, and some fungi be removed, but bacterial spores and some resistant microorganisms may remain (Table 3.1) [13].

Disinfectants and Methods for Transducer Decontamination

When choosing a disinfectant, there are several factors to take into account, with the most important being device classification. In the USA, the Food and Drug Administration (FDA) has not cleared disinfectant wipes and topical spray products for high-level disinfection [18]. There is a broad range of disinfectants available commercially, with all high-level disinfectants (HLD) requiring the probe to be immersed in a chemical solution. When choosing a disinfectant, there are several other considerations that should be taken into account as well:

- Level of decontamination necessary based on device classification
- Compatibility with probe and manufacturer guidelines
- Length of processing and disinfection time
- Need for ventilation and personal protective equipment
- Risk for transducer degradation
- Risk of toxic exposure to personnel and the patient
- Cost of installation and daily operation

Common high-level disinfectants include glutaraldehyde, hydrogen peroxide, and ortho-phthalaldehyde. Glutaraldehyde (e.g., Cidex®) is used very commonly in the healthcare setting to provide high-level disinfection. High-level disinfectants should not be used for noncritical devices due to its toxicity and relatively high cost [1]. These disinfectants can take anywhere from 5 minutes to 45 minutes of contact with the probe to achieve high-level disinfection. Caution should be used when selecting a HLD, as they are toxic and can cause respiratory or mucous membrane irritation [19]. Some high-level disinfectants may require a separate cleaning room, ventilation hood, and personal protective equipment to be used [20]. For example, installing a Cidex OPA station without a hood may require an adjustment in the total room air changes per hour in order to meet FDA and OSHA standards. Providers should coordinate such initiatives with their facility biomedical and infection control departments.

Another option to achieve HLD is through an automated, hydrogen peroxide mist device (e.g., Trophon® EPR). It requires the probe to be manually cleaned and placed in a self-contained unit for disinfection. Benefits of this include limiting user error related to immersion time and decreased exposure of personnel to the disinfectant [19]. This makes it a possible and, in some cases, an ideal point-of-care disinfecting solution. Experience in many training programs seems to carry a common thread; if left up to trainees to clean and care for transducers as well as manage infection control equipment maintenance, proper technique and maintenance quickly fall off. Automated devices, clear chains of responsibility, and involvement of full-time hospital staff for regular maintenance, cleaning, and upkeep are the best methods on ensuring quality and consistency.

Device manufacturers provide a list of compatible disinfectants for their devices. Some disinfectants can cause deterioration of the transducer, making it important to choose a compatible disinfectant. The depth to which a probe can be submerged in a solution varies between device manufacturers; therefore, the device manual should be referenced before submerging a transducer. It is very important to keep in mind that the entire probe is not electrically isolated and immersion of the portion from which the cord emanates can cause electric shock and equipment breakdown (Table 3.2) [18, 20].

Table 3.2 Chemical Disinfectants[a]

Sterilants	High-level disinfectants[b]	Low-level disinfectants
Ethylene oxide	Glutaraldehyde (e.g., Cidex®)	Ethanol or isopropyl alcohol
Hydrogen peroxide gas plasma	Hydrogen peroxide solution and mist (e.g., trophon)	Chlorine compounds
Peracetic acid	*ortho*-phthalaldehyde (e.g., Cidex® OPA)	Quaternary ammonium compounds
		Phenolics

[a]The device manufacturer chemical compatibility list should also be cross-referenced with your governmental regulatory agency (e.g., FDA) to determine compliance with approved standards

[b]Some high-level disinfectants can work as chemical sterilants with increased immersion times

Probe Cover Type: Sterile Sheaths Versus Condoms

The use of a protective cover has become a routine when performing transvaginal exams with the endocavitary probe (Fig. 3.2). One issue that has persisted is what level of decontamination is necessary when performing semi-critical exams if a cover is used. Low-level disinfection is commonly used, but risks of probe cover failure and persistent probe contamination by infectious microorganisms should be taken into account [14]. The use of a probe cover does not guarantee that the probe is protected from contamination by

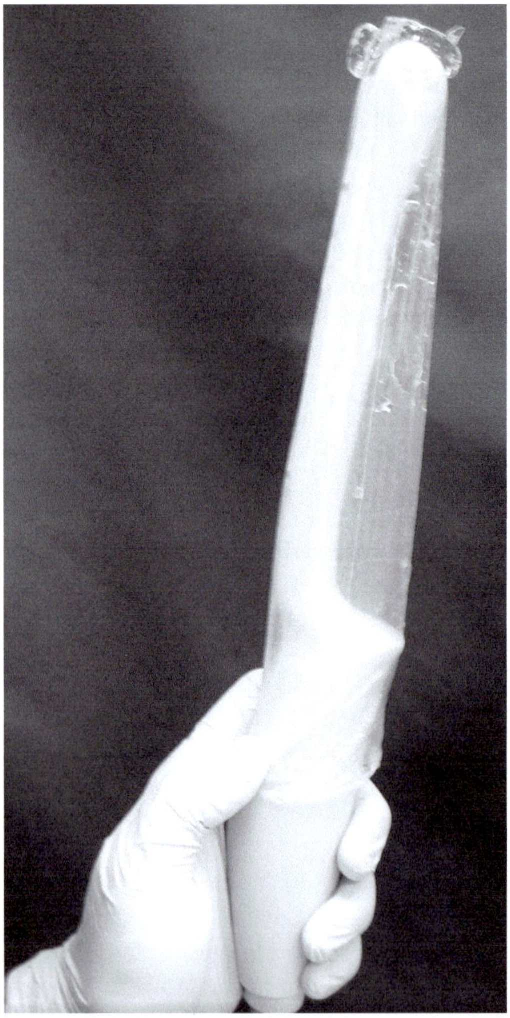

Fig. 3.2 Endocavitary probe with a protective cover

bodily fluids [21]. There is a chance that the probe cover may perforate during use or that bodily fluids can contaminate the probe near the edge of the cover [22]. Several studies have shown a 3% and 21% probe contamination rate by human papillomavirus (HPV) DNA after low-level decontamination despite use of a probe cover [23–25]. Whether the presence of HPV DNA is clinically significant is not known, as persistence of HPV DNA has been detected on other medical equipment despite proper disinfection procedures [24]. There are also no documented reports of disease transmission from a contaminated transvaginal ultrasound probe [26]. It is recommended that high-level disinfection be performed between examinations even when using a probe cover in semi-critical devices.

Several studies have compared the durability of probe covers versus condoms for endocavitary probe coverage. One benefit of condoms is that they are significantly cheaper compared to commercial probe covers. The perforation rates in condoms have been shown to be significantly lower compared to probe covers [27, 28]. Despite this, probe covers are still used more frequently. This may be from limited coverage of the probe by the condom. In addition, condoms are not designed for medical examination use, as in the case of performing a transvaginal ultrasound examination. Therefore, any complications or condom failure may cause unwanted, added liability on the provider.

Whether using a condom or a probe cover, the presence of any visualized defects in the cover should result in it being replaced prior to the exam. A patient's allergy profile should also be taken into account when choosing a cover. There are reports of anaphylactic reactions to latex probe covers in patients allergic to latex [29]. Additionally, an allergic reaction from a transesophageal echocardiogram has been reported. Powdered latex gloves were used to clean the transducer which was then contaminated with latex molecules [30].

Central venous line placement under ultrasound guidance exposes the transducer to blood and requires not only a commercial sterile sheath use but also HLD of the transducer by some interpretations of current standards (Figs. 3.3, 3.4, and 3.5) [12]. However, the only published point-of-care ultrasound guidelines relating to transducer care after central line placement recommend for low-level cleaning after each use as a noncritical device [17]. The recent explosion of peripheral vascular access under ultrasound guidance among nurses and technologists has led to

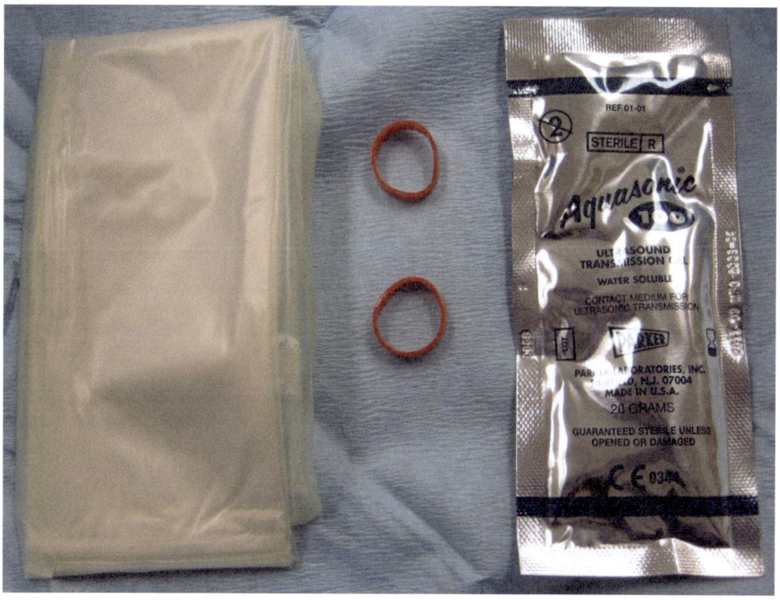

Fig. 3.3 Sterile sheath for ultrasound probe for central venous access

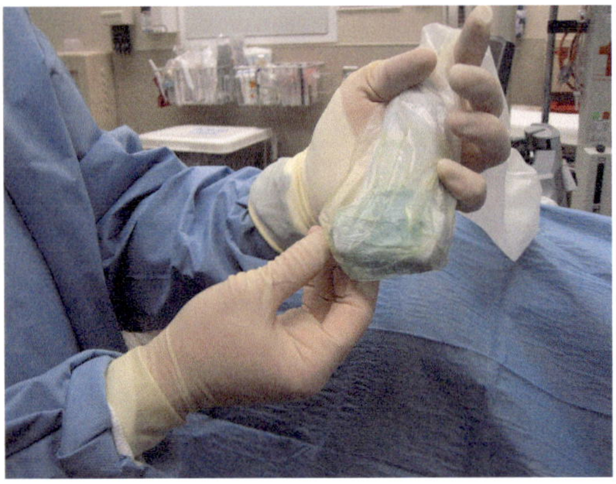

Fig. 3.4 Linear probe with a sterile sheath

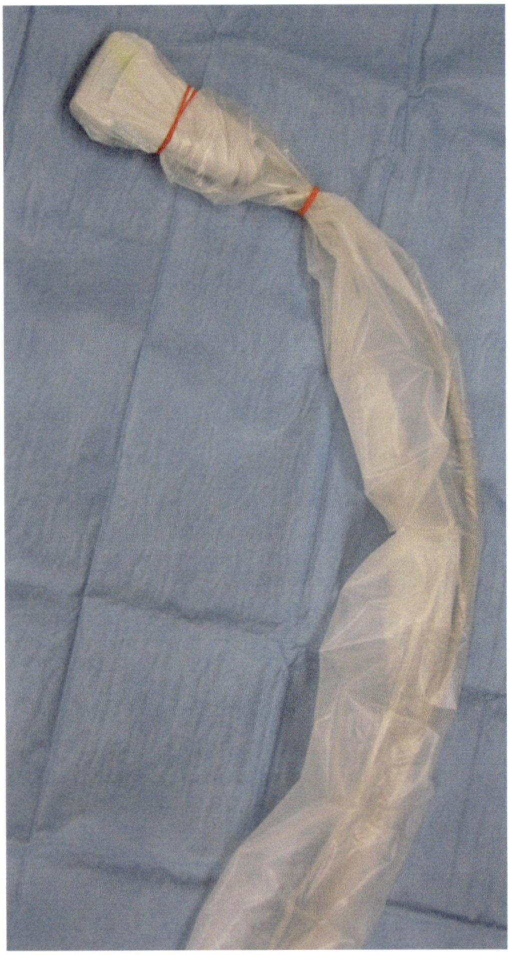

Fig. 3.5 Transducer with protective sheath in sterile field for central venous cannulation

increased use of coverings such as Tegaderm film for aseptic techniques. Similarly, injections and aspirations that are aseptic are often performed using these types of coverings. Their efficacy has been debated, although the scant data of their use in clinical settings showed no increased risk of infection [31].

Spaulding Classification Limitations and Other Risks

The use of ultrasound for peripherally invasive procedures like peripheral IV placement, musculoskeletal injections, and regional anesthesia is not generally thought of as requiring high-level disinfection of the probe. However, with these procedures, there is a chance for the probe to come into contact with blood or non-intact skin. General practice has been to not perform high-level decontamination of the probe. This can be related to time constraints and the cost of disinfection using HLD. This falls outside of the aforementioned recommendations and is not addressed by current guidelines. It has been reported that infection rates in peripheral IV lines placed with US had similar infection rates as IV lines placed traditionally [31]. This may signify that the development of infection with these procedures is low when using aseptic technique. One of the main concerns though is that disinfectant techniques between these procedures can vary widely among health practitioners [32]. *At a minimum, low-level disinfection should be performed between these types of examinations*, and general aseptic precautions should be taken during them.

There are several precautions that one can also take in addition to traditional aseptic techniques to decrease the risk of infection:

1. Clean the skin adjacent to where the gel and transducer will be applied in addition to the immediate area of the procedure. It is possible that gel from a contaminated area can be spread into the sterile field (Fig. 3.6) [33].

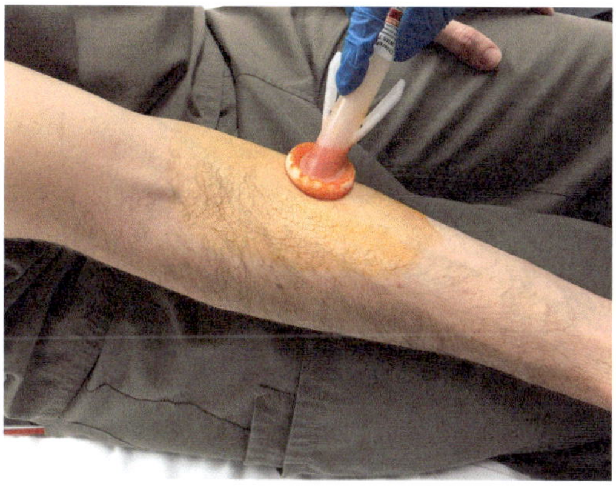

Fig. 3.6 A wide area is cleaned to prevent contamination from surrounding areas

2. Use a sterile, single-use gel packet for the examination. Nonsterile gel may be contaminated during the manufacturing process. Sterile, single-use gel packets may help to decrease the risk of infection [34]. Some providers disinfect the transducer with an approved wipe at this point to further decrease possible transducer surface contamination.
3. Apply a sterile, transparent adhesive dressing to the transducer head. Like a probe cover, this may serve as a barrier between the probe and patient, thus preventing cross contamination between the two. This should not significantly affect the image quality. One concern is that there may be residual adhesive on the probe head when the dressing is removed. The residual adhesive may become the foundation of a biofilm and be difficult to remove. Additionally, the adhesive may pull on the transducer surface with removal and over time lead to its breakdown [35]. A traditional probe cover can also be used (Figs. 3.7, 3.8, 3.9, and 3.10).

Pearls and Pitfalls

Pitfalls center on improper probe cleaning and infection control. With the wide availability of disinfecting wipes in many care settings which

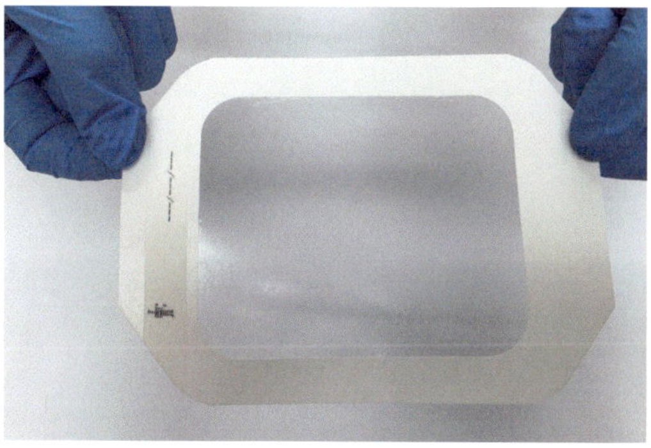

Fig. 3.7 Transparent adhesive dressing

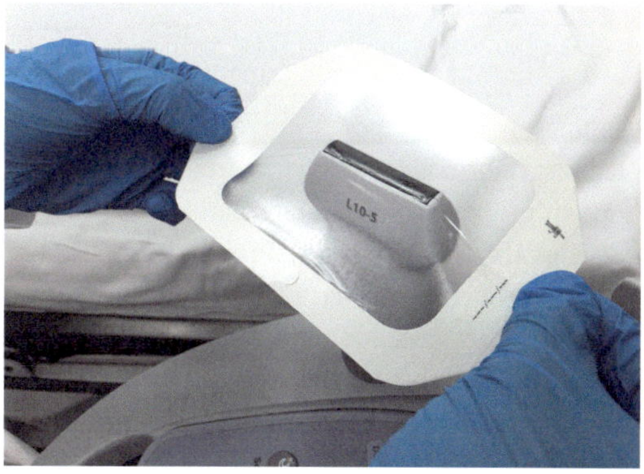

Fig. 3.8 Apply carefully to avoid forming air bubbles over the transducer

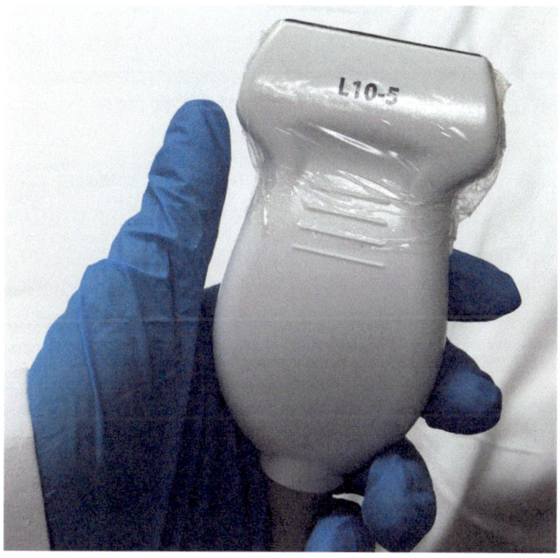

Fig. 3.9 The presence of air bubbles can reduce image quality

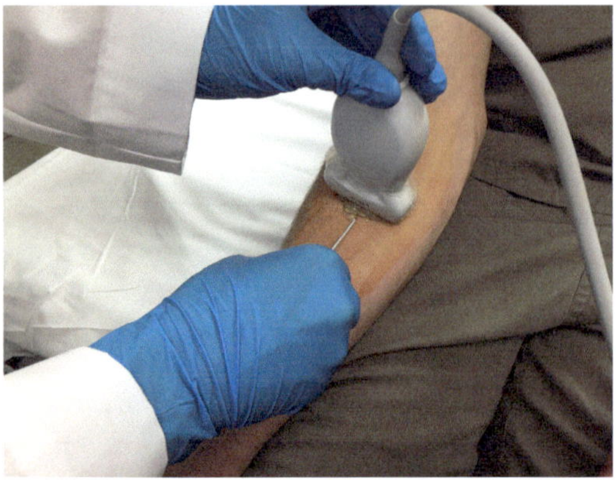

Fig. 3.10 Sterile gel is used in addition to prevent contamination

> **Key Points**
> - Know your hospital policies and relevant national guidelines and standards.
> - Probes have to be cleaned of macroscopic debris prior to further decontamination.
> - Establish cleaning and disinfection procedures and ensure compliance with those procedures.

eliminate all but spores on a surface, regular cleaning with such a wipe decreases the likelihood of probe surface contamination even further but adds little time or cost. Providers should not simply clean the surface of the transducer with the same chlorhexidine used to sterilize skin surface prior to a procedure and assume a sterile protective barrier is not required on the probe. When in doubt about level of decontamination needed, simply put yourself or a loved one in the place of the patient and then perform the level of cleaning and decontamination you would like to see in such a case.

Integration into Clinical Practice

It is imperative to make equipment cleaning and probe decontamination a part of regular routine when using ultrasound. This should be seen and taught as any standard infection control measure mandated by the hospital. Consider consulting with hospital infection control to make sure your procedures are consistent with their standards. Doing so would add a measure of protection in the unlikely chance an infection complication may occur and was traced back to an ultrasound-guided procedure. In larger practices, logs should be maintained regarding cleaning, maintenance of any disinfection stations and supplies, as well as periodic training and monitoring.

References

1. Centers for Disease Control and Prevention. Guideline for disinfection and sterilization in healthcare facilities, 2008. Centers for Disease Control and Prevention website; 2008. http://www.cdc.gov/hicpac/pdf/guidelines/Disinfection_Nov_2008.pdf. Accessed 26 Nov 2014.
2. Mirza W, Imam S, Kharal S, et al. Cleaning methods for ultrasound probes. J Coll Physicians Surg Pak. 2008;18(5):286–9.
3. Frazee B, Fahimi J, Lambert L, et al. Emergency department ultrasonographic probe contamination and experimental model of probe disinfection. Ann Emerg Med. 2011;58(1):56–63.
4. Backhouse S. Establishing a protocol for the cleaning and sterilization/disinfection of ultrasound transducers. Br Med Ultrasound Soc Bull. 2003;11(1):37–9.
5. Mullaney P, Munthali P, Vlachou P, et al. How clean is your probe? Microbiological assessment of ultrasound transducers in routine clinical use, and cost effective ways to reduce contamination. Clin Radiol. 2007;62:694–8.
6. Chu K, Obaid H, Babyn P, et al. Bacterial contamination of ultrasound probes at a tertiary referral university medical center. Am J Roentgenol. 2014;203:928–32.
7. Moran G, Krishnadasan A, Gorwitz R, et al. Methicillin-resistant S. aureus infections among patients in the emergency department. N Engl J Med. 2006;355(7):666–74.
8. Kumar N, David M, Boyle-Vavra S, et al. High S aureus colonization prevalence among patients with SSTIs and controls in an urban emergency department. J Clin Microbiol. 2014. https://doi.org/10.1128/JCM.03221-14.
9. Gillespie J, Arnold K, Noble-Wang J, et al. Outbreak of Pseudomonas aeruginosa infections after transrectal ultrasound-guided prostate biopsy. Urology. 2007;69:912–4.
10. Bancroft E, English L, Terashita D, et al. Letters to the editor: outbreak of Escherichia coli infections

associated with a contaminated transesophageal echocardiography probe. Infect Control Hosp Epidemiol. 2013;34(10):1121–2.
11. Weist K, Wendt C, Petersen L, et al. An outbreak of pyodermas among neonates caused by ultrasound gel contaminated with methicillin-susceptible Staphylococcus Aureus. Infect Control Hosp Epidemiol. 2000;21(12):761–4.
12. AIUM Official Statements. Guidelines for cleaning and preparing external- and internal-use ultrasound transducers between patients & safe handling and use of ultrasound coupling gel. https://aium.org/officialStatements/57.
13. Rutala W. APIC guideline for selection and use of disinfectants. Am J Infect Control. 1996;24:313–42.
14. Gray R, Williams P, Dubbins P, et al. Decontamination of transvaginal ultrasound probes: review of national practice and need for national guidelines. Clin Radiol. 2012;67:1069–77.
15. Hoyer R, Adhikari S, Amini R. Ultrasound transducer disinfection in emergency medicine practice. Antimicrob Resist Infect Control. 2016;5:12.
16. Miyague AH, Mauad FM, Martins Wde P, Benedetti AC, Ferreira AE, Mauad-Filho F. Ultrasound scan as a potential source of nosocomial and cross infection: a literature review. Radiol Bras. 2015;48(5):319–23.
17. ACEP Policy Statement. Guideline for ultrasound transducer cleaning and disinfection. Ann Emerg Med. 2018;72(4):e45–7.
18. GE Transducer Cleaning and Disinfection Guidelines. GE Healthcare 2013. http://www3.gehealthcare.com/static/ge-transducers/GEHC-Guidelines-Transducer_Cleaning_Disinfection_Guidelines.pdf. Accessed 13 Dec 2014.
19. Vickery K, Gorgis V, Burdach J, et al. Evaluation of an automated high-level disinfection technology for ultrasound transducers. J Infect Public Health. 2014;7:153–60.
20. Guidelines for cleaning and preparing external- and internal-use ultrasound probes between patients. American Institute of Ultrasound in Medicine; 2014. http://www.aium.org/officialStatements/57. Accessed 26 Nov 2014.
21. Jimenez R, Duff P. Sheathing of the endovaginal ultrasound probe: is it adequate? Infect Dis Obstet Gynecol. 1993;1:37–9.
22. Milki A, Fisch J. Vaginal ultrasound probe cover leakage: implications for patient care. Fertil Steril. 1998;69(3):409–11.
23. M'Zali F, Bounizra C, Leroy S, et al. Persistence of microbial contamination on transvaginal ultrasound probes despite low-level disinfection procedure. PLoS One. 2014;9(4):e93368. https://doi.org/10.1371/journal.pone.0093368.
24. Casalegno J, Carval K, Eibach D, et al. High risk HPV contamination of endocavity vaginal ultrasound probes: an underestimated route of nosocomial infection? PLoS One. 2012;7(10):e48137. https://doi.org/10.1371/journal.pone.0048137.
25. Ma S, Yeung A, Chan P, Graham C. Transvaginal ultrasound probe contamination by the human papillomavirus in the emergency department. Emerg Med J. 2012;30:472–5. https://doi.org/10.1136/emermed-2012-201407.
26. Johnson S, Proctor M, Bluth E, et al. Evaluation of a hydrogen peroxide-based system for high-level disinfection of vaginal ultrasound probes. J Ultrasound Med. 2013;32:1799–804.
27. Amis S, Ruddy M, Kibbler C, et al. Assessment of condoms as probe covers for transvaginal sonography. J Clin Ultrasound. 2000;28(6):295–8.
28. Rooks V, Yancey M, Elg S, Brueske L. Comparison of probe sheaths for endovaginal sonography. Obstet Gynecol. 1996;87(1):27–9.
29. Fry A, Meagher S, Vollenhoven B. Letters to the editor: a case of anaphylactic reaction caused by exposure to a latex probe cover in transvaginal ultrasound scanning. Ultrasound Obstet Gynecol. 1999;13:373–9.
30. Muller BA, Steelman VJ. Case report of latex aerosolization from a transesophageal echocardiogram machine. Allergy Asthma Proc. 2004;25(3):191–4.
31. Adhikari S, Blaivas M, Morrison D, Lander L. Comparison of infection rates among ultrasound-guided versus traditionally placed peripheral intravenous lines. J Ultrasound Med. 2010;29:741–7.
32. Charalambous C, Tryfonidis M, Sadiq S, et al. Septic arthritis following intra-articular steroid injection of the knee – a survey of current practice regarding antiseptic technique used during intra-articular steroid injection of the knee. Clin Rheumatol. 2003;22:386–90.
33. Sherman T, Ferguson J, Davis W, et al. Does the use of ultrasound affect contamination of musculoskeletal injection sites? Clin Orthop Relat Res. 2014. https://doi.org/10.1007/s11999-014-3909-4.
34. Provezano D, Liebert M, Steen B, et al. Investigation of current infection-control practices for ultrasound coupling gel: a survey, microbiological analysis, and examination of practice patterns. Reg Anesth Pain Med. 2013;38(5):415–24.
35. Chuan A, Tiong C, Maley M, et al. Decontamination of ultrasound equipment used for peripheral ultrasound-guided regional anaesthesia. Anaesth Intensive Care. 2013;41(4):529–34.

Ultrasound-Guided Airway Procedures

4

Abdullah Sulieman Terkawi, Ahmed Labib, Ashley Shilling, Andrew R. Bodenham, and Dimitrios Karakitsos

Introduction

The use of bedside ultrasound by nonradiologists, both for diagnosis and treatment, has revolutionized clinical practice. As ultrasound machines have become smaller, more portable, and cheaper, several specialties have begun to use ultrasound routinely in clinical practice [1]. While ultrasound utilization in airway management has lagged behind other common ultrasound applications (i.e., vascular applications, focused assessed sonography in trauma, lung sonography, etc.), the benefits of using ultrasound guidance for percutaneous dilation tracheostomy and cricothyrotomy have been well documented in literature [2]. Other potential uses include prediction of difficult laryngoscopy diagnosis of obstructive sleep apnea, endotracheal tube placement confirmation, diagnosis of acute epiglottitis, prediction of successful extubation, and ultrasound-guided superior laryngeal nerve block [3–5]. A thorough understanding of the sonoanatomy of upper airway and needle guidance principles is crucial to successfully perform ultrasound-guided upper airway procedures.

A. S. Terkawi (✉)
Department of Anesthesiology, Perioperative, and Pain Medicine, Stanford University, Stanford, CA, USA

Department of Anesthesiology, King Fahad Medical City, Riyadh, Saudi Arabia

Syrian Expatriate Medical Association - US (SEMA US), Santa Clara, CA, USA

A. Labib
Medical Intensive Care Unit, Hamad General Hospital, Doha, Qatar

A. Shilling
Department of Anesthesiology, University of Virginia, Charlottesville, VA, USA

A. R. Bodenham
Department of Anesthesia, Leeds General Infirmary, Leeds, UK

D. Karakitsos
Department of Internal Medicine, University of South Carolina, School of Medicine, Columbia, SC, USA

Advantages of Ultrasound Guidance

Traditionally, airway procedures such as tracheostomy and cricothyrotomy are performed by palpating anatomic landmarks. The success of these procedures is largely dependent on accurately identifying relevant anatomical landmarks (cricothyroid membrane, tracheal space) on palpation. However, digital palpation of surface landmarks is not always possible with excessive adipose tissue in the neck, less prominent thyroid cartilage, prior surgeries, radiation, etc. In an emergent situation, this technical difficulty can result in multiple unsuccessful attempts and hypoxia. Several studies have demonstrated the superiority of ultrasound-guided technique over

S. Adhikari, M. Blaivas (eds.), *The Ultimate Guide to Point-of-Care Ultrasound-Guided Procedures*, https://doi.org/10.1007/978-3-030-28267-7_4

the landmark method in identifying cricothyroid membrane and tracheal cartilages [6]. Ultrasound guidance increases procedure safety and operator confidence and decreases time in performing these procedures in emergent situations. With focused training in airway ultrasound, healthcare providers practicing in acute care settings can reliably use ultrasound guidance to perform these life-saving procedures.

Anatomy

The main anatomical structures of interest for upper airway ultrasound include:

1. *The tongue* consists of extrinsic and intrinsic muscles. The extrinsic muscles are the genioglossus, hyoglossus, styloglossus, and palatoglossus, while the intrinsic muscles include superior and inferior longitudinal muscles, verticalis, and transversus muscles. The tongue continues posteriorly as the epiglottis, while the valleculae results from the small depression between the tongue and the epiglottis. The mylohyoid muscles support the floor of the mouth, which extends between the mandibular rami as a hammock [3, 4, 7].
2. *The pharynx* is a collapsible tube that extends from the base of the skull down to the inferior border of the cricoid cartilage (around the C6 vertebral level), where it becomes continuous with the esophagus. It consists of three parts: the nasopharynx, oropharynx, and hypopharynx. The hypopharynx (laryngopharynx) extends from the upper border of epiglottis superiorly to the lower border of the cricoid cartilage inferiorly; it opens anteriorly to the larynx. The laryngeal inlet bulges into the hypopharynx leaving two recesses called the pyriform fossae, which are bounded by the aryepiglottic fold medially and the thyroid cartilage and thyrohyoid membrane laterally [3, 4, 7].
3. *The larynx* consists of the vocal cords and lies between the third and sixth cervical vertebrae. It is made up of muscles, ligaments, and a framework of cartilages. There are nine cartilages that support the larynx: three unpaired and three paired. The unpaired cartilages are (1) thyroid cartilage, which is connected to the hyoid bone by the thyrohyoid membrane; (2) cricoid cartilage, which is attached to the top of trachea and forms a complete ring to protect the upper airway from compression; and (3) the epiglottis, which closes the inlet of the trachea during swallowing. The paired cartilages include arytenoid, corniculate, and cuneiform cartilages. The true vocal cords are ligamentous structures that extend from the angle of the thyroid cartilage into the arytenoids. The triangular opening formed by the true vocal cards is the glottis. The larynx is innervated by the superior and recurrent laryngeal nerves. The former is the target for nerve blockade to facilitate awake intubation at it courses beside the hyoid bone. The internal division of the superior laryngeal nerve supplies the epiglottis, base of the tongue, and the supraglottic mucosa, while its external division provides sensation to the anterior subglottic mucosa and motor to cricothyroid muscle. The recurrent laryngeal nerve provides sensory innervation to the subglottic area and motor to all intrisic muscles of the larynx except cricothyroid [3, 4, 7].
4. *The trachea* is a tubular structure commencing at the lower border of the larynx (sixth cervical vertebra), at the level of cricoid cartilage, and bifurcates into the primary bronchi (fifth thoracic vertebra). It is flattened posteriorly and supported along its 10–15 cm length by 16–20 horseshoe-shaped cartilages (Fig. 4.1) [3, 4, 7, 8].

Sonoanatomy

Sonographically, bones like mandible and hyoid bone appear hyperechoic with a posterior anechoic shadowing. Fat is seen as hypoechoic lobules with echogenic septae. The thyroid and cricoid cartilages appear homogeneously hypoechoic on ultrasound. The muscles and connective tissue membranes are hypoechoic in structure but have a more heterogeneous striated appearance. Thyroid and salivary glands appear

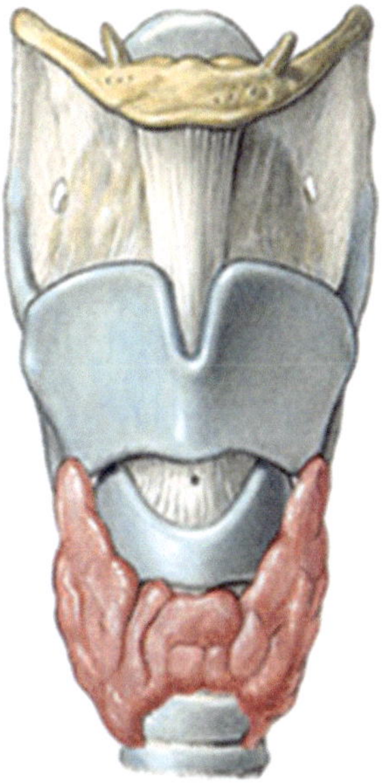

Fig. 4.1 Anatomy of upper airway (hyoid, thyroid cartilage, cricoid cartilage, trachea, thyroid). (Reproduced from Eur Arch Otorhinolaryngol (2011) 268:1357-1363-p. 1360)

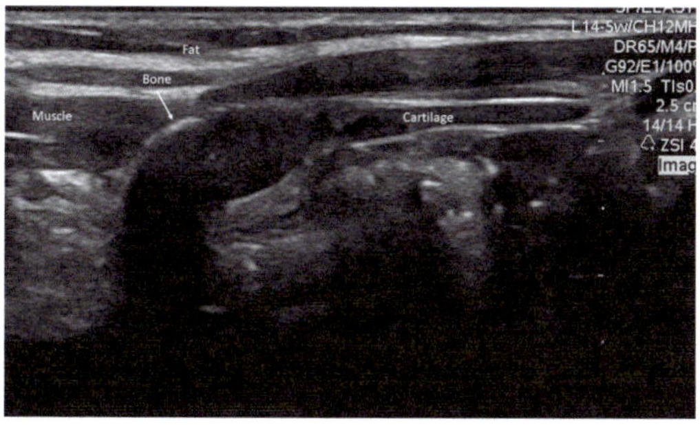

Fig. 4.2 Sonoanatomy of upper airway

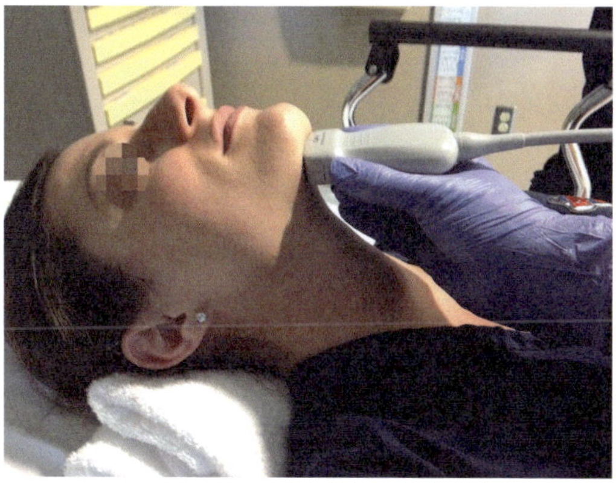

Fig. 4.3 Tongue and floor of mouth – transverse scanning plane. (Courtesy of Srikar Adhikari, MD)

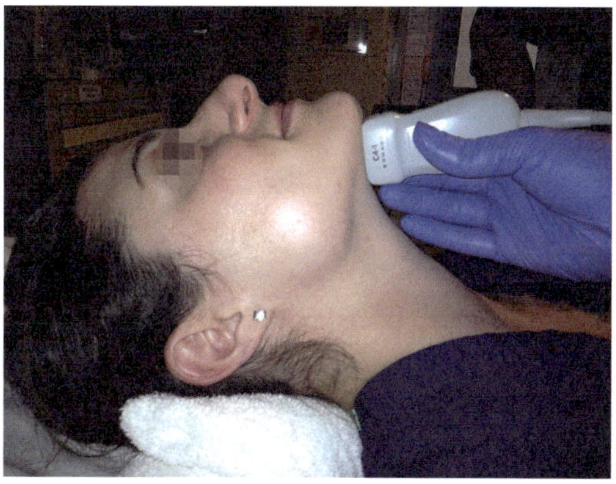

Fig. 4.4 Tongue and floor of mouth – sagittal scanning plane. (Courtesy of Srikar Adhikari, MD)

homogeneous and are more hyperechoic when compared to adjacent soft tissues and muscles. The interface between the upper airway mucosa and the intraluminal air which is called an air-mucosa interface appears as a bright hyperechoic line. Underneath the air-mucosa interface, air artifacts such as comet tail and reverberation artifacts are usually seen as multiple white lines. Air within the lumen of trachea impedes visualization of posterior wall of the trachea, posterior pharynx, and posterior commissure (Fig. 4.2).

Upper airway ultrasound is performed by orienting ultrasound probe in three planes: sagittal, parasagittal, and transverse with patient in sniffing position. An upper airway scanning protocol should include structures from floor of the mouth to the suprasternal notch. In order to best visualize the structures within the mouth including the tongue, a curvilinear probe should be used (Figs. 4.3 and 4.4). Due to the depth of the tongue, when imaging submentally, a lower-frequency transducer provides better penetration of the soft and bony structures. The mandible appears as a hyperechoic structure with acoustic shadowing posteriorly. The geniohyoid, genioglossus, and hyoglossus muscles are the extrinsic muscles generally seen on ultrasound. The geniohyoid muscle is seen as a thick hypoechoic band of tissue, and

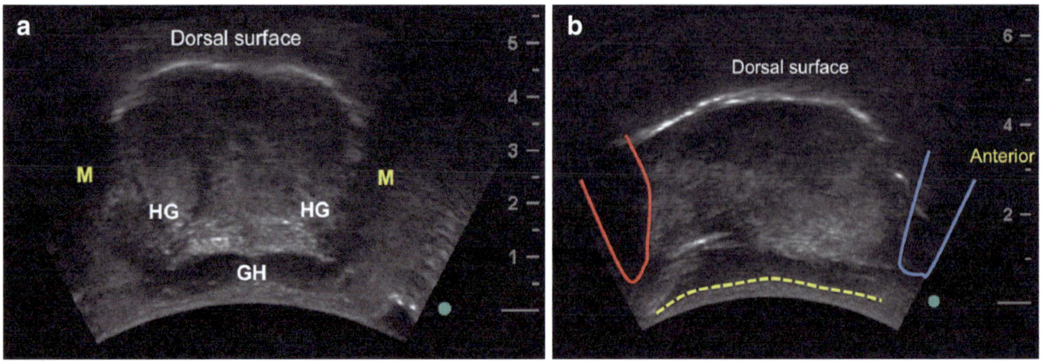

Fig. 4.5 B-mode image of tongue: (**a**) transverse view and (**b**) sagittal view using the curvilinear transducer. The mandible (M) contains the tongue bilaterally. The mentum is demarcated by blue, the hyoid bone in red, while the lower border of the muscles in the mouth floor is in dashed yellow. *GH* geniohyoid muscle,. *HG* hyoglossus muscles

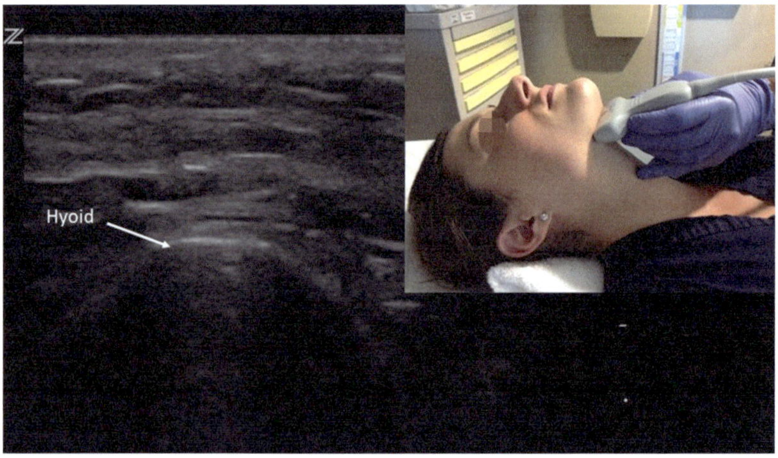

Fig. 4.6 Hyoid bone in transverse axis seen as an echogenic inverted U-shaped curvilinear structure with posterior acoustic shadowing. (Courtesy of Srikar Adhikari, MD)

the genioglossus muscles are found deep to the geniohyoid muscle on either side of the lingual septum and have hypoechoic and striated appearance (Fig. 4.5). The bony structures (mandible and the mastoid) prevent sonographic visualization of other extrinsic muscles of the tongue. The dorsal surface of the tongue is hyperechoic in appearance due to the air-mucosa interface. Typically a high-frequency linear array probe is used to visualize the rest of the upper airway anatomical structures. The hyoid bone serves as an important sonographic landmark that divides the upper airway into the suprahyoid and infrahyoid regions. It also serves as a landmark view when trying to locate the superior laryngeal nerve. The hyoid bone is seen as an echogenic inverted U-shaped curvilinear structure with posterior acoustic shadowing in short axis and a narrow hyperechoic curved structure with an acoustic shadow in sagittal and parasagittal planes (Figs. 4.6 and 4.7). The thyrohyoid membrane is seen as a hypoechoic rectilinear structure extending between the caudal border of the hyoid and the cephalad border of the thyroid cartilage. The epiglottis appears as a hypoechoic curvilinear structure through the thyrohyoid membrane on ultrasound. It has an inverted "C" appearance on transverse view. A hyperechoic preepiglottic space is seen anterior to epiglottis, and a bright linear air-mucosa interface is visualized posterior to epiglottis (Fig. 4.8). Identification of the epiglottis can be facilitated by tongue protrusion and swallowing. Thyroid cartilage is visualized as a hypoechoic inverted V-shaped structure in the

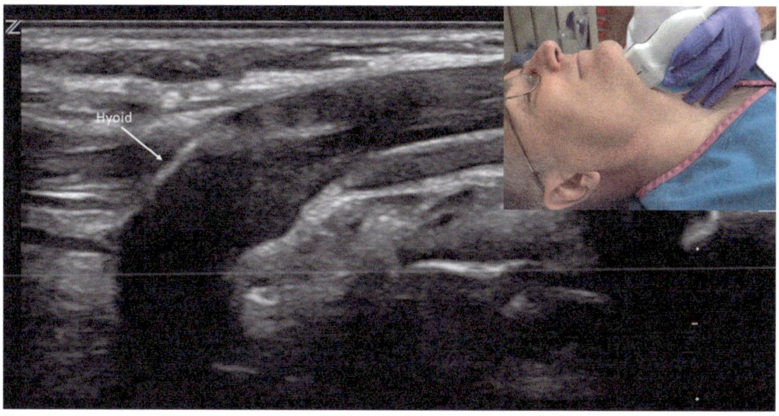

Fig. 4.7 Hyoid bone in long-axis narrow hyperechoic curved structure with an acoustic shadow. (Courtesy of Srikar Adhikari, MD)

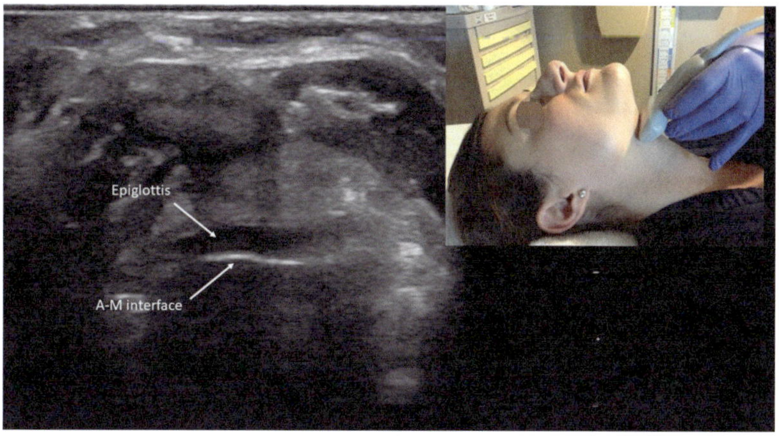

Fig. 4.8 B-mode image of epiglottis in transverse view seen as hypoechoic curvilinear structure (A-M interface-air-mucosa interface). (Courtesy of Srikar Adhikari, MD)

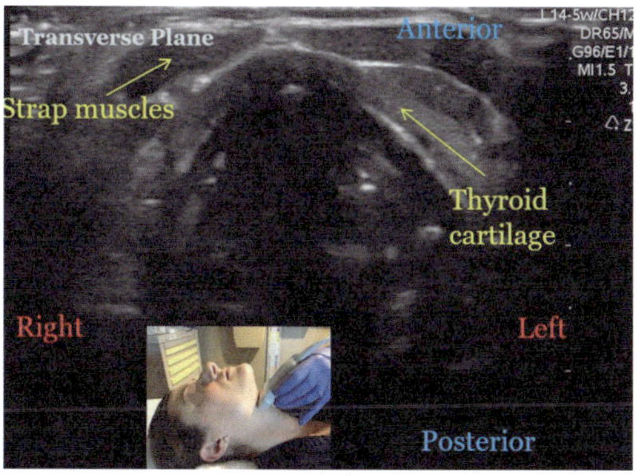

Fig. 4.9 Thyroid cartilage in transverse plane-hypoechoic inverted V-shaped structure. (Courtesy of Srikar Adhikari, MD)

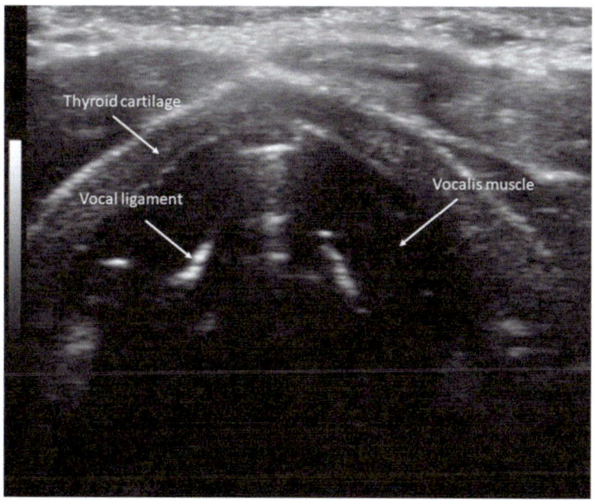

Fig. 4.10 B-mode image of true vocal cords seen as hypoechoic structures outlined medially by echogenic vocal ligaments. (Courtesy of Srikar Adhikari, MD)

transverse plane (Fig. 4.9). Vocal cords are seen deep to the thyroid cartilage. The triangular true vocal cords appear hypoechoic and are outlined medially by echogenic vocal ligaments (Fig. 4.10). The false vocal cords are found parallel and cephalad to the true vocal cords and are more hyperechoic in appearance due to increased fat content in the false vocal cords (Fig. 4.11). The cricothyroid membrane is seen as a hyperechoic band that runs between the hypoechoic thyroid and cricoid cartilages in sagittal and parasagittal planes (Fig. 4.12). The hypoechoic cricoid cartilage is cuboid in shape in short axis with a bright air-mucosa interface and reverberation artifacts from intraluminal air posteriorly (Fig. 4.13). The hypoechoic tracheal rings have inverted U appearance in transverse plane with hyperechoic air-mucosa interface and reverberation artifacts posteriorly. The isthmus of the thyroid gland is seen at the level of the second or third tracheal rings, and in the parasagittal plane, the tracheal rings resemble a "string of beads" (Figs. 4.14 and 4.15). Just lateral to the trachea, the anechoic carotid artery and internal jugular vein are identified. In the transverse plane, esophagus is seen as round or elliptical structure typically posterior and lateral to the trachea and has a "bull's eye" appearance at the level of the suprasternal notch (Fig. 4.16). Identification of the esophagus can be confirmed by asking the patient to swallow and observing the peristaltic movement and the intraluminal movement of the contents swallowed [8].

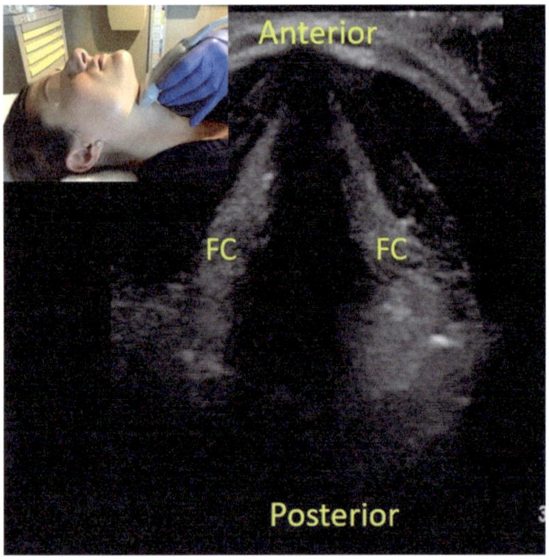

Fig. 4.11 Hyperechoic false vocal cords (FC). (Courtesy of Srikar Adhikari, MD)

Procedures

Percutaneous Dilation Tracheostomy (PDT)

Percutaneous dilation tracheostomy (PDT) is a commonly performed bedside surgical procedure. Refinement of equipment design, increased experience, and better training have led to enhanced safety of the procedure. However, complications such as perforation of the posterior wall of the trachea, puncture of the esophagus,

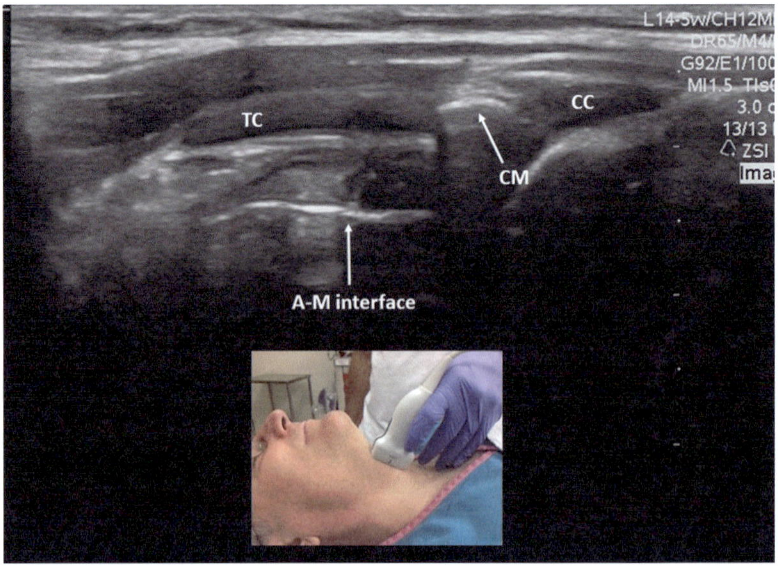

Fig. 4.12 Cricothyroid membrane (CM) seen as a hyperechoic band between the hypoechoic thyroid cartilage (TC) and cricoid cartilage (CC) in sagittal plane (A-M interface-air-mucosa interface). (Courtesy of Srikar Adhikari, MD)

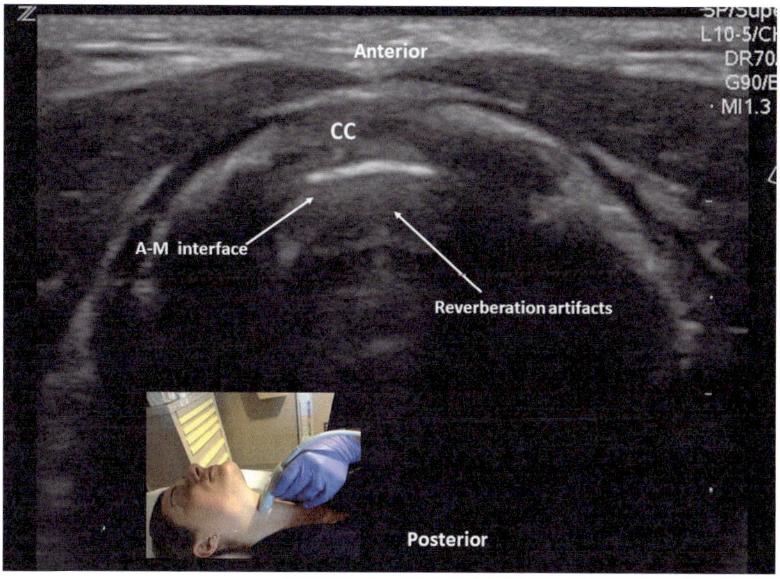

Fig. 4.13 Hypoechoic cricoid cartilage in short axis with a bright air-mucosa interface (A-M interface) and reverberation artifacts. (Courtesy of Srikar Adhikari, MD)

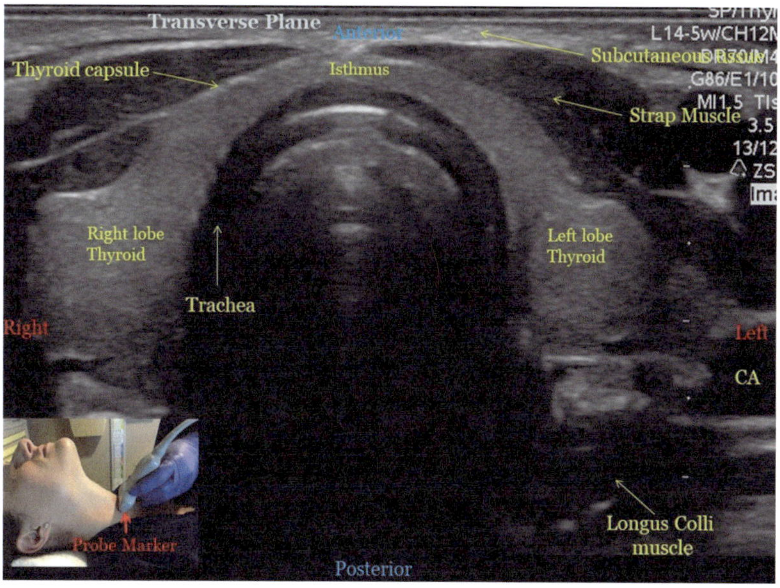

Fig. 4.14 Hypoechoic tracheal rings – inverted U appearance in transverse plane with hyperechoic air-mucosa interface and reverberation artifacts posteriorly. The isthmus of the thyroid gland is seen in this image. (Courtesy of Srikar Adhikari, MD)

tracheal ring injury, and vocal cord injury can still occur. Ultrasound can help avoid some of the aforementioned complications, improve safety, and increase the success rate of the procedure especially in the challenging patient [2, 3]. The optimum puncture level for PDT is usually guided by manual palpation of the anatomical landmarks of the anterior neck and endoscopic fiberoptic monitoring. However, this approach has several limitations. Ultrasound scanning of the neck prior to PDT and real-time guided penetration of the trachea may offset some of these shortfalls particularly when anatomical landmarks are not easily identifiable (e.g., in patients with previous tracheostomy, scar tissue, previous surgery or when neck mobility is limited during cervical spine precautions, and morbid obesity) [9, 10].

Abnormal cervical anatomy and obscure landmarks are associated with a higher incidence of peri- and post-procedural complications [11].

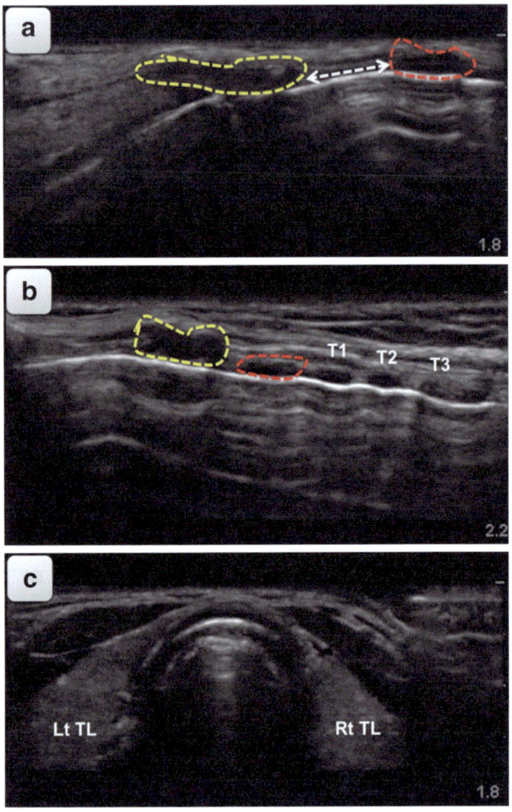

Fig. 4.15 Trachea, cricothyroid cartilage, and cricothyroid membrane scanning using a linear transducer (**a**) upper mid-sagittal plane, (**b**) lower mid-sagittal plane, and (**c**) transverse plane. The white hyperechoic line represents the tissue/air interface, while all echoes below it represent artifacts. The thyroid and cricoid cartilages are lined by yellow and red, respectively, and the arrow between them represents the cricothyroid membrane. T1, T2, and T3 indicate the first three tracheal rings; Lt TL and Rt TL indicate the left and right thyroid lobes

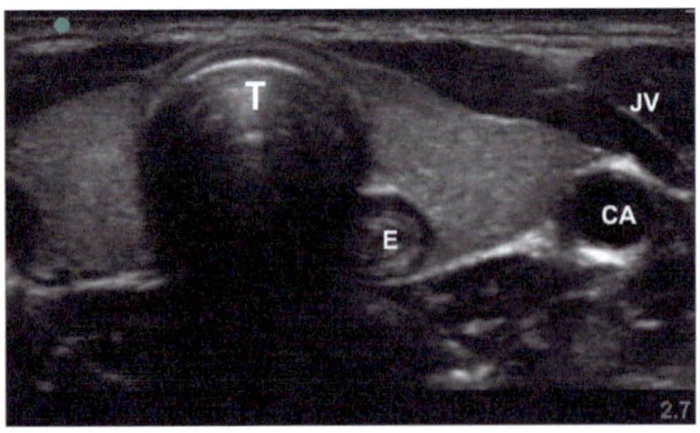

Fig. 4.16 Transverse view of the anterior neck depicting the trachea (T), the thyroid lobes, the esophagus (E), the carotid artery (CA), and external jugular vein (JV)

Even the use of endoscopic guidance could not avoid tracheostomy tube misplacement above or below the intended insertion site in a quarter of patients signaling poor correlation between actual insertion levels and palpated external landmarks [12].Obese patients undergoing PDT were five times more likely to suffer severe complications despite fiberoptic guidance [13].

Endoscopy offers direct and nearly continuous visualization of the advancing needle, guidewire, dilator, and tube position. However, it does not identify or reveal at-risk vascular structures, thyroid tissue, difficult cervical anatomy, or tracheal depth. Furthermore, endoscopy requires specialized equipment, training, and expertise which are all less likely to be available in any setting than a point-of-care ultrasound machine. Bleeding was observed in 4.8% of PDT patients in one series, and the authors suggested the use of ultrasound to minimize hemorrhagic complications [14]. Kollig et al. changed the planned puncture site in 24% of their patients following ultrasound assessment [15].

Real-time ultrasound-guided PDT was found to be safe in a small series of acute brain injury patient with cervical spine precautions [9]. Obese patients scheduled for PDT present various challenges. A short, thick neck and anatomical difficulties can render the ability to identify relevant external landmarks. Hence, PDT is relatively contraindicated in the morbidly obese patient. In contrast, ultrasound scanning of the obese patient requires considerable experience due to a short thyromental distance, thick pretracheal tissue, limited neck mobility, excessive subcutaneous fat, and poor anatomical landmarks. These factors make image acquisition and interpretation more challenging [10]. Nevertheless, in experienced hands scanning the anterior neck will provide the operator valuable information.

In a recent prospective study, Guinot et al. reported that real-time ultrasound-guided PDT in critically ill obese patients is safe and feasible. The incidence and severity of complications, as well as the time of completion of the procedure, did not differ significantly between obese and non-obese groups. The planned tracheal puncture point was changed in 50% of cases. Of note, ultrasound guidance and identification of cervical anatomy were described as being “difficult” in ten patients (20%), four of which were non-obese [10]. In the TARGET study, patients were randomized to undergo traditional landmark or real-time ultrasound-guided PDT. Ultrasound guidance was associated with significantly higher first needle pass success rate and more accurate tracheal puncture site placement. Fewer complications were observed in the ultrasound group [16].

Indications

The most common indication for PDT is respiratory failure and the need for continued mechanical ventilation. Other indications include upper airway obstruction from trauma, angioedema, malignancy, and obstructive sleep apnea, to facilitate weaning in difficult-to-wean patients and to aid in tracheobronchial toileting.

Contraindications

1. Infection at the site of insertion
2. Unstable patient
3. Infants
4. Unstable cervical spine injury
5. Uncontrollable coagulopathy

Equipment/Probe Selection (Fig. 4.17)

- High-frequency (12–5 MHz or higher) linear array probe
- A low-frequency (5–1 MHz) probe
- Percutaneous dilatational tracheostomy kit (22 gauge needle and syringe; 11 F short punch dilator; 1.32 mm guidewire; 8 F guiding catheter; 18 F, 21 F, 24 F, 28 F, 32 F, 36 F, and 38 F dilators; Shiley no. 8 double-cannula tracheostomy tube)

Preparation/Preprocedural Evaluation

1. The operator stands on the right side of the patient, and the ultrasound monitor is positioned on the opposite side at the appropriate height.
2. The operator should follow sterile precautions.
3. The patient is positioned supine and the neck is extended when possible.
4. Palpate the neck and identify landmark structures; the thyroid cartilage and sternal notch are palpable even in the morbidly obese.
5. Place the transducer transversely in the midline over the thyroid cartilage, and move caudally toward the suprasternal notch. This will

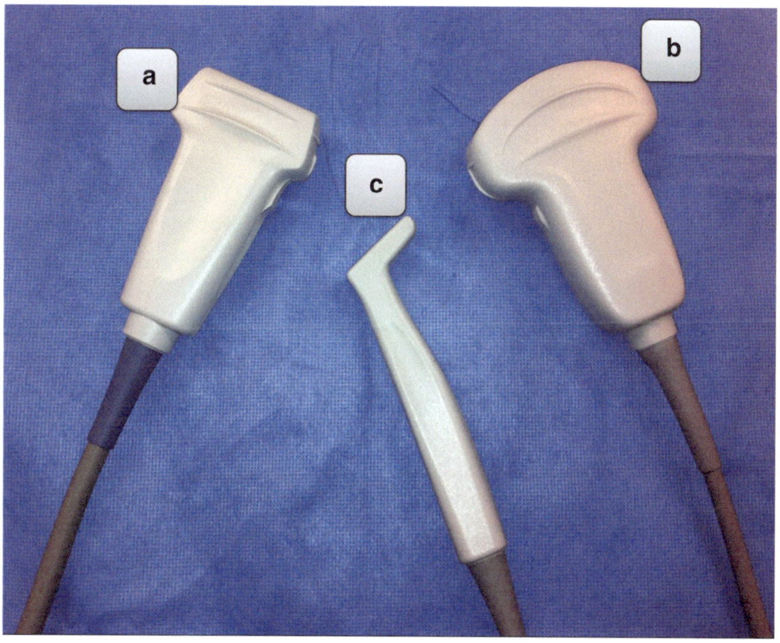

Fig. 4.17 (a) Linear, (b) curvilinear, and (c) hockey-stick transducers

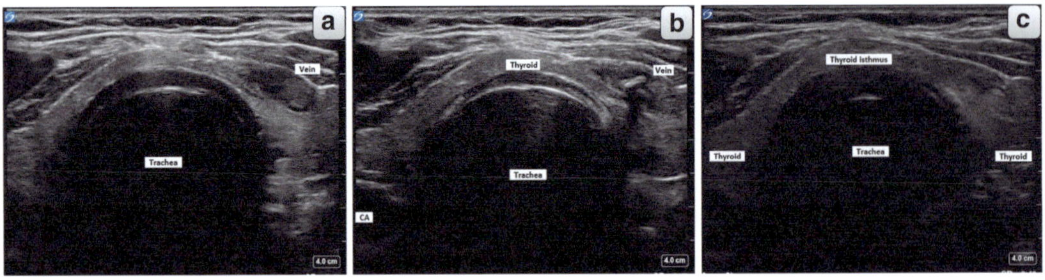

Fig. 4.18 A transverse scan using a linear probe at the level of the second tracheal ring. An off-midline vein is not uncommon (**a**). Note the effect of transducer compression upon the vein (**b** and **c**)

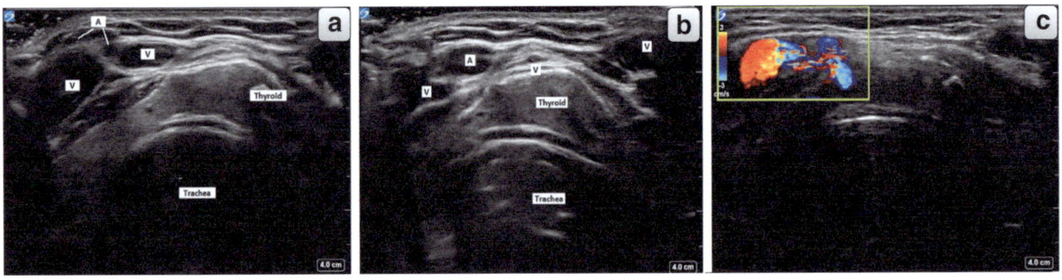

Fig. 4.19 Transverse scan of the neck with a linear transducer at the level of the third tracheal ring. Images (**a**) and (**b**) depict a number of "risk" vessels including a small vein at the possible needle penetration point (observe the probe compression in image **b**). (**c**) Color Doppler differentiating artery (pulsating flow) versus vein (orange shadow)

reveal the hypoechoic cartilaginous skeleton of the larynx and trachea with overlying thyroid isthmus (Fig. 4.14). Note that cartilages are uniformly hypoechoic, whereas striated muscles and connective tissue produce less homogeneous echoes. However, cartilages may become calcified and thus appear hyperechoic in the elderly. The thyroid gland and other glandular tissue usually appear as slightly hyperechoic (brighter) structures.

6. Select the highest resolution and adjust the image depth, so that the trachea could be seen at the bottom of the screen. The operator should measure the depth of the trachea from the skin, with the neck in a neutral position. This is particularly important when an extended-length tracheostomy tube is to be considered. Tracheal diameter and axis are also evaluated.
7. To obtain a sagittal/longitudinal view, the operator slides the transducer laterally on the neck (either side) while maintaining the edge of the transducer on the tracheal midline and then rotates the transducer 90° onto the sagittal plan. Subtle tilting of the transducer may be needed to optimize image acquisition. The resultant image is described as "pearls on a string" and represents the hypoechoic cricoid cartilage and individual tracheal rings anterior to the hyperechoic air-mucosa interface (Fig. 4.15). The operator should check for vascular structures with color Doppler within the area of interest at the midline to avoid those structures accordingly (Figs. 4.18 and 4.19). Then the optimum puncture site can be marked on the skin.

Procedure

1. Dynamic ultrasound guidance enables the visualization of the advancing needle and guidewire, mimicking ultrasound-guided vascular access and locoregional anesthetic procedures.
2. Static preprocedural ultrasound mapping of the neck is performed to provide preliminary information as discussed above.
3. The patient is prepared in a standard method (positioning, anesthesia, local anesthetic,

oxygenation and ventilation, monitoring, muscle relaxation, and drapes).

4. The operator should follow full aseptic technique, including sterile transducer sheath and gel.
5. An assistant adjusts the position of the tip of the endotracheal tube (ETT) under direct laryngoscopy, so that the tip is just inferior to the vocal cords. Alternatively, the ETT is replaced with a supraglottic airway device; however, this technique remains debatable as the airway is no longer protected or secured.
6. Hold the transducer in the nondominant hand and obtain a transverse view of the trachea.
7. Select optimum puncture level as discussed mentioned above, ideally between the first and fourth tracheal rings, avoiding vessels or a vascular isthmus in the path of the needle (Figs. 4.20).
8. Insert the tracheostomy puncture needle attached to a saline-filled syringe in the midline perpendicular to the skin, in an out-of-plane approach, and observe the ultrasound monitor for the characteristic acoustic shadow and artifacts due to tissue displacement caused by the advancing needle (Figs. 4.21 and 4.22). As with any needle guidance by ultrasound, an in-plane approach is preferred for its greater precision and safety. However, in some cases space may be limited, and an out-of-plane approach may be necessary as it can be in central line placement on occasion. Anterior tracheal wall indentation is sometimes observed. Typically, with out-of-plane approach, identification and discerning of the needle tip from the shaft can be challenging due to low angle of insinuation.
9. Stop advancing the needle when the needle is seen to penetrate the anterior tracheal wall. This is associated with an obvious change of resistance and a "give." Aspiration of air confirms intraluminal tip position. Tilt the needle slightly caudally to avoid retrograde passage of the wire guide.
10. Insert guidewire and remove the needle.
11. The guidewire is visualized on transverse and particularly longitudinal views as a distinct hyperechoic signal (Fig. 4.14). Ideal puncture is as close as possible to the midline [17]. Endoscopic examination at this stage will confirm wire entry point and rule out tracheal ring fracture or posterior wall injury. This further enhances the safety of the procedure.
12. Thereafter, proceed with PDT as per standard practice [17].

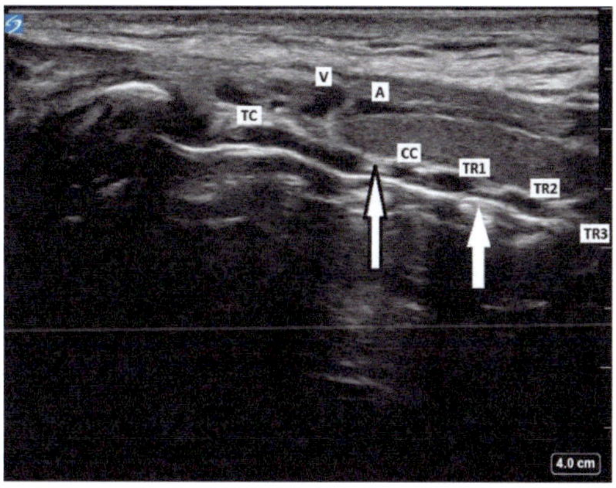

Fig. 4.20 Parasagittal plane of the trachea using a linear probe. Note the superficial airway structures (<2 cm beneath the skin) and the bright, hyperechoic air-tissue interface. Artifacts caused by air can be seen deeply to this interface, while the posterior wall of the trachea cannot be visualized. The thyroid, cricoid, and individual rings can be seen, and optimum puncture site can be chosen. Note the small vessels superior to the thyroid gland. The thyroid isthmus is seen overlying the 1st–3rd tracheal rings

Complications

- Transient hypoxia
- Major/minor bleeding
- Infection
- Posterior tracheal wall damage
- Tracheo-cutaneous, tracheo-innominate, and tracheo-esophageal fistula

Integration into Clinical Practice

Percutaneous dilatational tracheostomy is often performed in the intensive care setting. Ultrasound has been shown to reduce the incidence of vascular injury and assist with accurate placement of the cannula in the midline position at the optimum level. Some institutions have already implemented the adjunctive use of ultrasound during PDT as a safety measure. The number of ultrasound-guided PDT one has to perform to achieve

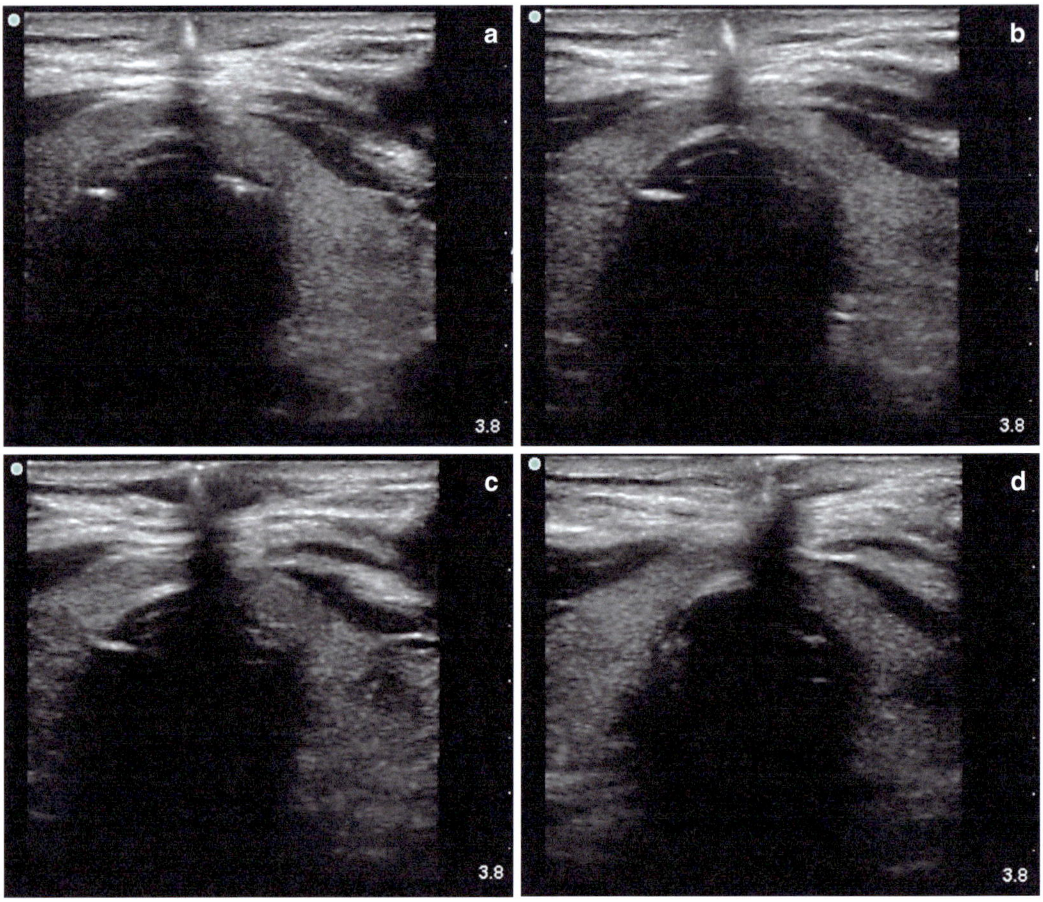

Fig. 4.21 Axial view using a linear probe of real-time ultrasound-guided PDT. Note the hyperechoic needle tip (**a**) and the acoustic shadow of the advancing needle (**b**). Observe the indentation of the anterior tracheal wall following needle penetration (**c** and **d**)

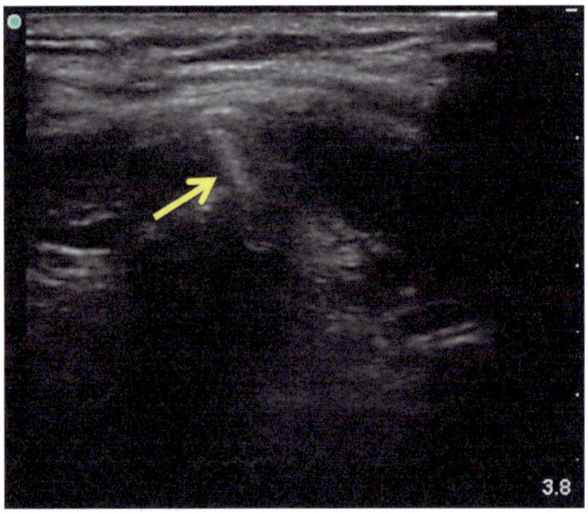

Fig. 4.22 Axial view using a linear probe depicting the guidewire position within the trachea

competency has not been determined. However, this point-of-care ultrasound application is not very challenging for providers with experience in using ultrasound guidance for other procedures. Ultrasound should be routinely used to perform PDT in patients who are morbidly obese or have difficult airway anatomy. In addition, ultrasound should be used for the identification of pretracheal vascular structures to avoid bleeding during PDT especially in patients on anticoagulants or at risk for bleeding from coagulopathy.

Pearls/Pitfalls

The ultrasound technique has its own inherent limitations, mainly inability to visualize the posterior wall of the trachea, which may risk inadvertent posterior wall puncture, subsequent perforation, and tube malposition. In the out-of-plane approach, identifying and discerning the needle tip from the shaft and tracking the entire needle can be challenging. As mentioned above, the sagittal plane and thus an in-plane needle guidance technique has the advantage of giving the operator a "birds-eye" view of the upper airway anatomy and is the ideal view in choosing the site of the tracheal puncture. Ultrasound remains largely an operator-dependent technique.

Evidence

In critically ill patients, especially in patients with morbid obesity and spinal damage, real-time ultrasound-guided PDT has been shown to be safe and cost-effective [18, 19]. Recent evidence suggests that the complications are ten times less in patients who receive ultrasonography-guided PDT when compared to patients who undergo landmark-guided PDT [20–22]. In a meta-analysis, ultrasound-guided PDT has been shown to be safe with decrease in complication rate when compared to the anatomical landmark-guided PDT. In addition, the complication rate was found to be comparable to the bronchoscopy-guided PDT [23]. The success rates were also higher, and time taken to successfully cannulate was shorter with ultrasound-guided PDT when compared to the conventional landmark methods [24].

Key Points

- Recent evidence supports the use of real-time ultrasound during PDT.
- Real-time ultrasound guidance can improve the rate of first-pass puncture and accuracy of site of puncture.
- Ultrasound guidance during PDT can decrease complication rate including bleeding from inadvertent puncture of adjacent vascular structures.
- Knowledge of upper airway sonoanatomy and a good understanding of fundamentals of needle guidance are crucial to perform ultrasound-guided PDT.

Ultrasound-Guided Cricothyrotomy

Direct access to the trachea via the cricothyroid membrane (CM) by emergent cricothyrotomy is the recommended rescue technique for "can't intubate, can't ventilate" (CICV) scenario with worsening hypoxia [25]. Cricothyrotomy is a time-critical, life-saving infrequently performed procedure, and successful outcome necessitates swift and precise identification of the CM and appropriate cannula or tube insertion through the CM. The CM spans the inferior border of the thyroid cartilage and the superior border of the cricoid cartilage. The average CM dimensions are 8 mm (width) × 11 mm (height) [26, 27].

In a major recent UK study, small-bore needle CT was cited as the preferred airway rescue technique, albeit with 63% failure rate. Failure to secure the airway with CT was reported at 64%. In the same report, a majority of needle CT performed in the intensive care unit and the emergency department (6 out of 8 procedures) failed to secure the airway. The authors recommended regular procedural training with particular emphasis on CM identification in obese and critically ill patients. The report calls for more research into equipment design and techniques including ultrasound [28].

Reliance on manual palpation and external anatomical landmark may be inadequate for correct identification of CM. Misidentification is more common in females. Without ultrasound assistance, CM was incorrectly identified 70% of the time, and in only 10% of cases did operators accurately identify the midline [29]. In morbidly obese patients with short thick necks and increased pretracheal tissue thickness and neck circumference, anatomical landmarks are more challenging, and careful airway assessment is recommended. Pregnancy and distorted neck anatomy warrant the same considerations.

Ultrasound guidance enabled rapid and accurate endotracheal access in a recent cadaveric study. A median time to identify the CM in less than 4 seconds and median time to complete CT in 26 seconds suggest that US-guided CT could be performed quickly and may not cause delays in airway rescue [30].

Indications

The emergency cricothyrotomy is generally indicated in any can't intubate, can't oxygenate (CICO) situation. Few examples of this scenario are listed below:

- Oral or maxillofacial trauma
- Cervical spine trauma
- Profuse oral bleeding
- Copious vomiting
- Anatomic abnormalities that prevent endotracheal intubation

Contraindications

There are no absolute contraindications to emergent cricothyrotomy. Relative contraindications include prior tracheal surgery, fractured larynx, laryngotracheal trauma and disruption, and children. Cricothyrotomy is a relative contraindication in children because of the funnel shape of the pediatric airway and increased risk of subglottic stenosis.

Equipment/Probe Selection

- Ultrasound system with a high-frequency (15–5 MHz, approximate range) linear array transducer
- Yankauer suction
- Scalpel (preferably #20 blade)
- Gum elastic bougie
- Cuffed tracheostomy tube 6.0
- 10 ml syringe
- Ventilator and tubing

Preparation/Preprocedural Evaluation

Preprocedural scanning is recommended to identify CM on ultrasound. On sagittal and parasagittal scanning planes, CM is visualized as a hyperechoic band bridging the hypoechoic thyroid above and cricoid cartilage below (Fig. 4.23). On the transverse view, the prominent thyroid cartilage is easily recognized as a triangular hypoechoic structure. Sliding the transducer caudally, a horizontal hyperechoic line caused by air-tissue interface defines the CM. Inferior to the CM, the cricoid cartilage is identified as an ovoid hypoechoic structure.

Procedure

Two techniques have been described: the longitudinal "String of Pearl" (SOP) technique and the transverse "Thyroid-Airline-Cricoid-Airline" (TACA) technique. The SOP technique is the most extensively studied and has been shown to be superior over palpation method. It also allows the identification of optimal site for tracheostomy tube placement. We recommend using string of pearl technique (Fig. 4.24) except in patients with short

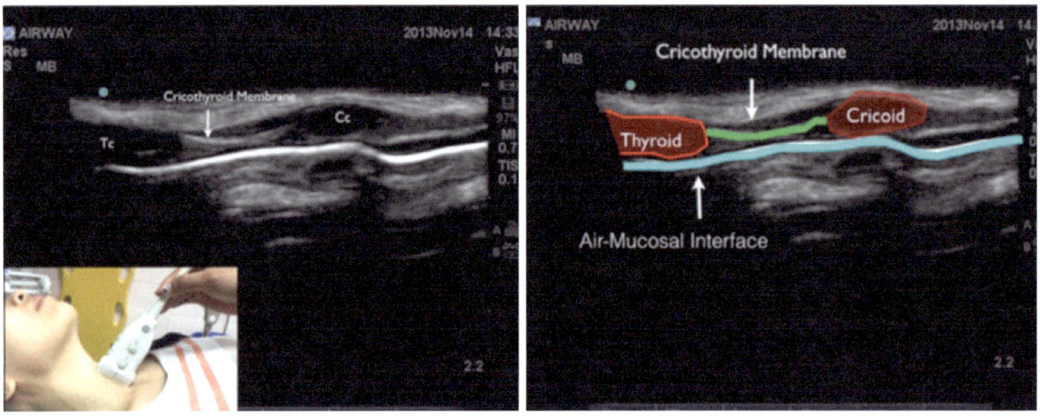

Fig. 4.23 Cricoid cartilage, thyroid cartilage, and cricothyroid membrane in longitudinal plane. Cc cricoid cartilage, Tc thyroid cartilage. (Reproduced with permission from Journal of Intensive Care (2016) 4:52- Role of upper airway ultrasound in airway management-p. 2)

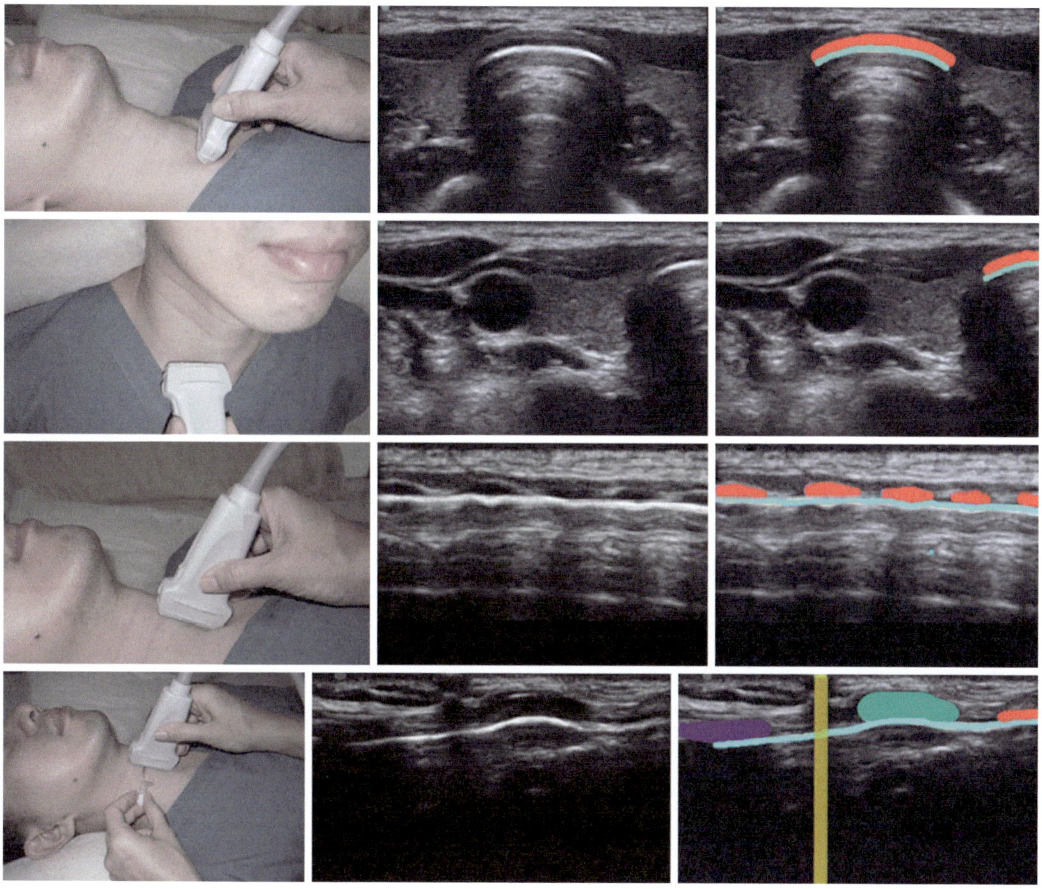

Fig. 4.24 Longitudinal "string of pearl" (SOP) technique for identifying the cricothyroid membrane and the interspaces between tracheal rings. Orange-red = tracheal ring; light blue = the tissue-air border; green = the cricoid cartilage; purple = the distal end of the thyroid cartilage. Yellow = the shadow from the needle slid in between the transducer and the skin. (Reproduced with permission from You-Ten et al. [6])

neck or flexion deformity of the neck that would make it difficult to place the ultrasound transducer in the longitudinal plane.

1. The operator stands on the right side of the patient and positions the ultrasound monitor at appropriate height at head end of the patient.
2. A linear-array high-frequency transducer (12–5 MHz) is ideal.
3. Place the transducer in transverse plane on the patient's neck just above the suprasternal notch to visualize the trachea which is seen as inverted U hypoechoic structure with hyperechoic reverberation artifacts posteriorly.
4. Slide the transducer toward the patient's right side of the neck (toward the operator) so that the right edge of the transducer is positioned in the midline of the trachea.
5. Maintain the right edge of the transducer over the midline of the trachea, and rotate the left end 90° into the sagittal plane to visualize trachea in long axis. A number of hypoechoic rings will be visualized anterior to the white echogenic line similar to "string of pearls." The dark hypoechoic "pearls" are the anterior portions of the tracheal rings.
6. Slide the transducer cephalad longitudinally in the midline until the cricoid cartilage (cuboid

in shape) is visualized. Slide further the cephalad to see thyroid cartilage. The echogenic CM is cephalad to the cricoid cartilage between thyroid and cricoid cartilages (Fig. 4.24).
7. While holding the transducer with nondominant hand, use the other hand to slide a needle between the transducer and the patient's skin until the needle's shadow is seen midway between the caudal border of the thyroid cartilage and the cephalad border of the cricoid cartilage. The needle marks the center of the cricothyroid membrane, and the rest of the procedure can be performed similar to traditional cricothyrotomy [2].

Complications

- Infection
- Bleeding
- Hypoxia
- Tracheal perforation
- Lacerations of tracheal cartilage, thyroid, cricoid, or tracheal rings
- Creation of a false tract (passage of the endotracheal tube into an area other than the trachea)

Pearls/Pitfalls

- The center of the CM can be marked with a pen, and the procedure can be performed without transducer in place.
- In some cases, an in-plane needle guidance approach and sagittal/longitudinal scanning plane cannot be utilized. Some patients have short neck and there won't be enough space to place the ultrasound transducer in a transverse plane. The out-of-plane approach should be used in these patients.
- The longitudinal scanning approach can provide additional information including the localization of the cricotracheal interspace and of the tracheal ring interspaces. This approach will be useful in smaller children, in patients with tumors overlying the CM, and in cases with subglottic obstruction.
- Focused training in airway ultrasound is helpful to achieve proficiency.
- Ultrasound-guided marking of the CM is generally unaffected by change in neck position.

Integration into Clinical Practice

Prior to rapid sequence induction, a quick ultrasound assessment of the anterior neck and confirmation of CM position and cricothyrotomy puncture site will reduce time and complications. In addition, identification of potentially difficult CM access may help clinician prepare better in handling a difficult airway. When there is significant airway concerns, preparation of the ultrasound machine with a sterile sleeve applied with gel and a needle cricothyrotomy kit at hand may prevent deleterious outcomes. Appropriate training in airway anatomy and needle guidance techniques are essential to successfully perform this emergency procedure.

Evidence

In studies comparing the identification of CM with palpation versus ultrasonography by a heterogeneous group of clinicians, successful identification of the CM with palpation alone was 67% in lean subjects, 46% in a mixed BMI cohort, and 37% in the morbidly obese, whereas with ultrasound, it improved to 69% in lean subjects, 100% in mixed BMI subjects, and 83% in morbidly obese subjects [31–33]. Curtis et al. demonstrated the feasibility of performing ultrasound-guided bougie-assisted cricothyroidotomy that may assist emergency physicians with identification of CM during difficult airway management [30]. In a randomized cadaver study done by Siddiqui et al. comparing digital palpation versus ultrasonography, injuries to the airway were three times lower in the ultrasound-guided group [34].

Key Points

- Accurate sonographic identification of the cricothyroid membrane is crucial in preparation for emergency airway management.
- "String of pearl" (SOP) technique is the preferred approach.
- Ultrasound-guided cricothyrotomy can result in higher success rates and decreased complications.

Ultrasound-Guided Endotracheal Intubation

Endotracheal tube (ETT) positioning can be confirmed both directly and indirectly. Direct visualization of the tube passing through trachea can be observed during real-time transverse ultrasound scanning of the neck at the level of the suprasternal notch or vocal cords (widening of the vocal cords). An indirect method of confirming ETT placement can be performed by lung sonography when placing the probe in the midaxillary line and observing the "sliding sign" bilaterally during ventilation. Endotracheal intubation is a critical procedure which relies upon being properly performed in the shortest duration of time possible to prevent poor patient outcomes. In patients with difficult anatomy, direct visualization of the endotracheal tube (ETT) inserted between the vocal cords may not be possible. Other ways to confirm placement of the ETT is chest wall rise during ventilation, flexible bronchoscope, capnometry, capnography, and chest radiograph. However, none of these methods provide real-time procedural guidance, and each of these methods has unique challenges for the provider. Ultrasound-guided endotracheal intubation can provide immediate information, and bedside ultrasound can also assist with subsequent tube position confirmation. Unlike capnography, there is also no need for lung ventilation with ultrasound. Confirmation of tube placement with ultrasound is faster compared to chest radiography [33].

Real-time endotracheal intubation can be visualized in three main areas of the upper airway: thyroid cartilage, tracheal rings, and the region above the suprasternal notch to visualize the trachea and esophagus simultaneously. In younger adults, the cartilage has not yet calcified, allowing visualization of the underlying vocal cords. Successful intubation through the vocal cords under ultrasound will be seen as a change in the air-mucosa interface, described as a "flickering" or "fluttering." Below the thyroid cartilage are the subglottic region and the tracheal rings. The trachea and the esophagus can be visualized together in the transverse axis under ultrasound. The esophagus lies more laterally, typically to the left of the patient's trachea, as it approaches the suprasternal notch. Transverse ultrasound views are preferred because sagittal views will only allow one to see the trachea or the esophagus and not both at the same time.

Indications

- Patients with difficult upper airway anatomy or trauma preventing direct visualization of ETT passing through vocal cords.
- Patients in which capnography is unreliable, i.e., poor pulmonary blood flow (e.g., pulmonary embolism), cardiopulmonary arrest, airway obstruction, etc. [34].
- Patients who are presumed to present with full stomachs, such as trauma patients, where insufflation of the stomach with gastric contents can cause vomiting and/or aspiration [35].
- Patients with limited cervical mobility [36].
- Delay or lack of other confirmatory mechanisms, such as capnography/capnometry, chest radiography, etc.
- Resource limited settings and austere environment.

Contraindications

- Patients with open anterior neck injuries
- Surgical airway
- Patients with short necks and technically difficult to perform ultrasound

Equipment and Probe Selection

- Ultrasound system with linear array probe and curved array probe, if ultrasound of the diaphragm is performed. A phased array transducer will work well for diaphragmatic assessment as well, but performs poorly for imaging the upper airway.
- Second operator other than the person intubating the patient to operate the machine and transducer (if performing real-time guidance)
- Ultrasound gel
- Laryngoscope blade and handle
- Endotracheal tube
- Syringe
- Equipment to capture capnography, ventilator, ETT tube securing kit, and appropriate monitor and ventilator set-up
- Wall suction set-up

Preparation and Preprocedural Evaluation

If time permits, assess the upper airway anatomy with ultrasound, especially if there is upper airway infection or trauma. As mentioned above, if real-time ultrasound guidance is pursued, a second individual is required to operate the machine and transducer. Focus on three regions for visualization: thyroid cartilage/vocal cords, tracheal rings, and the simultaneous view of the trachea and esophagus in transverse axis just above the suprasternal notch. Adjust the gain and the depth prior to the intubation, so visualization can be optimal.

Procedure

A transverse view of the airway structures is preferred. Place the ultrasound probe over the thyroid cartilage. As the ETT is passed through the vocal cords deep to the thyroid cartilage, disruption of the air-mucosa interface will cause a "flicker." Once you see the flicker, slide the ultrasound probe down to the tracheal rings to follow the change in the air-mucosa interface. Lastly, to have a side-by-side view of the trachea and the esophagus, slide the probe down to just above the suprasternal notch. In a successfully endotracheally intubated patient, you will see the reverberation artifact of the inflated ETT cuff in the trachea (Figs. 4.25 and 4.26), with an adjacent collapsed esophagus. In an esophageal intubation, a "double-tract sign" is seen (Fig. 4.27), meaning there are two air-mucosa interfaces with reverberation artifact, one from the trachea and the other from the distended esophagus with an inflated ETT cuff. To improve visualization of the cuff, fill the cuff with water instead of air so an anechoic circle can appear and elucidate the cuff's position. If esophageal intubation has occurred, then the ETT should be removed as

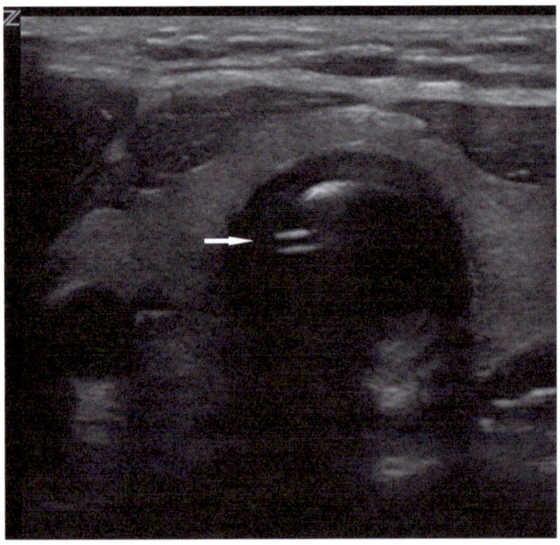

Fig. 4.25 Transverse view of endotracheal tube (arrow) in trachea. (Courtesy of Srikar Adhikari, MD)

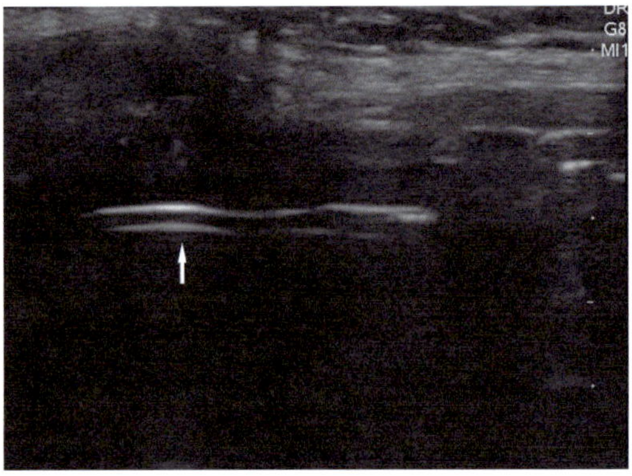

Fig. 4.26 Longitudinal view of endotracheal tube (arrow) in the trachea. (Courtesy of Srikar Adhikari, MD)

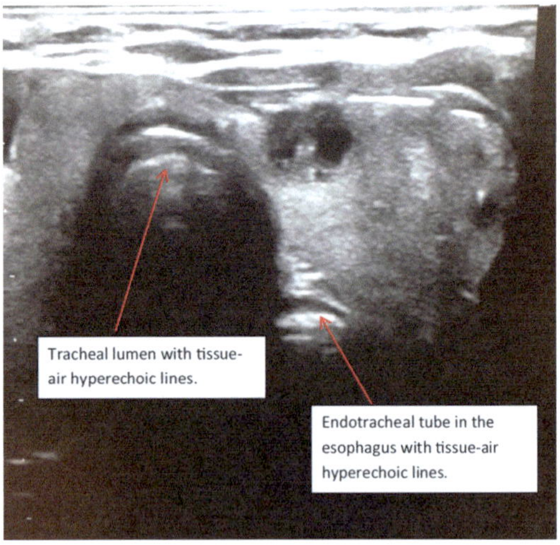

Fig. 4.27 Esophageal intubation. Transverse view just above the suprasternal notch and to the left of the trachea. The tissue-air hyperechoic lines are visualized in the trachea and esophagus (because of esophageal intubation), which is referred to as the "double-tract sign". (Reproduced with permission from You-Ten et al. [6])

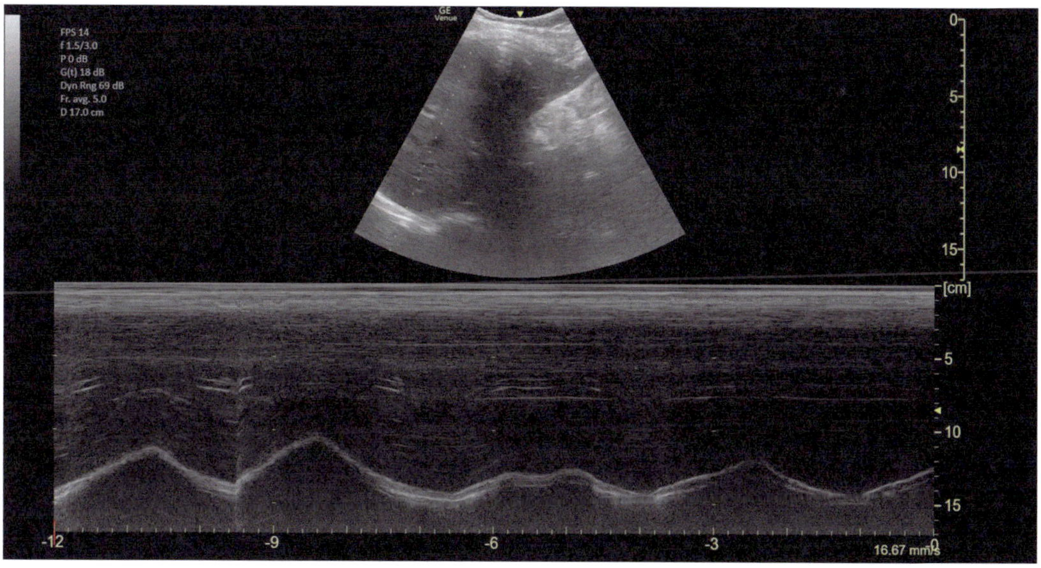

Fig. 4.28 M-mode image showing diaphragmatic excursion. (Courtesy of Srikar Adhikari, MD)

soon as possible, and another attempt at endotracheal intubation should ensue.

After intubation, tube placement confirmation can also be performed. With the patient lying supine, locate the most anterior portion of the patient's chest wall, typically the third or fourth intercostal space. Using the linear array probe, direct the probe indicator toward the patient's head, and place it in the most anterior intercostal space to search for pleural sliding on the right. Repeat on these steps on the left. If there is pleural sliding on both sides, then the depth of the ETT placement is adequate for bilateral lung ventilation. If there is only lung sliding on the right and none on the left, the ETT may be in the right main stem. Carefully retract the ETT in small intervals and repeat the thoracic ultrasound until you see lung sliding on the left, but pay careful attention to prevent extubation. If there is persistently no lung sliding on the left, then there may be a left-sided pneumothorax.

Diaphragmatic ultrasound imaging can also assist with tube placement confirmation. Instead of using the linear array probe, use the curved array probe to find the diaphragm on the right lower lateral chest wall. The diaphragm will appear as a hyperechoic strip coursing directly cephalad over the liver. To see the up and down movement of the diaphragm more clearly, M-mode can be used to trace the movement by placing the M-mode sampling line over the arch of the diaphragm (Fig. 4.28). Repeat these steps over the left side of the diaphragm, above the spleen.

Complications

The main complications will arise from operator experience. The operator will need to be competent with at least the main sonographic views of the upper airway for ETT guidance. Errors in either false-positive or false-negative confirmations can be catastrophic and will require other more traditional mechanisms of confirmation, which may delay discovery of an esophageal intubation. Other complications would be patient discomfort or the rare skin irritation from ultrasound gel.

Pearls/Pitfalls

There are challenges to performing real-time ultrasound-guided endotracheal intubation. This ultrasound application requires a second individual to perform the ultrasound, which is not always possible. With the increasing portability of ultrasound and its ubiquity, incorporation of this skill into pre-hospital medicine may be limited by the need of a second individual. Also, because of the placement of the ultrasound probe, it can be in the direct path of the laryngoscope handle, limiting the mobility of the person intubating the patient [37]. However, even with one person, ultrasound can still be used to confirm ETT placement through the methods discussed above.

Visualization of airway structures may not be possible. Ultrasound images can be obscured by multiple reasons: difficult patient anatomy, subcutaneous emphysema, and calcifications of the thyroid cartilage or tracheal rings.

Integration into Clinical Practice

Endotracheal intubation is a common procedure, and the success of the procedure is critical to protect the patient's airway and prevent further clinical decompensation. Ultrasound guidance of this procedure is relatively simple to learn, and it is noninvasive. Especially in emergent situations, real-time guidance can assist with patients with difficult anatomy, upper airway infections, trauma, etc. and in situations where capnography is limited in its reliability. Confirmation of intubation is also facile, frequently able to be performed before chest radiography equipment is available. Knowledge of upper airway sonographic anatomy will translate into diagnosis of airway pathologies and assist with directing/planning cricothyrotomies in patients with difficult to palpate anatomy.

Evidence

Das et al. published a systematic review and meta-analyses in 2015 on using transtracheal ultrasound to verify endotracheal tube placement [33]. The final analysis included 11 studies and 969 intubations, revealing a pooled sensitivity of 98% and specificity of 98%. In emergent intubations and ETT verifications, the sensitivity was 98% and specificity was 94%. It shows that this ultrasound skill is achievable, even among varied experienced operators.

Studies have shown the time required to perform ultrasound verification of intubation is short, ranging from 5 to 45 seconds [38–40]. Pfeiffer et al. produced two studies which compared the timeliness of ultrasound to capturing capnography and found that the median time for verification was much shorter with ultrasound [37, 38]. Muslu et al.'s study showed that their sonographer was able to determine tracheal or esophageal intubation in real time within 3 seconds of intubation [41]. These studies once again highlight the benefit of bedside ultrasound and the benefits of incorporating ultrasound into common procedures, giving the provider immediate information for medical decision making.

Key Points

- Real-time ultrasound-guided endotracheal intubation is noninvasive and fast and has multiple benefits over the current gold standard of capnography.
- Even if real-time guidance cannot be performed because of lack of a second operator during intubation, ultrasound confirmation of tracheal intubation and bilateral lung ventilation (via thoracic ultrasound or diaphragmatic ultrasound) can still be performed.
- If time permits, prescan the patient's upper airway anatomy, especially in the setting of trauma, upper airway infection, or possible obstruction.
- Ultrasound images can also be obscured by multiple reasons: difficult patient anatomy, subcutaneous emphysema, and calcifications of the thyroid cartilage or tracheal rings.

Superior Laryngeal Nerve (SLN) Block

There are anecdotal reports of a successful visualization and blockade of SLN using a 5–10 MHz linear probe for awake endotracheal intubation [42]. Recently, another study reported a successful "field" SLN block facilitating awake endotracheal intubation (Fig. 4.29) [43].

Barberet et al. [44] in 100 patients, using a 4 cm width 12 MHz linear probe, could not visu-

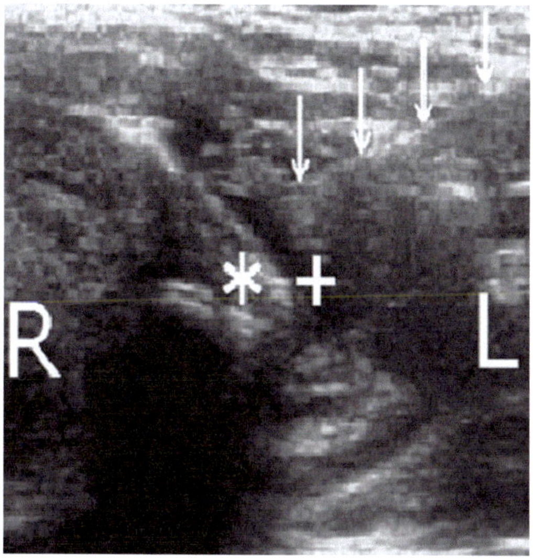

Fig. 4.29 Superior laryngeal nerve block. Transverse view at the level of the hyoid bone demonstrating an in-plane technique. Arrows indicates the entry of the needle from the 2 o'clock direction;* indicates the greater horn of the hyoid; + indicates the injected anesthetic agent. (Reproduced with permission from J Anesth (2013) 27:309–310 Ultrasound-guided superior laryngeal nerve block and translaryngeal block for awake tracheal intubation in a patient with laryngeal abscess-p. 310)

alize the SLN as the nerve is small sized (1 mm). However, they suggested that the nerve could be localized in a space named SLN space. The space contains the internal branch of the nerve (contributing to sensory innervation to the airway) and is formed by the hyoid bone superiorly, the thyroid cartilage inferiorly, the thyrohyoid muscle anteriorly, and the thyrohyoid membrane and the preepiglottis space posteriorly. When all of thyrohyoid muscle, preepiglottis space, hyoid bone, thyroid cartilage, and thyrohyoid membrane are seen in the ultrasound image, then it considered an optimal image. But when all of the previous structures other than the thyrohyoid membrane are seen, then this is a suboptimal image and poor in all other cases. Notably, Kaur et al. [45] in 20 volunteers, using a hockey stick-shaped 15–8 MHz probe, were able to visualized the nerve clearly in 1/3 of the cases, equivocally visualized the nerve in another 1/3, and could not visualize it in the remaining 1/3 of cases. The superior laryngeal artery was visualized in 10% of the scans. Kaur et al. suggested method to localize the hyoid bone in a sagittal position first and then to rotate the transducer obliquely until you get a consistent image of the SLN, as the nerve travels medially and caudally toward the thyrohyoid membrane. The nerve can be traced until it pierces the thyrohyoid membrane to confirm the finding. The mean distance from the internal branch of the SLN to the greater horn of the hyoid bone is 2.4 mm. While visualization of SLN is not possible to all sonographers, this does not preclude the use of ultrasound in performance of a successful nerve block.

References

1. Terkawi AS, Karakitsos D, Elbarbary M, Blaivas M, Durieux ME. Ultrasound for the anesthesiologists: present and future. Sci World J. 2013;2013:683685.
2. Osman A, Sum KM. Role of upper airway ultrasound in airway management. J Intensive Care. 2016;4:52.
3. Kristensen MS. Ultrasonography in the management of the airway. Acta Anaesthesiol Scand. 2011;55: 1155–73.
4. Kristensen MS, Teoh WH, Graumann O, Laursen CB. Ultrasonography for clinical decision-making and intervention in airway management: from the mouth to the lungs and pleurae. Insights Imaging. 2014;5:253–79.
5. Adhikari S, Zeger W, Schmier C, Crum T, Craven A, Frrokaj I, et al. Pilot study to determine the utility of point-of-care ultrasound in the assessment of difficult laryngoscopy. Acad Emerg Med. 2011;18:754–8.
6. You-Ten KE, Siddiqui N, Teoh WH, Kristensen MS. Point-of-care ultrasound (POCUS) of the upper airway. Can J Anaesth. 2018;65(4):473–84.
7. Rajagopal MR, Paul J. Applied anatomy and physiology of the airway and breathing. Indian J Anaesth. 2005;49(4):251–6.
8. Singh M, Chin KJ, Chan VW, Wong DT, Prasad GA, Yu E. Use of sonography for airway assessment: an observational study. J Ultrasound Med. 2010; 29(1):79–85.
9. Rajajee V, Fletcher JJ, Rochlen LR, Jacobs TL. Real-time ultrasound-guided percutaneous dilatational tracheostomy: a feasibility study. Crit Care. 2011; 15:R67.
10. Guinot PG, Zogheib E, Petiot S, Marienne JP, Guerin AM, Monet P, et al. Ultrasound-guided percutaneous tracheostomy in critically ill obese patients. Crit Care. 2012;16:R40.
11. Massick DD, Powell DM, Price PD, Chang SL, Squires G, Forrest LA, et al. Quantification of the learning curve for percutaneous dilatational tracheotomy. Laryngoscope. 2000;110:222–8.

12. Walz MK, Schmidt U. Tracheal lesion caused by percutaneous dilatational tracheostomy–a clinico-pathological study. Intensive Care Med. 1999;25:102–5.
13. Byhahn C, Lischke V, Meininger D, Halbig S, Westphal K. Peri-operative complications during percutaneous tracheostomy in obese patients. Anaesthesia. 2005;60:12–5.
14. Muhammad JK, Major E, Wood A, Patton DW. Percutaneous dilatational tracheostomy: haemorrhagic complications and the vascular anatomy of the anterior neck. A review based on 497 cases. Int J Oral Maxillofac Surg. 2000;29:217–22.
15. Kollig E, Heydenreich U, Roetman B, Hopf F, Muhr G. Ultrasound and bronchoscopic controlled percutaneous tracheostomy on trauma ICU. Injury. 2000; 31:663–8.
16. Rudas M, Seppelt I, Herkes R, Hislop R, Rajbhandari D, Weisbrodt L. Traditional landmark versus ultrasound guided tracheal puncture during percutaneous dilatational tracheostomy in adult intensive care patients: a randomised controlled trial. Crit Care. 2014;18:514.
17. Rashid AO, Islam S. Percutaneous tracheostomy: a comprehensive review. J Thorac Dis. 2017;9(Suppl 10):S1128–38.
18. Joelsons D, Ho YL, Park M. Ultrasound-guided percutaneous tracheostomy: a feasible alternative for tetanus patients. Crit Care. 2014;18(3):441.
19. Mehta Y. Percutaneous dilatational tracheostomy: guided well with real-time ultrasound. Indian J Crit Care Med. 2013;17(6):335–6.
20. Kate OR. Ultrasound: the new standard of care for percutaneous dilatational tracheostomy? J Clin Anesthesiol. 2014;40:3.
21. Dinh VA, Farshidpanah S, Lu S, Stokes P, Chrissian A, Shah H, et al. Real-time sonographically guided percutaneous dilatational tracheostomy using a long-axis approach compared to the landmark technique. J Ultrasound Med. 2014;33(8):1407–15.
22. Ziyaeifard M, Azarfarin R. Ultrasound is a new and reliable technique for central venous cannulation. Res Cardiovasc Med. 2014;3(3):e24653.
23. Gobatto ALN, Besen BAMP, Cestari M, Pelosi P, Malbouisson LMS. Ultrasound-guided percutaneous dilational tracheostomy: a systematic review of randomized controlled trials and meta-analysis. J Intensive Care Med. 2018;885066618755334.
24. Dinsmore J, Heard AM, Green RJ. The use of ultrasound to guide time critical cannula tracheotomy when anterior neck airway anatomy is unidentifiable. Eur J Anaesthesiol. 2011;28(7):506–10.
25. Apfelbaum JL, Hagberg CA, Caplan RA, Blitt CD, Connis RT, Nickinovich DG, et al. Practice guidelines for management of the difficult airway: an updated report by the American Society of Anesthesiologists Task Force on Management of the Difficult Airway. Anesthesiology. 2013;118:251–70.
26. Dover K, Howdieshell TR, Colborn GL. The dimensions and vascular anatomy of the cricothyroid membrane: relevance to emergent surgical airway access. Clin Anat. 1996;9:291–5.
27. Elliott DS, Baker PA, Scott MR, Birch CW, Thompson JM. Accuracy of surface landmark identification for cannula cricothyroidotomy. Anaesthesia. 2010;65:889–94.
28. Socity TRCoAaTDA. Major complications of airway management in the UK. 4th National Audit. 2011.
29. Campbell M, Ash S, Royds J, et al. The accuracy of locating the cricothyroid membrane by palpation – an intergender study. BMC Anesthesiol. 2014;14(1):108.
30. Curtis K, Ahern M, Dawson M, Mallin M. Ultrasound-guided, Bougie-assisted cricothyroidotomy: a description of a novel technique in cadaveric models. Acad Emerg Med. 2012;19:876–9.
31. Kristensen MS, Teoh WH, Rudolph SS, et al. Structured approach to ultrasound-guided identification of the cricothyroid membrane: a randomized comparison with the palpation method in the morbidly obese. Br J Anaesth. 2015;114:1003–4.
32. Barbe N, Martin P, Pascal J, Heras C, Rouffiange P, Molliex S. Locating the cricothyroid membrane in learning phase: value of ultrasonography? Ann Fr Anesth Reanim. 2014;33:163–6. Siddiqui N, Arzola C, Friedman Z, Guerina L, You-Ten KE. Ultrasound improves cricothyrotomy success in cadavers with poorly defined neck anatomy: a randomized control trial. Anesthesiology. 2015;123(5):1033–41.
33. Yildiz G, Göksu E, Şenfer A, Kaplan A. Comparison of ultrasonography and surface landmarks in detecting the localization for cricothyroidotomy. Am J Emerg Med. 2016;34:254–6. Das SK, Choupoo NS, Haldar R, Lahkar A. Transtracheal ultrasound for verification of endotracheal tube placement: a systematic review and meta-analysis. Can J Anesth/J Can Anesth. 2014; 62(4):413–23.
34. Cook TM, Nolan JP. Use of capnography to confirm correct tracheal intubation during cardiac arrest. Anaesthesia. 2011;66:1183–4.
35. Zechner PM, Breitkreutz R. Ultrasound instead of capnometry for confirming tracheal tube placement in an emergency? Resuscitation. 2011;82:1259–61.
36. Moustafa MA, Arida EA, Zanaty OM, El-tamboly SF. Endotracheal intubation: ultrasound-guided versus fiberscope in patients with cervical spine immobilization. J Anesth. 2017;31(6):846–51.
37. Pfeiffer P, Rudolph SS, Borglum J, Isbye DL. Temporal comparison of ultrasound vs. auscultation and capnography in verification of endotracheal tube placement. Acta Anaesthesiol Scand. 2011;55:1190–5.
38. Pfeiffer P, Bache S, Isbye DL, Rudolph SS, Rovsing L, Borglum J. Verification of endotracheal intubation in obese patients – temporal comparison of ultrasound vs. auscultation and capnography. Acta Anaesthesiol Scand. 2012;56:571–6.
39. Chou HC, Tseng WP, Wang CH, et al. Tracheal rapid ultrasound exam (T.R.U.E) for confirming endotracheal tube placement during emergency intubation. Resuscitation. 2011;82:1279–84.

40. Adi O, Chuan TW, Rishya M. A feasibility study on bedside upper airway ultrasonography compared to waveform capnography for verifying endotracheal tube location after intubation. Crit Ultrasound J. 2013;5:7.
41. Muslu B, Sert H, Kaya A, et al. Use of sonography for rapid identification of esophageal and tracheal intubation in adult patients. J Ultrasound Med. 2011; 30:671–6.
42. Manikandan S, Neema PK, Rathod RC. Ultrasound-guided bilateral superior laryngeal nerve block to aid awake endotracheal intubation in a patient with cervical spine disease for emergency surgery. Anaesth Intensive Care. 2010;38:946–8.
43. Iida T, Suzuki A, Kunisawa T, et al. Ultrasound-guided superior laryngeal nerve block and translaryngeal block for awake tracheal intubation in a patient with laryngeal abscess. J Anesth. 2013;27:309–10.
44. Barberet G, Henry Y, Tatu L, Berthier F, Besch G, Pili-Floury S, et al. Ultrasound description of a superior laryngeal nerve space as an anatomical basis for echoguided regional anaesthesia. Br J Anaesth. 2012;109:126–8.
45. Kaur B, Tang R, Sawka A, Krebs C, Vaghadia H. A method for ultrasonographic visualization and injection of the superior laryngeal nerve: volunteer study and cadaver simulation. Anesth Analg. 2012;115:1242–5.

Ultrasound-Guided Cardiac Procedures

5

Timothy Faust and J. Matthew Fields

Transvenous Pacemaker

Introduction

In an emergent setting, cardiac pacing is used as a temporary stabilizing measure in patients with dysfunctional cardiac electrical activity resulting in bradycardia and hemodynamic instability. There are multiple modes of providing temporary pacing, but the most common methods in the emergency department are transcutaneous and transvenous pacing [1]. This section will focus on transvenous pacing with ultrasound guidance to facilitate the procedure and avoid potential complications (Figs. 5.1 and 5.2).

Advantages of Ultrasound Guidance

The use of bedside ultrasound will provide benefits during various stages of placing a transvenous pacemaker. It should be noted that the first step in placing a transvenous pacemaker is obtaining central venous access in order to facilitate advancement of a pacemaker catheter into the right ventricle. As noted in the central venous access chapter, utilizing ultrasound guidance for placing central venous catheters significantly decreases complications and increases success rates.

For the placement of a transvenous pacemaker, continuous real-time ultrasound guidance can be utilized to visualize proper placement and propagation of a cardiac pacing catheter and avoid potential complications, which may include advancement into the pulmonary artery, damage to the myocardium, or coiling in the right atrium. Ultrasound visualization of the inferior vena cava (IVC) is also useful for evaluation of catheter malposition.

Bedside ultrasound can additionally be beneficial in assessing for capture in both transcutaneous [2] and transvenous pacing. The standard cardiac views will be used to evaluate for cardiac activity after each of these procedures has been performed. This may be a valuable adjunct in addition to the clinical signs which are typically used to evaluate the effectiveness of temporary pacing. Bedside echocardiographic evaluation before and after pacemaker implantation can demonstrate the effectiveness of the procedure. Additionally, ultrasound can be repeated to assess for continued effectiveness given any changes in the clinical picture.

Anatomy

The preferred sites for placement of a transvenous pacemaker are the right internal jugular vein and left subclavian vein. These sites provide the most direct course to the right atrium, via the

T. Faust · J. M. Fields (✉)
Department of Emergency Medicine, Thomas Jefferson University Hospital, Philadelphia, PA, USA

S. Adhikari, M. Blaivas (eds.), *The Ultimate Guide to Point-of-Care Ultrasound-Guided Procedures*, https://doi.org/10.1007/978-3-030-28267-7_5

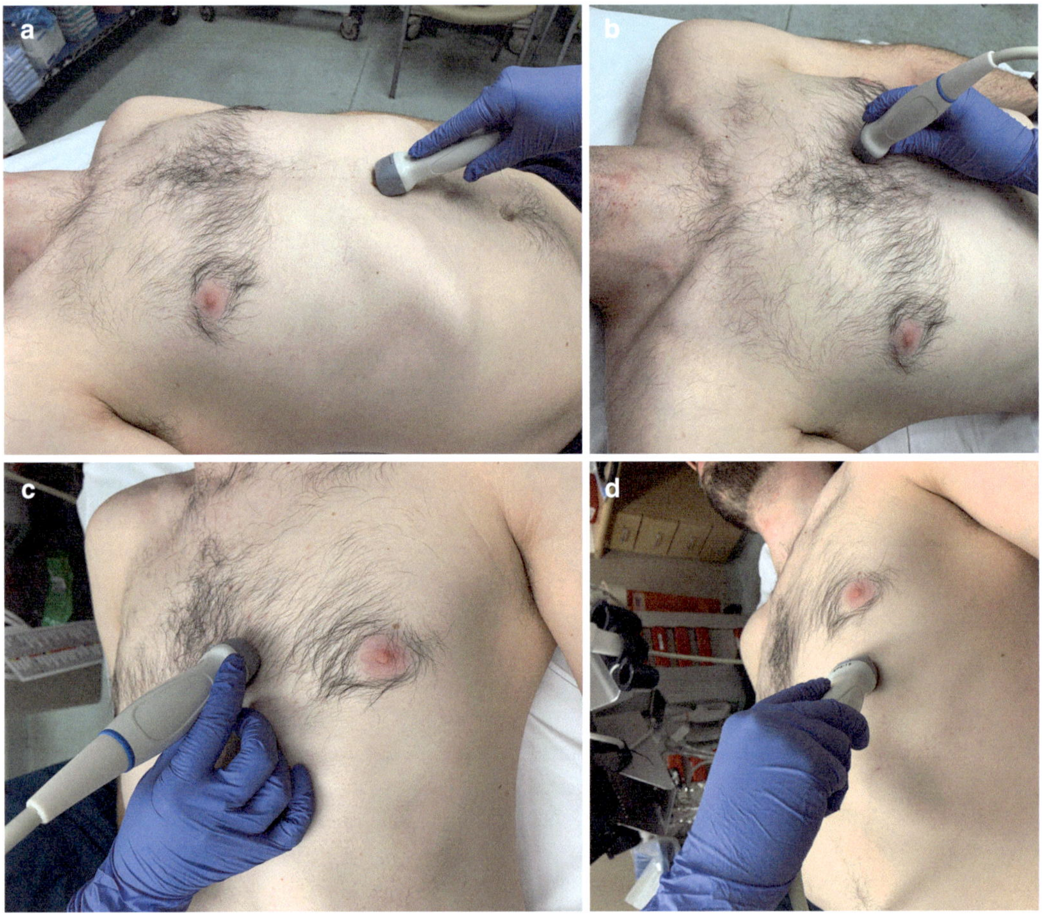

Fig. 5.1 Probe positioning for cardiac views: (**a**) Subxiphoid (**b**) Parasternal long (**c**) Parasternal short (**d**) Apical

superior vena cava, and limit the potential for malpositioning [1]. The right internal jugular vein is typically recommended as the site for temporary transvenous pacemaker placement, because the left subclavian vein is typically utilized for patients requiring permanent catheter placement.

Once a central venous catheter is placed, the pacing catheter will be directed through the central venous line, known as the introducer sheath. The introducer sheath will terminate in the SVC, and the transvenous pacing catheter will be advanced further with the goal of traversing the right atrium, through the tricuspid valve, and ultimately terminating in the right ventricle. The ultrasound views will include the standard subxiphoid, parasternal, and apical views with focus on obtaining views which will optimize visualization of the right atrium and ventricle (typically the subxiphoid and apical), allowing for advancement of the pacing catheter under dynamic ultrasound visualization.

Indications

Emergent cardiac pacing is indicated in multiple clinical scenarios which result in interruption or dysfunction of normal cardiac electrical activity. Common causes include SA node dysfunction, AV block, electrolyte or metabolic disorders, overdose or drug-associated dysrhythmias, and infection-related dysrhythmias. Cardiac pacing in an emergent setting is typically performed until a permanent pacemaker can be implanted or until the underlying etiology can be treated. Emergent pacing is generally provided via the transcutaneous or transvenous methods. A typical clinical scenario includes initiation of transcutaneous pacing with subsequent placement of a

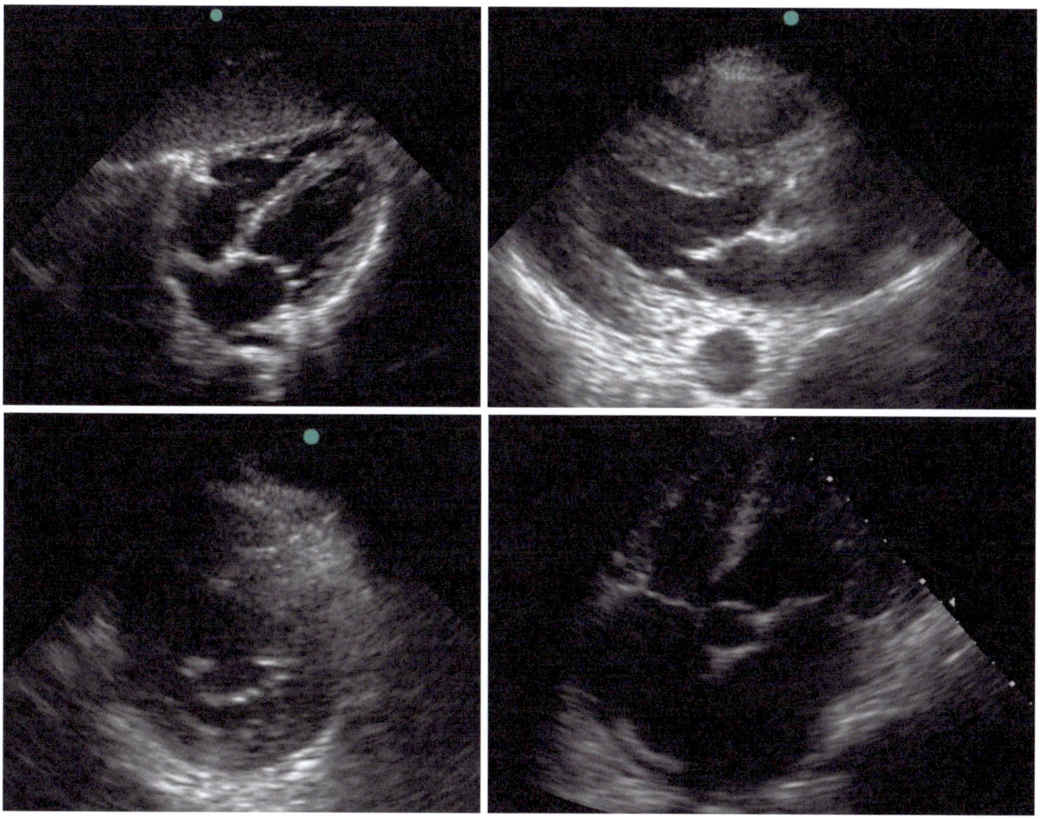

Fig. 5.2 Ultrasound images for cardiac examination: subxiphoid (top left); parasternal long axis (top right); parasternal short axis (bottom left); apical four chamber (bottom right)

transvenous pacemaker. Transvenous pacing is generally better tolerated by the patient and more effective at obtaining capture, though it is more invasive and takes longer to initiate.

Contraindications

Placement of a transvenous pacemaker should be avoided when the cause of bradycardia can be corrected by immediate alternative measures. This is true in the case of hypothermia, in which the appropriate treatment would be active rewarming. Other examples included drug toxicity where an antidote is readily available or electrolyte abnormalities that can be easily corrected.

Emergent transvenous pacing is contraindicated when bradycardia is not associated with hypotension or signs of end-organ dysfunction. Many patients may have bradycardia of little to no clinical significance in whom pacemaker placement can safely be delayed. Having the equipment to perform this procedure at bedside is important for any patient in which the possibility of hemodynamic compromise is anticipated. In addition, contraindications to central venous access similarly apply to this procedure.

Equipment/Probe Selection

For initial central venous access, a high-frequency linear probe will be utilized to identify appropriate anatomy and visualize advancement of the needle tip as described in the central venous access chapter. During placement of the transvenous pacemaker, a phased array (or curvilinear) probe will be used to obtain cardiac and IVC views.

Equipment (Fig. 5.3)

- Antiseptic (chlorhexidine gluconate, betadine, etc.)
- Local anesthetic (1% lidocaine)
- Gauze
- 25 gauge needle for anesthetic infiltration
- 18 gauge introducer needle
- Syringes (3 cc, 10 cc)
- Needles for anesthetic (18 gauge, 25 gauge)
- Sterile drapes
- Sterile gown, sterile gloves, mask
- Sterile ultrasound probe cover
- J-shaped guidewire
- Dilator
- 11 blade scalpel
- Introducer catheter (larger in diameter than pacemaker catheter). A critical point about the cordis introducer sheath diameter is that not only does it have to be larger than the diameter of the pacemaker catheter, but also it has to be just slightly larger. Most pacemaker catheters will have specific introducer sheaths for them or at least list what diameter/French the cordis should be. Placing the pacemaker catheter through even a slightly larger one, than indicated on the packaging, will result in persistent leakage of blood from the insertion point. The greater the diameter disparity, the greater the leak.
- Sterile cap for introducer catheter
- Large Tegaderm
- Cardiac monitoring equipment
- Pacemaker catheter with (+) and (−) leads
- Sterile transparent sheath for pacing catheter
- Pacer generator (Fig. 5.4)
- Battery with backup, new battery

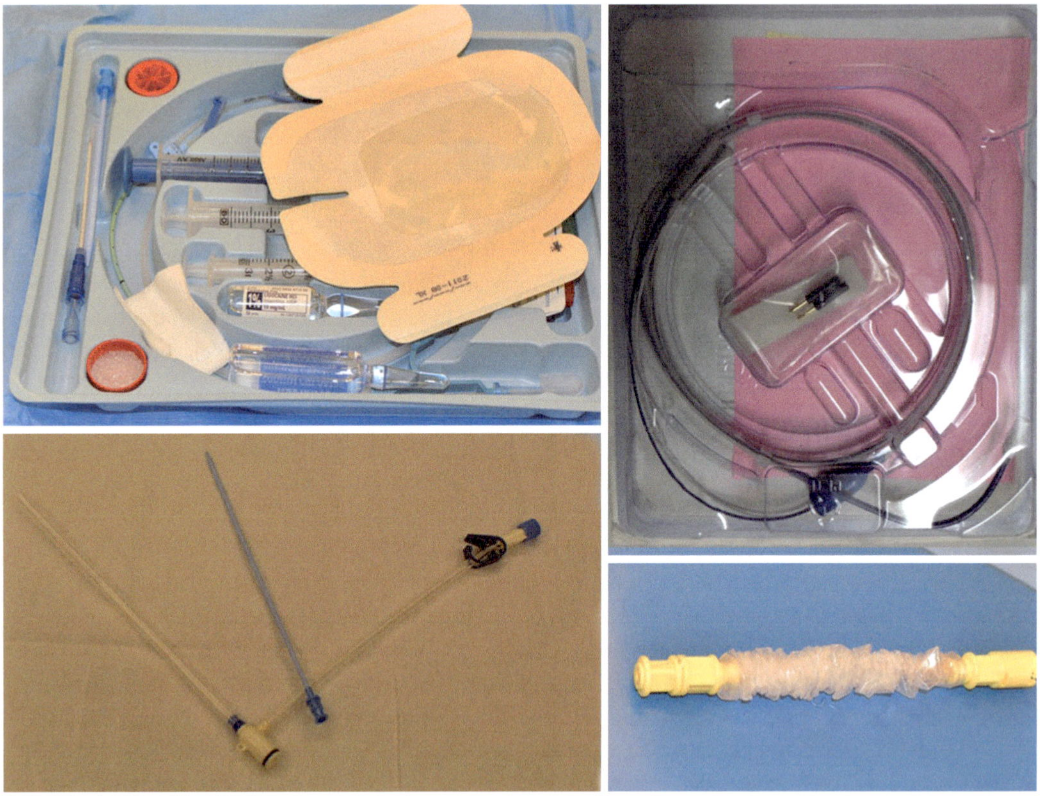

Fig. 5.3 Transvenous pacemaker equipment: central line kit (top left); pacing catheter with electrodes (top right); introducer catheter w/ dilator (bottom left); sterile sheath (bottom right)

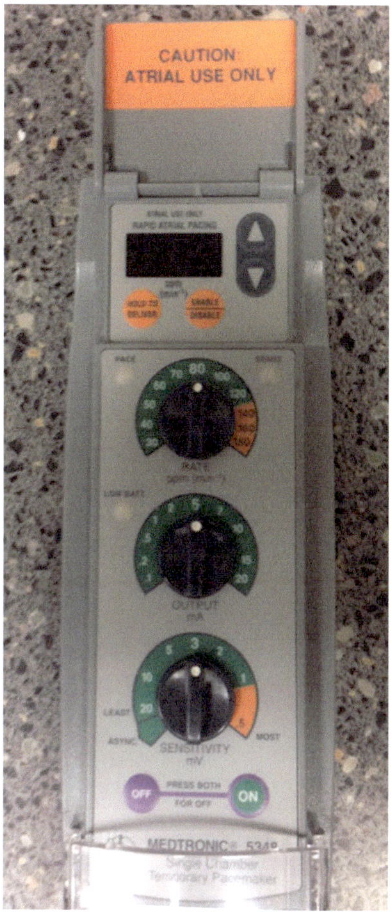

Fig. 5.4 Pacemaker generator

Preparation/Preprocedural Evaluation

As with any invasive procedure, the insertion of a transvenous pacemaker begins with patient consent and preparation. Informed consent should be obtained whenever possible. In the emergent setting, when the patient or a next of kin is unable to provide timely consent, implied consent may be necessary. The procedure should be performed under sterile conditions with proper skin preparation, local anesthesia at site of catheter insertion, full drape and gown, gloves, and mask for the provider performing the procedure. Generally, central venous access is to be obtained to facilitate placement of the pacing catheter. Often a kit containing the equipment both for central venous access and for pacing can be found in a single transvenous pacemaker kit. The additional equipment required for the pacemaker portion include sterile transparent sheath, the pacing catheter, pacing generator with battery, and backup battery.

Adequate preparation involves ensuring all the necessary equipment is available and working. Evaluate the patency of the pacer catheter balloon by filling balloon with 1.5 mL of sterile saline and inspecting for leaks. A nonsterile assistant will be necessary to connect the electrode connectors to the pacing generator, and operate the ultrasound during guidance of pacing catheter placement. Additionally, since advancement of the pacing catheter should be performed under and directed by real-time ultrasound visualization of the heart, a sterile assistant is important who can feed the sheath-covered pacing catheter into the cordis introducer sheath one to several centimeters at a time.

Procedure

The first step is insertion of the central venous catheter (introducing catheter), as described in the central venous access chapter. Once central venous access is obtained, connect the transparent catheter sheath to the introducing catheter hub, and insert the pacing catheter through the sheath and into the introducing catheter hub. Advance the pacing catheter about 10 cm to assure the distal tip lies beyond the length of the introducing catheter. At this time, 1.5 mL of sterile saline can be used to inflate the balloon to facilitate proper advancement. The proximal electrode tip can be connected to the positive (+) connector terminal of the pacer generator. While critical for blind placement of temporary transvenous pacemakers, alligator clips connected to distal electrodes will be of lesser value when using ultrasound guidance and may make the procedure more cumbersome. Real-time cardiac ultrasound will allow visualization and guidance of the pacing catheter tip into its ideal destination at the apex of the right ventricle. Traditionally, adequate positioning of the pacing wire would be confirmed by observing a left bundle branch block ECG pattern [1]. Relying on this method is not only time consuming, but also has the potential for inaccurate interpretation and is impossible to justify in the setting of real-time ultrasound guidance of pacing catheter placement directly into the right ventricle. Previous descriptions of this procedure have also indicated the use of fluoroscopy to visualize proper placement in real time. This has the obvious disadvantage of using large, bulky equipment (most of which is typically not available in clinical settings), taking the time necessary to obtain this equipment and the associated radiation for the patient and those performing and assisting with the procedure.

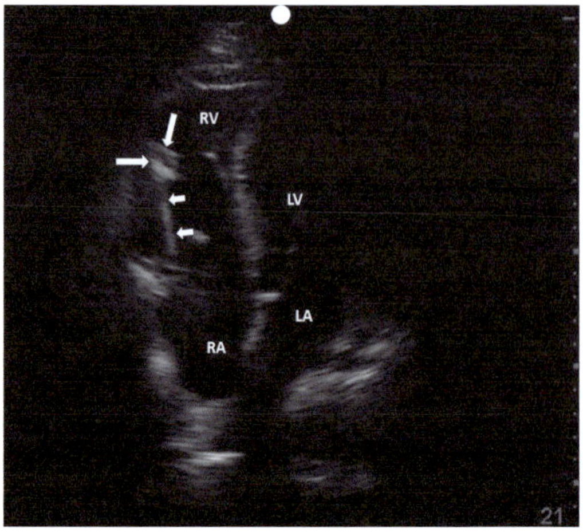

Fig. 5.5 Pacer catheter (small arrows) and balloon (large arrows) are seen approaching the apex of the right ventricle in this apical view. *RV* right ventricle, *LV* left ventricle, *RA* right atrium, *LA* left atrium. (Courtesy of Michael Blaivas, MD, MBA)

Using bedside ultrasound, the progression of the pacemaker catheter can be visualized in the right atrium and through to the right ventricle. The best views for visualizing the regions are the subxiphoid and apical four chamber and are typically the most useful for ultrasound-guided transvenous pacemaker placement (Figs. 5.5 and 5.6). However, it should be noted that a parasternal long-axis view with a tilt to visualize the right ventricular inflow tract and right atrium can provide an excellent vantage point for visualizing and guiding pacer balloon entry when other options are limited. As in many real clinical scenarios and settings, perfect images and an availability of three or more clear windows to the heart are unrealistic and rare. Thus, being aware of more than one option for pacer balloon guidance is critical. The preference for which view to obtain relies on which will provide the best image available to assure adequate placement. If the pacer tip is not visualized initially, fanning of the probe may be required for adequate visualization [3, 4]. Additionally, inflating and deflating the balloon will often make it more obvious. Finally, inflating the balloon with saline from a 10 ml syringe in which 9 ml of fluid and 1 ml of air are mixed through vigorous syringe agitation can create a hyperechoic spherical object that may stand out even in the most limited images.

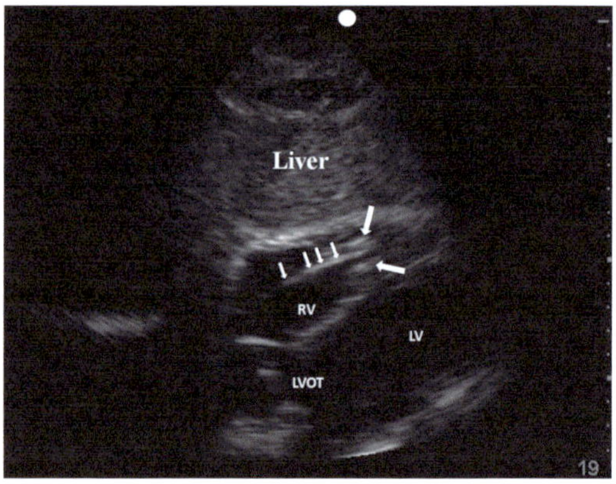

Fig. 5.6 This slightly oblique subxiphoid view reveals a pacemaker catheter balloon (large arrows) approaching the apex of the right ventricle. Pacing catheter: small arrows, *RV* right ventricle, *LV* left ventricle, *LVOT* left ventricular outflow tract. (Courtesy of Michael Blaivas, MD, MBA)

Once the transvenous pacemaker is in appropriate position, the pacing generator can be turned on. In the setting of peri-arrest or hemodynamic compromise, the initial settings include a rate of 80–100 bpm, maximum output (typically 5 mA), and sensitivity of 3 mV. Observe for capture and for clinical improvement. Palpate for peripheral pulses once capture is noted. Bedside echocardiogram with ECG lead attachments can additionally be utilized at this time to evaluate for proper capture of pacing beats. The output can then be decreased until capture is no longer appreciated. This is known as the threshold output. Output should be set to 2–3× the threshold output. In nonemergent situations, the initial output can be set low and gradually increased until capture is appreciated. Following proper placement and appreciation of capture, the balloon should be deflated, the pacing catheter can be secured into place, the sterile sheath can be advanced over the external portion of the pacer wire, and a sterile dressing can be applied.

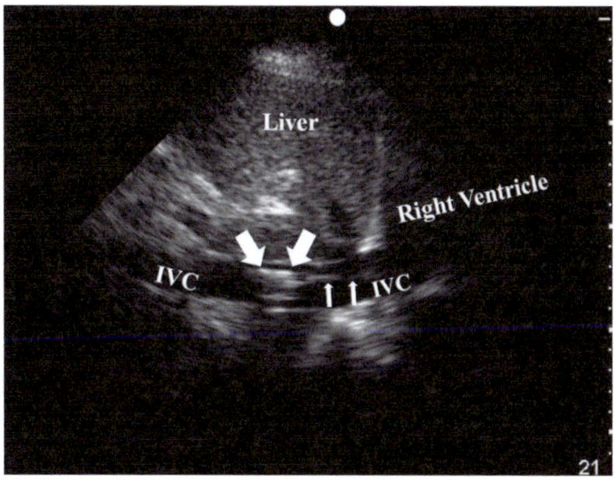

Fig. 5.7 Long-axis view of inferior vena cava (IVC) shows the pacemaker catheter (small arrows) and balloon (large arrows) passing into the IVC from the superior vena cava (SVC). (Courtesy of Michael Blaivas, MD, MBA)

Complications

There are multiple complications which can occur throughout various stages of this procedure of which the provider should be aware. The intrinsic complications associated with obtaining venous access have the potential to occur during the initial step of inserting the introducer catheter. These include pneumothorax, vascular injury, cannulation of the associated artery, thrombus formation, and infection.

Failure to adequately obtain cardiac capture is another complication and one which may occur for various reasons. Malpositioning, such as in the pulmonary artery, right atrium, or IVC, of the pacing catheter may result in failure to capture, which can be determined by bedside ultrasound. If the pacing catheter cannot be identified in the right atrium or right ventricle despite appropriate advancement, the tip may lie in the IVC. Simply switching ultrasound views from a cardiac view to a view of the IVC (Fig. 5.7) will allow for possible identification of the pacing catheter [5]. If this is the case, the catheter should be withdrawn, and additional attempts of advancement with the inflated balloon should be made. The pacing catheter may lie in the right atrium and meet resistance at the level of the tricuspid valve, preventing proper placement in the right ventricle. This can be diagnosed by identifying the tip of the pacing catheter in the right atrium via ultrasound. The potential for placement of the pacing catheter in either the IVC or right atrium increases in the setting of hemodynamic compromise and poor forward blood flow [1]. In the case of a pacing catheter in the right atrium, advancement of the catheter during a visualized diastolic cycle may aid in appropriate placement. In some patients, guiding the balloon into the right atrium proves to be exceedingly difficult. Twisting the pacer catheter at the hub clockwise and then counterclockwise slowly while advancing the catheter may facilitate balloon entry into the right atrium. If the pacing catheter has been advanced into the pulmonary circulation, it will need to be retracted and the tip of the catheter properly situated in the right ventricle. Cases of catheter tip over advancement into the pulmonary circulation illustrate the importance of using ultrasound for direct visualization during the procedure.

Additional complications include ventricular arrhythmias and ventricular injury. The most serious of ventricular injuries would involve perforation of the right ventricle. The potential for this complication is reduced by proper direct visualization under ultrasound with the focus on appropriate placement and continued assessment of where the tip of the pacing catheter lies. More importantly, the operator should never force advancement of a catheter. If resistance is met, the operator can try to determine the cause with ultrasound or try withdrawing and re-manipulating the catheter before attempting further advancement. In the setting of ventricular perforation, close hemodynamic monitoring and repeat bedside echocardiograms will be important to evaluate for signs of hemopericardium and tamponade. A common ventricular arrhythmia encountered during this procedure is non-sustained ventricular tachycardia, though persistent ventricular tachycardia or ventricular fibrillation may be encountered. Patients requiring this procedure often have myocardium which is more sensitive to dysrhythmias. Therefore, continuous cardiac monitoring should be maintained throughout the procedure. Magnesium can help stabilize myocardial cell membranes, and 2 grams can be infused in as little as 20 minutes when needed. If significant myocardial irritability is noted or suspected and time allows, magnesium infusion may significantly decrease the risk of ventricular tachycardia or fibrillation without dropping heart rate or blood pressure further.

If proper placement of the catheter is visualized via ultrasound, failure to capture may occur for alternative reasons. The procedure itself may be successful, but electromechanical dissociation may persist. Ultrasound is useful in determining this [6]. The patient's underlying medical condition may prevent appropriate capture or proper functioning of the myocardium despite pacing. It is always important to consider treatment of the underlying cause as the definitive therapy and frequent reassessments should be made to assure clinical improvement. This is especially true in the case of metabolic or toxicologic etiologies.

Reevaluation of the pacing equipment should be made as well if encountering problems in providing appropriate pacing. This includes checking functionality of the power source, changing to a new battery for the pacer generator, and checking for appropriate connectivity of all leads.

Pearls/Pitfalls

- Cardiac images via bedside ultrasound may be limited by patient body habitus, bowel gas, positioning, or the clinical scenario which may require multiple simultaneous interventions.
- Subxiphoid and apical four-chamber views tend to best visualize the right ventricle and transvenous wire.
- Two providers are required to insert a transvenous pacemaker under direct ultrasound guidance. The provider operating the ultrasound should be proficient in obtaining and interpreting cardiac views. This can be difficult to achieve in a busy clinical setting but is important to optimize success of the procedure.
- Failure to appreciate the pacemaker catheter in the right ventricle may simply be the result of the catheter lying out of plane of the ultrasound field of view. Fanning of the probe to allow full visualization of the right ventricle may reveal the tip of the catheter [3, 4].

Integration into Clinical Practice

The placement of a temporary transvenous pacemaker has proven to be an important skill in acute care settings and one in which emergency physicians have shown to be proficient in performing [7]. There are inherent risks to this procedure; however, the use of bedside ultrasound as an adjunct has shown the ability to assess for correct positioning and potentially reduce the time taken to perform the procedure [4, 5].

Key Points

- Transvenous pacing provides better cardiac capture and is better tolerated when compared to transcutaneous methods.
- Bedside ultrasound improves placement of a transvenous pacemaker by allowing direct visualization of the pacing catheter and observation of cardiac function after placement, while helping to avoid the potential complications of the procedure.
- The subxiphoid and apical views provide the best visualization of the right atrium and right ventricle allowing for dynamic catheter guidance.
- Placement of a transvenous pacemaker

can be time consuming. Treatment of underlying cause, constant hemodynamic monitoring, and temporary transcutaneous pacing should all be employed, or considered, during preparation and performance of the procedure.

Pericardiocentesis

Introduction

Pericardiocentesis is a critical procedure in acute care settings performed in the presence of suspected or anticipated cardiac tamponade caused by a pericardial effusion. Pericardial effusions can accumulate quickly or gradually depending on the underlying etiology and may be large or small in size before resulting in compromise of cardiac function. The determination of hemodynamic compromise is more closely related to the rate of accumulation as opposed to the size of the effusion. Rapid identification and treatment of cardiac tamponade can be lifesaving. This section will discuss the use of bedside ultrasound in detection of pericardial effusion, signs of cardiac tamponade, and the steps in performing a pericardiocentesis.

Advantages of Ultrasound Guidance

The advantage of ultrasound use is clear in detection of pericardial effusion, in evaluation for cardiac tamponade, and in aiding pericardiocentesis. Cardiac tamponade is a life-threatening condition which presents with signs and symptoms which may be consistent with several other cardiopulmonary disorders. The symptoms described by the patient may include chest pain, shortness of breath, lightheadedness, generalized fatigue, and syncope. Signs of cardiac tamponade include distended neck veins, muffled heart sounds, hypotension, and shock. The classic Beck's triad (hypotension, muffled heart sounds, and JVD) is a late finding and unreliable for practical clinical use. A strong clinical suspicion must be maintained for those at risk for developing a pericardial effusion. This includes those with risk factors such as a history of cancer, renal disease, chronic inflammatory conditions, infections (including Lyme disease, TB, and HIV), recent cardiothoracic surgery, or thoracic trauma. Evaluation with chest X-ray or ECG may reveal signs of pericardial effusion but may not do so unless there is a large effusion or until later in the disease course [8].

The use of bedside ultrasound plays a very important role in evaluating for pericardial effusion and should be performed in any patient with concern for possibility of a pericardial effusion, especially those with signs of hemodynamic compromise. Ultrasound assessment of right ventricular diastolic collapse is considerably more accurate than the physical examination for a pulsus paradoxus [9]. Bedside ultrasound is a modality which can be easily learned and utilized by clinicians for this purpose [10]. The use of bedside ultrasound can allow for early detection of a pericardial effusion while also allowing for evaluation of the size of the effusion, the location of the effusion, and the evaluation of the physiologic effects on cardiac function (i.e., tamponade). There are several signs of pericardial tamponade including right atrial collapse with progression to right ventricular collapse during diastole (Figs. 5.8 and 5.9). In the setting of a normal right

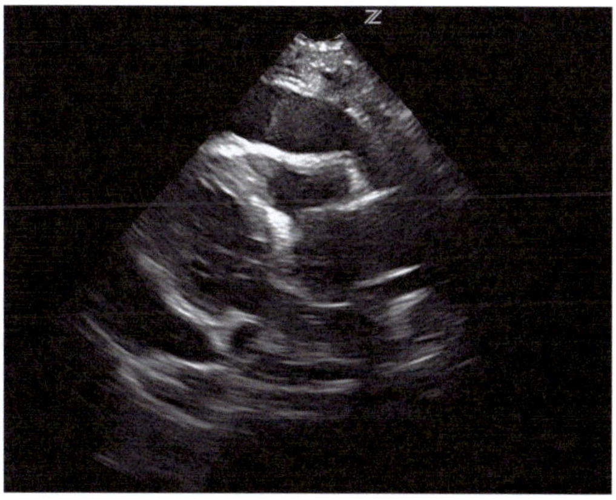

Fig. 5.8 Parasternal view of pericardial effusion with tamponade. There is right ventricle wall collapse during diastole

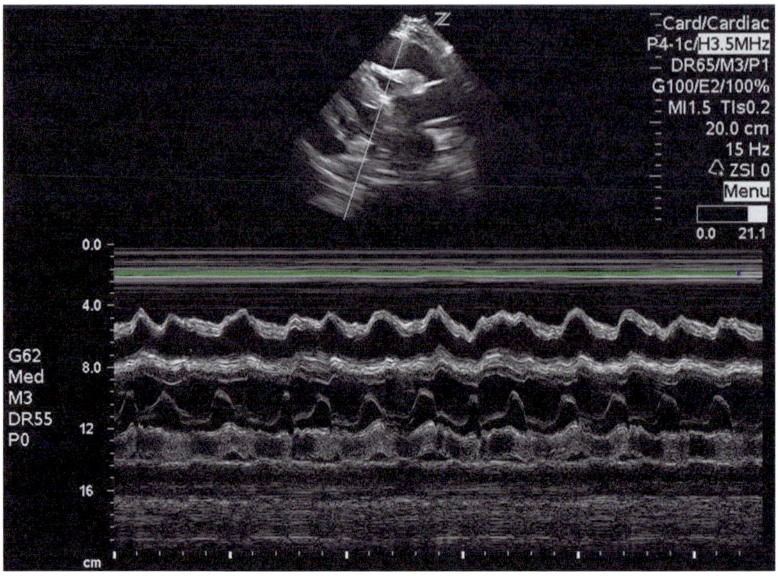

Fig. 5.9 M-mode demonstrating diastolic right ventricular collapse suggesting pericardial tamponade

ventricular compliance and function, diastolic collapse is indicative of pericardial pressures that have exceeded right ventricular diastolic pressure. This finding is specific for physiologic changes seen with pericardial tamponade. When right atrial collapse in systole lasts for more than one third of systole, pericardial tamponade is also suggested. Increases in right ventricular diastolic filling during inspiration cause the septum to shift and result in lower left ventricular diastolic filling and therefore volume. The opposite is seen with expiration. Pulsed-wave Doppler can be used to interrogate the tricuspid and mitral inflow velocities in diastole and will show increased diastolic inflow velocity in the right ventricle but decreased diastolic inflow in through the mitral valve. A dilated IVC that shows minimal or no collapse with inspiration is a nonspecific but very sensitive marker for tamponade physiology.

Bedside ultrasound subsequently can be utilized to assist pericardiocentesis. Ultrasound allows for determination of the appropriate anatomic site for needle insertion, visualization of the needle path during the procedure, identification of surrounding anatomic structures, and ultimate decrease in the known complications of the procedure. Echocardiographic evaluation can be performed postprocedure as well to evaluate for physiologic improvement of tamponade [11].

Anatomy

The pericardium is a fibrocollagenous layer which surrounds the heart. Physiologically, there may normally be a trace amount of pericardial fluid. This minimal amount of fluid will not affect cardiac function; however, in the setting of multiple different disease processes, additional fluid may accumulate in this space. Pericardial effusions related to chronic medical conditions typically tend to accumulate slowly over long periods of time. The pericardium has elastic properties and will exhibit a compensatory stretch as the effusion grows. This allows for larger effusions to gradually accumulate without generating pressures on the myocardium, which would result in hemodynamic compromise, until later in the disease course. Conversely, effusions secondary to trauma or pericardial disruption may result in a pericardial effusion which accumulates too rapidly to allow for compensatory stretch of the pericardium.

Indications

The indication to perform a pericardiocentesis by the clinician is for appreciation of a pericardial effusion which has resulted in hemodynamic compromise or in which impending hemodynamic compromise is expected. Drainage of a pericardial effusion in a stable patient should be done within coordination and consultation with a cardiologist or cardiothoracic surgeon.

Contraindications

Excluding patient refusal, there are no absolute contraindications to performing a pericardiocentesis once cardiac tamponade has been diagnosed [12]. As noted above, drainage of an effusion without signs of tamponade or hemodynamic instability should be done in coordination with a specialist. Considerations should be taken in performing this procedure on patients with bleeding diathesis.

Effusions resulting from a traumatic etiology or via ascending aortic aneurysm are preferably repaired surgically, and emergent pericardiocentesis is not generally indicated. In Type A aortic dissections, hemopericardium will tend to rapidly reaccumulate if drainage is attempted, and while in some patient attempts at relieving pericardial pressure may prove futile, in many cases they will be lifesaving. A large bore catheter such as a cordis introducer sheath should be introduced to allow easier drainage of thick fluid (blood) which may be partially clotted. As in all cases of pericardiocentesis, a catheter should not only be used for drainage but should be left in place and sewn in to allow for additional drainage as needed. In cases of tamponade from aortic dissection, repeated drainage may have to be performed in short intervals while definitive surgical care is pending. Emergent pericardiocentesis is an established and often successful temporizing measure in settings in which trauma surgery or cardiothoracic surgery is not readily available or in which there is significant hemodynamic compromise secondary to tamponade[13, 14].

Equipment/Probe Selection

Bedside ultrasound with a phased array probe is ideal for evaluation of an effusion, evaluating for tamponade, and guidance of pericardiocentesis. A linear, high-frequency probe should be used for needle tip guidance during the procedure [8, 15]. Alternatively, a curvilinear transducer capable of good resolution or a high-resolution microconvex probe such as a neonatal transducer can also be utilized. Use of the phased array transducer for needle guidance should be avoided due to very poor near-field resolution.

Equipment for Pericardiocentesis

- Antiseptic (chloroprep, betadine)
- Local anesthetic (1% lidocaine)
- Gauze
- 25 gauge needle for anesthetic infiltration
- 16 gauge or 18 gauge long needle
- Syringes (5 cc, 10 cc, 60 cc)
- Sterile drapes
- Sterile gown, sterile gloves, mask
- Sterile ultrasound probe cover
- ECG machine
- Cardiac monitoring equipment
- Three-way stopcock
- J-shaped guidewire
- Dilator
- 11 blade scalpel
- Pigtail catheter with side and end holes. When other options are limited, a triple or quadruple central line can be used. When a bloody or viscous effusion is encountered, a 7.5 or 8 French cordis introducer sheath may be the only way to effect fluid drainage.

Preparation/Preprocedural Evaluation

Ideally, pericardiocentesis would be performed with the patient in a semi-recumbent position with the head of the bed elevated to 35 to 40 degrees. However, if the patient is in extremes, the procedure can be performed with the patient supine. Small effusions may be difficult to aspirate, as they become dependent. When tolerated, the left lateral decubitus position may improve success by causing the effusion to accumulate around the apex of the heart and displacing the left lung laterally.

Preparation for this procedure includes ensuring all the appropriate equipment is available at the bedside and is appropriately functional.

Bedside echocardiography should be used to evaluate the effusion, and appropriate needle insertion site should be determined. The needle insertion site should be chosen based on the site at which the effusion lies closest to the skin and which avoids vital structures. The modern standard of care calls for a parasternal approach whenever possible as supported by clear-cut literature on the topic [16]. Secondary location is apical or subxiphoid approaches. The expected needle path should be determined during this preparation time. Movement of the patient will require reassessment of the effusion and needle path [16]. Topical antiseptic should be applied to the subxiphoid and left parasternal region. Sterile drapes should be applied over the patient. Sterile precautions should be applied, and sterile ultrasound cover should be applied to the phased array ultrasound probe. Local anesthetic should be administered subcutaneously and along the expected needle path. Negative pressure should be held during insertion of the needle used for local anesthesia to avoid intravenous injection of anesthetic.

Procedure

The steps for performing a pericardiocentesis have been described both with and without bedside ultrasound. Performing a pericardiocentesis without the use of ultrasound is considered a "blind" procedure, and the advantages of using ultrasound are discussed above. Additionally, the "static" ultrasound method is described as a method in which anatomical landmarks are first determined with the use of ultrasound and then the procedure is performed in the standard "blind" fashion with needle insertion performed without real-time ultrasound guidance. While this method is an improvement over the truly "blind" method in which ultrasound was not used at all, it is strongly recommended to utilize ultrasound to continuously guide needle placement to minimize complications.

Pericardiocentesis, under ultrasound guidance, can be performed from the subxiphoid, parasternal, and apical approach. However, the parasternal approach should be chosen whenever possible. It proves the safest, shallowest, and most direct path to the pericardial space. As an effusion enlarges, lung is pushed out of the way, and even typically poor parasternal windows suddenly become adequate. When performing a pericardiocentesis without ultrasound, most providers opt for a subxiphoid approach. This technique is described as inserting the needle just left of the xiphoid process, in the notch between the xiphoid and left subcostal area. The needle is then directed toward the left shoulder with negative pressure held on the syringe until the pericardium is entered and pericardial fluid is aspirated. Ultrasound guidance for the subxiphoid approach is achieved by placing the phased array ultrasound probe directly inferior to the xiphoid process and aimed toward the left thoracic cavity. This may require pressure to be placed on top of the probe, over the patient's superior abdomen, and lowering of the angle so the back end of the probe is approximating the patient's abdomen. The probe marker will typically be to the patient's right (note: this is assuming the screen marker is also located on the left). Appropriate visualization allows identification of the pericardial effusion and underlying myocardium. Needle guidance is very difficult in the subxiphoid compared to the ease encountered in a parasternal approach, but ideally, the needle can then be inserted to the right (patient's left) of the probe and directed toward the effusion, with continuous observation of the needle tip as it is advanced. This may involve directing the needle through a portion of the liver, which will be visualized on the subxiphoid ultrasound evaluation. A known complication of this approach is liver and diaphragmatic injury. Realistically, accurate needle guidance using a phased array is nearly impossible in the near field in a high-pressure clinical setting. When coupled with needle passage through the liver and diaphragm and difficulty in accessing the pericardial space when compared to a parasternal approach, the subxiphoid window (like the apical) should only be utilized in cases of some degree of effusion loculation leaving too little fluid parasternally for safe needle and catheter insertion or another absolute barrier to the parasternal approach.

The apical techniques may be preferred to minimize complications over the subxiphoid but in many patients still prove much more challenging and dangerous than utilizing the preferred parasternal window. The apical view can be obtained by placing the probe over the point of maximal impulse, typically in the fifth intercostal space over the anterior axillary line, with the probe marker pointing toward the left shoulder and screen indicator on the right side as per cardiology convention. The parasternal approach is typically performed under visualization with the parasternal long view. This is obtained by placing the high-resolution linear, curvilinear, or microconvex transducer over the anterior chest, just to the left of the sternum. The probe marker is oriented toward the patient's right shoulder with probe indicator marker on the right side of screen as per cardiac scanning convention. In reality, probe and screen marker orientation can be considered irrelevant as long as the provider will have optimal imaging and not be confused about where the needle will appear on the ultrasound machine screen. To further ensure this, verify needle entry location just prior to needle insertion by depressing the chest with a sterile gloved finger adjacent to the probe's long axis, and watch for soft tissue deformation on the screen. This will be where the needle and catheter will appear for in-plane guidance.

Along these views, the needle can be inserted directly next to the long axis of the ultrasound probe (Figs. 5.10 and 5.11) and advanced toward the effusion, along the expected needle path, with continuous visualization of the needle tip (Figs. 5.12 and 5.13). Insertion of the needle should be performed with consideration to avoid damage to the left internal mammary artery, which lies about 3–5 cm lateral to the sternum, and the neurovascular bundles, which run over the inferior portion of each rib.

Once pericardial fluid begins to be aspirated, sterile saline should be flushed while the transducer is held in the parasternal window. Ideally

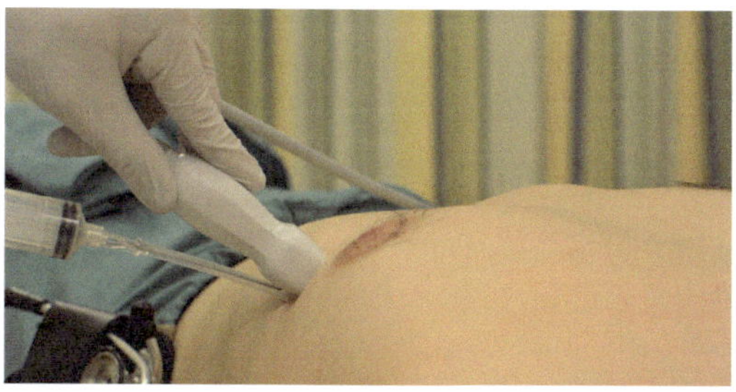

Fig. 5.10 Apical approach for pericardiocentesis

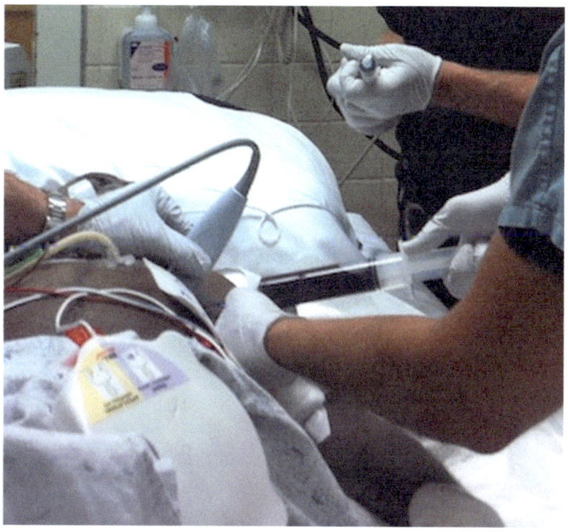

Fig. 5.11 Pericardiocentesis from the apical approach with the use of ultrasound

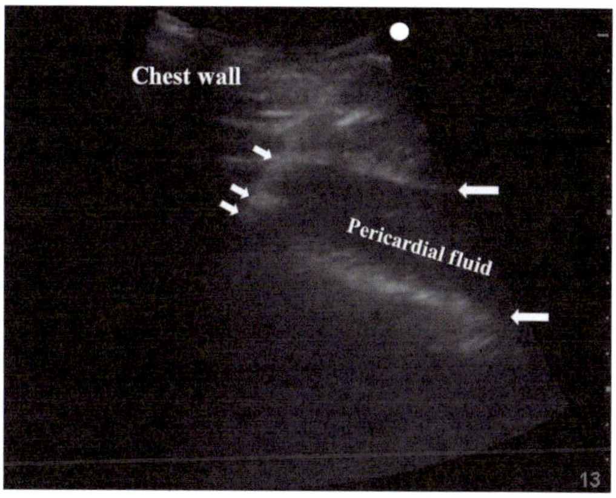

Fig. 5.12 Ultrasound-guided pericardiocentesis using a curvilinear transducer during a sudden cardiac arrest in a chest pain patient who was actually having an aortic root dissection. The introducer needle (small arrows) from a cordis introducer sheath kit is seen entering through the pericardial space (large arrows show pericardium) chest wall in the parasternal approach. The patient immediately improved after drainage of 80 cc of thick, clotting blood and survived a 4 hour transfer to cardiothoracic surgery, ICU, and then eventually home with full recovery. (Courtesy of Michael Blaivas, MD, MBA)

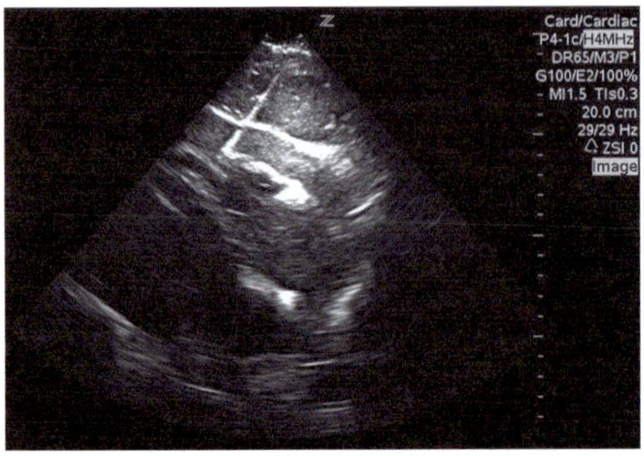

Fig. 5.13 Ultrasound-guided pericardiocentesis. Echogenic needle seen using phased array probe

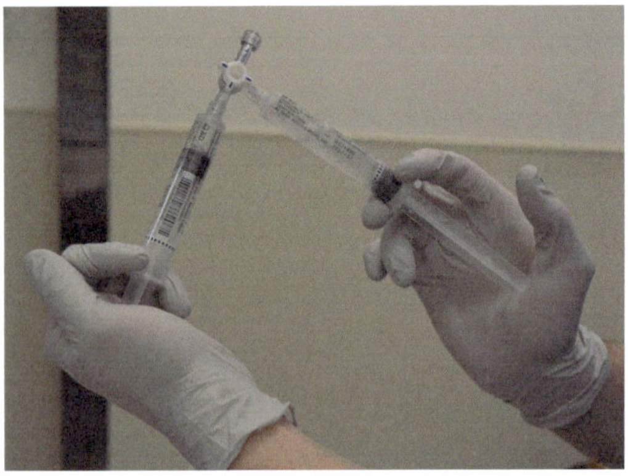

Fig. 5.14 Making agitated saline with two syringes and three-way stopcock

prepared prior to the procedure, agitated saline is created by connecting a 10 ml syringe filled with saline and a 10 ml syringe filled with air to a three-way stopcock. With the syringes open to each other, via the stopcock, the saline is flushed back and forth between each syringe (Fig. 5.14). The agitated saline can be aspirated into the single syringe to be used for initial pericardial space access or be put into a syringe, which will then be connected to the pericardiocentesis needle via the stopcock [3]. If the needle tip is in correct position, a swirl of bright echoes should be seen within the pericardial space. Monitor the needle tip, making sure it does not begin to make contact with the myocardium. If a catheter is already loaded over the needle, advance it into the pericardium while watching on ultrasound. If not, a guidewire should be inserted and over it an appropriate diameter catheter for ongoing and later drainage. The catheter should be sewn in to prevent dislodgement.

As mentioned above, placing a drain may be done using the Seldinger technique, with a guidewire, or by using a needle with an overlying angiocatheter, which can be advanced after entering the pericardium. If using a guidewire, advancement of the guidewire, through the needle, into the pericardium, can be visualized sonographically. Once the guidewire is identified in the pericardium, the dilator can be used to make a tract through the skin and subcutaneous layer. A pigtail or other catheter can then be advanced over the guidewire, into the pericardial space. As with central line placement, one hand should always remain on the guidewire during the procedure, and the wire is to be removed after placement of the catheter drain. The catheter must then be sewn into the skin and appropriately dressed with sterile coverings. After initial drainage, subsequent drainage of effusion should occur intermittently as dictated by the clinical situation.

Complications

Complications of performing a pericardiocentesis include damage to surrounding structures when attempting to enter pericardium with the needle. In the preferred parasternal location, this can include the lung, internal mammary artery, neurovascular bundles of the ribs, coronary arteries, and myocardium. In the subxiphoid and apical approaches, the liver, diaphragm, and gastrointestinal tract can be damaged. The apical approach can potentially put all of the above listed structures at risk depending on heart size, location, and patient's body morphology and habitus. Avoidance of these structures is optimized by the use of ultrasound for identification and guidance of needle placement, as well as with awareness of the associated anatomy. Bedside ultrasound will also allow for a needle path which is shortest in distance to minimize potential for damage to surrounding structures. If

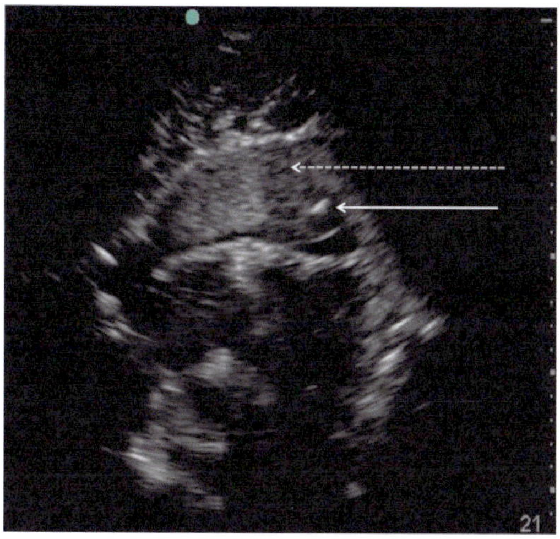

Fig. 5.15 Subxiphoid view of clotted hemopericardium. Needle tip visualized within hemopericardium (solid arrow) and surrounding clotted blood (dotted arrow)

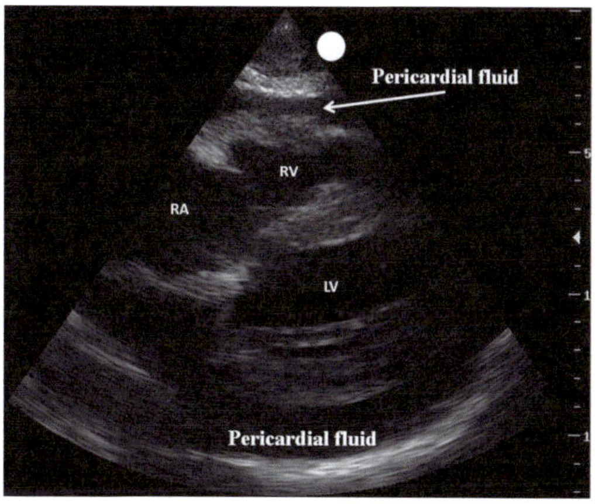

Fig. 5.16 A subcostal view of the heart with a pericardial effusion seen in near and far field. *RV* right ventricle, *LV* left ventricle, *RA* right atrium. (Courtesy of Michael Blaivas, MD, MBA)

using the subxiphoid approach, decompression of the stomach with an oral/nasogastric tube can decrease the incidence of perforation, but may not be feasible in an emergent situation.

Failure to drain the pericardial effusion is an additional complication of this procedure. The use of ultrasound is important if pericardial fluid cannot be aspirated. Identification of the needle tip and assurance of placement within the pericardium suggest procedural placement is not the problem. Focus can be taken to evaluate for possible clogging of the needle bore or presence of hemopericardium with clotted blood (Fig. 5.15). In this case, placement of a large bore such as an 8 French cordis introducer sheath is likely the only way to drain the thickening blood besides performing a thoracotomy. This can be surprisingly effective as a temporizing measure, and such patients have little to lose and much to gain unless cardiothoracic surgery is immediately available.

Pearls/Pitfalls

- Failure to maintain visualization of the needle tip during advancement of the needle may lead to the complications noted above. This may be aided by use of a linear array, high-frequency probe [8, 15], or injection of agitated saline to assess placement.
- Attempted drainage of hemopericardium may result in attempted aspiration of clotted blood. This may obstruct the needle bore or prevent proper aspiration and relief of tamponading effects. Use large diameter drainage catheters such as 8 French cordis introducer sheaths in cases of clotting blood or other highly viscous fluid such as pus.
- A pericardial fat pad may also be mistaken for a pericardial effusion. It should be noted, however, that this scenario should not result in sonographic signs of tamponade or the reason for hemodynamic compromise. In this case, pericardiocentesis would not be indicated, and alternative diagnostic efforts should be made in the case of hemodynamic compromise. The single best maneuver to differentiate between a fat pad and pericardial effusion is to change the subcostal window probe orientation (Fig. 5.16) to the IVC inlet view (Fig. 5.17). Fat pads (Fig. 5.18) do not extend circumferentially around the heart and will disappear in this location leaving the normal appearance of the right ventricle moving directly adjacent to the diaphragm (Fig. 5.19). In the absence of this, pericardial effusion is almost certainly present (Fig. 5.18).

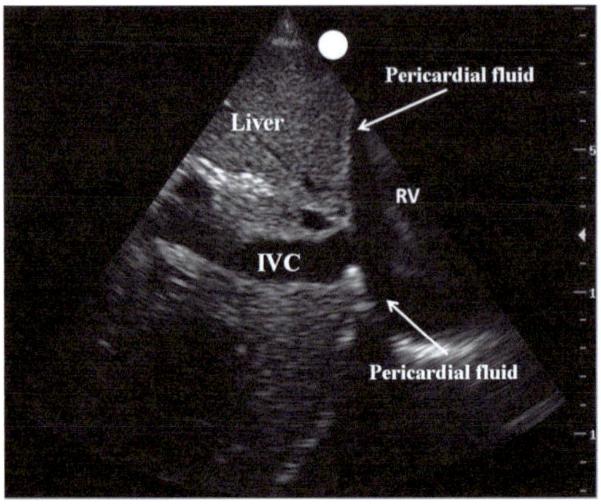

Fig. 5.17 An IVC inlet view of the same patient as Fig. 5.16 obtained during the same cine loop shows a clear stripe of anechoic fluid representing pericardial effusion between the diaphragm and right ventricle (RV). (Courtesy of Michael Blaivas, MD, MBA)

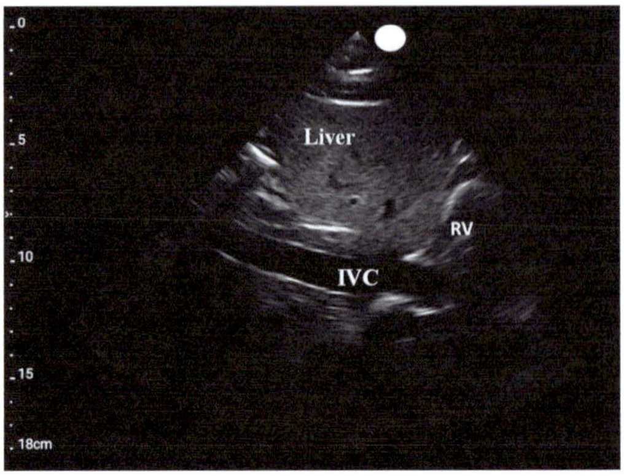

Fig. 5.19 An IVC inlet view on the same patient as in Fig. 5.18, captured during the same cine loop. The image shows the right ventricle abutting the diaphragm directly indicating that the echogenic collection noted in Fig. 5.18 was a fat pad, not a pericardial effusion. (Courtesy of Michael Blaivas, MD, MBA)

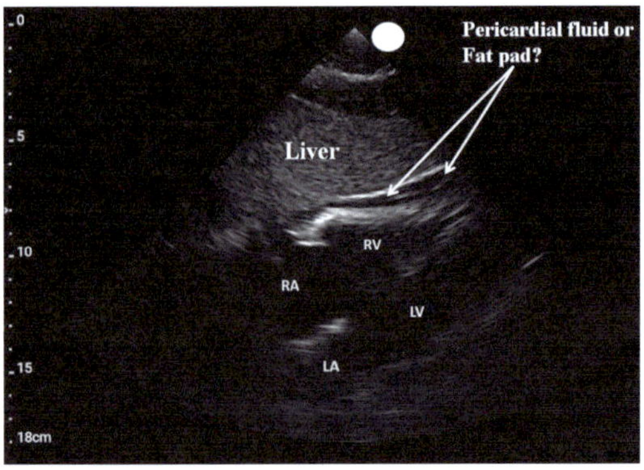

Fig. 5.18 A subcostal four-chamber view of the heart in a patient with sharp, tearing chest pain radiating to the back and bilateral arm tingling and numbness. An echogenic collection is seen just near field to the right ventricle. *RV* right ventricle, *LV* left ventricle, *RA* right atrium, *LA* left atrium. (Courtesy of Michael Blaivas, MD, MBA)

Integration into Clinical Practice

Cardiac tamponade secondary to the accumulation of a pericardial effusion can result in significant hemodynamic compromise and is a cardiac emergency. Pericardiocentesis is a lifesaving procedure in this instance. There are several methods which have been described to perform this procedure including under fluoroscopic guidance and with the guidance of ECG monitoring. These techniques are all associated with the complications inherent to the procedure of performing a pericardiocentesis. The use of bedside ultrasound allows for identification of an effusion with tamponade physiology, guidance of the needle during pericardiocentesis, and postprocedure cardiac evaluation. Ultrasound guidance is important for minimizing the known complications of this procedure and increasing its success rate and is especially effective in the parasternal approach. It should be used when pericardiocentesis is necessary [8, 11, 16].

Key Points

- Pericardial effusions may develop for multiple reasons and may result in tamponade at any size depending on etiology.
- Pericardiocentesis may be a lifesaving procedure, critical in the practice of Medicine.
- The parasternal approach is the far preferred method with excellent literature support for its superiority and safety.
- Multiple approaches can be taken and should be chosen to avoid known complications and optimize success rate/clinical improvement for the patient.

- Ultrasound guidance significantly improves success rates and minimizes known complications. Ultrasound is recommended for both evaluation of pericardial effusion/tamponade as well as for performance of pericardiocentesis.
- Accurate orientation of the probe is crucial for procedural guidance (i.e., aligning the probe indicator with the marker on the monitor).
- Operator has to pay close attention to the trajectory of the needle tip on ultrasound to reduce error.

References

1. Harrigan RA, Chan TC, Moonblatt S, Vilke GM, Ufberg JW. Temporary transvenous pacemaker placement in the Emergency Department. J Emerg Med. 2007;32:105–11.
2. Holger JS, Lamon RP, Minnegan HJ, Gornick CC. Use of ultrasound to determine ventricular capture in transcutaneous pacing. Am J Emerg Med. 2003; 21:227–9.
3. Ma OJ, Mateer JR, Blaivas M. Emergency ultrasound. New York: McGraw-Hill Medical; 2007.
4. Aguilera PA, Durham BA, Riley DA. Emergency transvenous cardiac pacing placement using ultrasound guidance. Ann Emerg Med. 2000;36:224–7.
5. Blanco P, Nomura JT. An atypical misplacement of a temporary pacing catheter diagnosed and resolved by ultrasound. Am J Emerg Med. 2014;32:1296.e1–3.
6. Macedo W Jr, Sturmann K, Kim JM, Kang J. Ultrasonographic guidance of transvenous pacemaker insertion in the emergency department: a report of three cases. J Emerg Med. 1999;17:491–6.
7. Birkhahn RH, Gaeta TJ, Tloczkowski J, Mundy T, Sharma M, Bove J, et al. Emergency medicine--trained physicians are proficient in the insertion of transvenous pacemakers. Ann Emerg Med. 2004;43:469–74.
8. Hatch N, Wu TS, Barr L, Roque PJ. Advanced ultrasound procedures. Crit Care Clin. 2014;30:305–29, vi.
9. Singh S, Wann LS, Klopfenstein HS, Hartz A, Brooks HL. Usefulness of right ventricular diastolic collapse in diagnosing cardiac tamponade and comparison to pulsus paradoxus. Am J Cardiol. 1986;57:652–6.
10. Mandavia DP, Hoffner RJ, Mahaney K, Henderson SO. Bedside echocardiography by emergency physicians. Ann Emerg Med. 2001;38:377–82.
11. Nagdev A, Mantuani D. A novel in-plane technique for ultrasound-guided pericardiocentesis. Am J Emerg Med. 2013;31:1424.e5–9.
12. Roberts JR, Hedges JR. Roberts and Hedges' clinical procedures in emergency medicine. Philadelphia: Elsevier Health Sciences; 2013.
13. Lee TH, Ouellet J-F, Cook M, Schreiber MA, Kortbeek JB. Pericardiocentesis in trauma: a systematic review. J Trauma Acute Care Surg. 2013;75:543–9.
14. Cruz I, Stuart B, Caldeira D, Morgado G, Gomes AC, Almeida AR, et al. Controlled pericardiocentesis in patients with cardiac tamponade complicating aortic dissection: Experience of a centre without cardiothoracic surgery. Eur Heart J Acute Cardiovasc Care. 2015;4(2):124–8.
15. Fields JM, Paziana K, Vuljaj N, Fischer J, Ku BS. Emergency ultrasound-guided pericardiocentesis using a high-frequency linear array transducer to improve needle tip visualization. Acad Emerg Med. 2012;19:e16.
16. Tsang TSM, Freeman WK, Sinak LJ, Seward JB. Echocardiographically guided pericardiocentesis: evolution and state-of-the-art technique. Mayo Clin Proc. 1998;73:647–52.

Ultrasound-Guided Central Venous Access

6

Azeem Tajani, Arthur Au, and J. Matthew Fields

Introduction

Central venous access is a commonly performed procedure in a variety of acute care settings. The use of real-time ultrasound guidance for cannulation has been shown to improve success rates and decrease mechanical complications when compared to traditional landmark-based techniques. Multiple studies have demonstrated the benefits of using ultrasound guidance for central venous access in internal jugular and subclavian veins. Real-time needle visualization results in fewer needle pass attempts, increased first-pass success, and decreased complications. Understanding sonographic anatomy and basic principles of needle guidance is crucial to successfully perform central venous cannulation using ultrasound guidance. Ultrasound-guided needle placement can be performed in an "in-plane" or "out-of-plane" or "oblique" technique. Once the guidewire is inserted, ultrasound can be used to ensure the correct placement of the wire. It is critical to confirm wire location prior to dilation and central line placement. The diameter of the typical introducer needle and guidewire ensures minimal complications in the case of arterial penetration in comparison to dilation and cannulation with a central line catheter. Following catheter placement, ultrasound can be used to confirm catheter position using a saline flush test in combination with cardiac sonography.

A. Tajani · A. Au · J. M. Fields (✉)
Department of Emergency Medicine,
Thomas Jefferson University Hospital,
Philadelphia, PA, USA

Advantages of Ultrasound Guidance

Ultrasound provides real-time visualization of the needle and needle tip in relation to the target vessel and other surrounding vital anatomic structures leading to improvements in success rates and decreases in complications over traditional landmark techniques. The benefit of ultrasound has been extensively demonstrated for placement of CVCs in the internal jugular vein. A recent Cochrane review found a 71% reduction in complications and a 57% increase in first-stick success when using ultrasound guidance for internal jugular CVC placement compared to anatomic landmark techniques [1]. Another similar review also showed a reduction in complications with ultrasound-guided subclavian CVC placement and an improved success rate for femoral vein CVC placement [2]. Ultrasound guidance for internal jugular venous access is currently recommended by multiple organizations including the Agency for Healthcare Research and Quality [3].

Another advantage to ultrasound is the ability to evaluate the patency of a vein prior to cannulation. The operator can ensure the vein distends adequately without evidence of stenosis, throm-

S. Adhikari, M. Blaivas (eds.), *The Ultimate Guide to Point-of-Care Ultrasound-Guided Procedures*, https://doi.org/10.1007/978-3-030-28267-7_6

bus, or variant anatomy. After cannulating the vessel, ultrasound can visualize guidewire entry and confirm successful catheter placement.

Anatomy

The internal jugular and subclavian veins are commonly used for ultrasound-guided central venous access. The internal jugular vein exits the skull via jugular foramen; then descends down the neck, lateral to the carotid artery within the carotid sheath; and eventually joins the subclavian vein. It is the most superficial in the upper part of the neck and lies underneath the sternocleidomastoid muscle at the level of the thyroid cartilage. At the level of the sternoclavicular joint, the internal jugular vein joins the subclavian vein to form the brachiocephalic vein. Since it is not concealed by bone, it is an ideal vein to visualize using ultrasound. The subclavian vein is a continuation of the axillary vein, lying anterior to the subclavian artery and runs from the lateral border of the first rib to the medial border of the anterior scalene muscle. It joins the internal jugular vein posterior to the sternoclavicular joint and forms the brachiocephalic vein. Since the subclavian vein runs for a significant distance under the clavicle which generates an acoustic shadow on ultrasound, it is technically challenging to perform ultrasound-guided cannulation compared to internal jugular vein cannulation. The common femoral vein is found medial to the common femoral artery below the inguinal ligament. In the proximal thigh, the femoral and deep femoral veins join to form the common femoral vein. Below the inguinal ligament, the greater saphenous vein joins the common femoral vein anteromedially. The common femoral vein becomes the external iliac vein as it ascends posterior to the inguinal ligament.

It is crucial to distinguish the sonographic appearance of veins from arteries to perform ultrasound-guided central venous access. Veins and arteries are typically identified by their size, shape, ability to be compressed with pressure, color Doppler characteristics, and spectral Doppler waveforms. Both structures have an anechoic lumen, while the artery is round in appearance, has a thick hyperechoic wall, and demonstrates visible pulsations. Veins have relatively thin hypoechoic wall, are oval in appearance, are easily compressible with pressure, and demonstrate phasic flow (Figs. 6.1, 6.2, 6.3, and 6.4). Pulsed-wave Doppler is the only reliable method of confirming vessel identify in almost

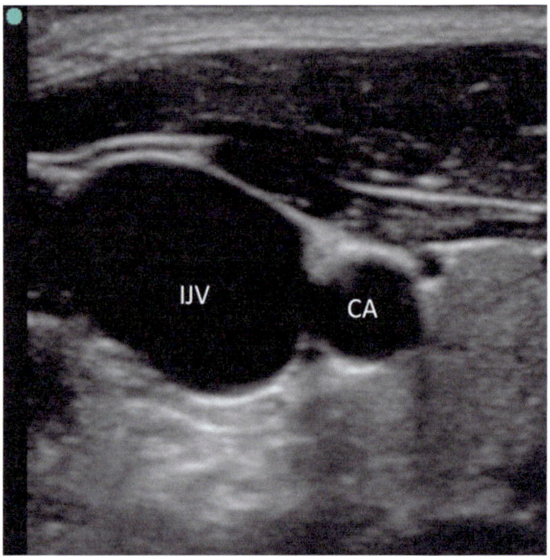

Fig. 6.1 B-mode image of oval internal jugular vein (IJV) and round carotid artery (CA). (Courtesy of Srikar Adhikari, MD)

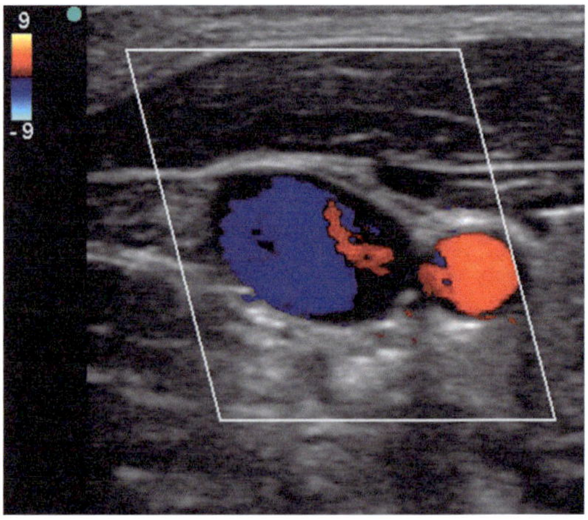

Fig. 6.2 Color Doppler image of internal jugular vein and carotid artery demonstrating the differences in the direction of flow. (Courtesy of Srikar Adhikari, MD)

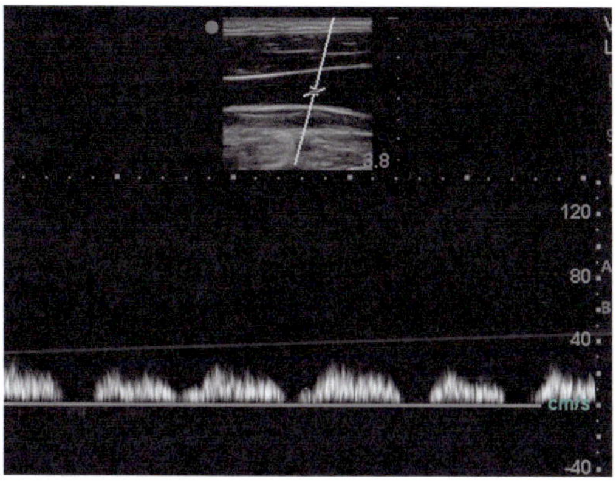

Fig. 6.3 Spectral Doppler image of internal jugular vein showing phasic flow. (Courtesy of Srikar Adhikari, MD)

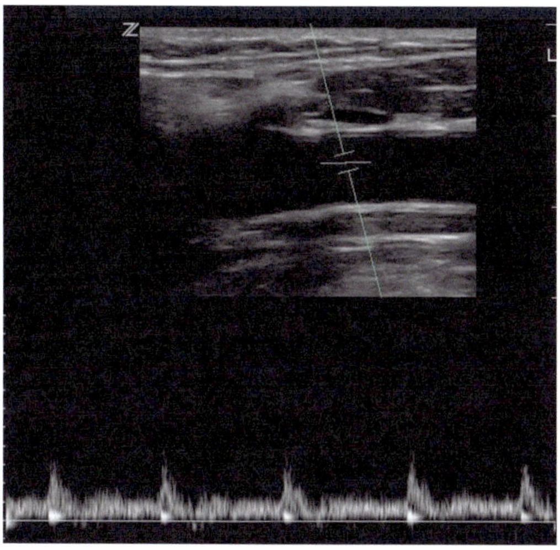

Fig. 6.4 Spectral Doppler image of common carotid artery showing pulsatility. (Courtesy of Srikar Adhikari, MD)

all conceivable situations as various combinations of conditions can lead to confusion between artery and vein when relying solely on compression and color Doppler assessment.

Indications

- Providing medications that are caustic to smaller vessels, i.e., vasopressors, certain antibiotics, and long-term electrolyte replacement
- Large volume resuscitation (Cordis line)
- Hemodynamic monitoring
- Transvenous cardiac pacing
- Hemodialysis/plasmapheresis
- Difficult venous access

Contraindications

A CVC should not be placed in an area with overlying cellulitis or where it will be difficult to maintain site sterility. A CVC should not be placed in a clotted or stenotic vein or if there is known or suspected venous injury. Coagulopathic and obese patients should be approached with great care as there is an increased risk of complications. If a patient is in need of dialysis or is to have an arteriovenous (AV) fistula placed, the central line should not be placed in the vein that the AV fistula or temporary catheter will be placed.

Equipment and Probe Selection

Probe Selection

A high-frequency linear probe (Fig. 6.5) should be used as it provides the best resolution for superficial structures such as the veins that require cannulation as well as the needle tip. Typical modern broadband transducers now range from approximately 15–6 MHz, but exact frequencies and bandwidth can vary widely.

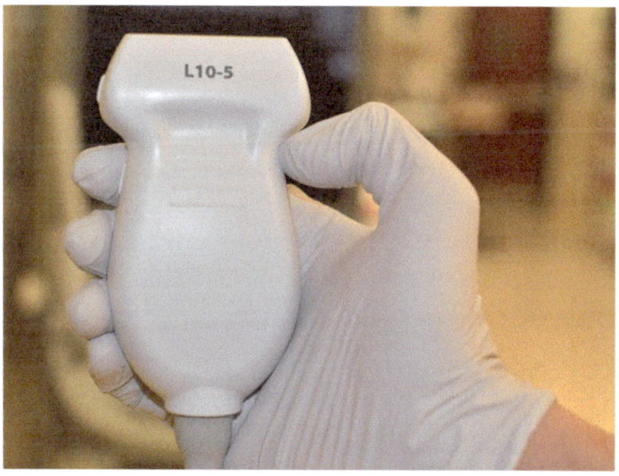

Fig. 6.5 High-frequency linear array probe

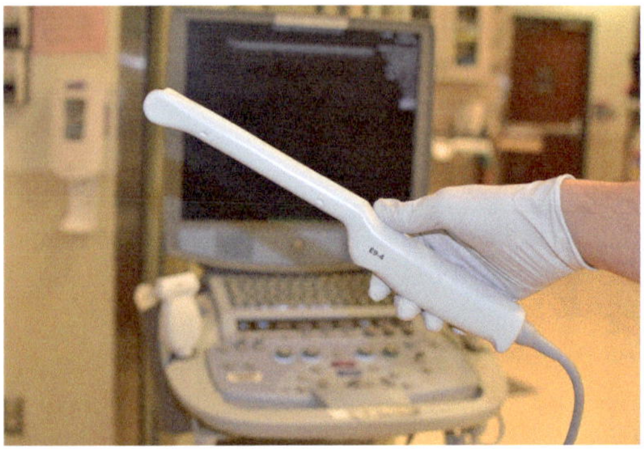

Fig. 6.6 Endocavitary probe

While attempting a supraclavicular subclavian line, the endocavitary probe (Fig. 6.6) or other small footprint high-frequency probe can be used as this provides better access to the supraclavicular fossa.

Equipment

Antiseptic (chlorhexidine gluconate, betadine, etc.)
Local anesthetic (1% lidocaine)
Gauze
25 gauge needle for anesthetic infiltration
18 gauge introducer needle
Syringes (3 cc, 10 cc)
Needles for anesthetic (18 gauge, 25 gauge)
Sterile drapes, gown, gloves, mask, and hat
Sterile ultrasound probe cover
J-shaped guidewire
Dilator
11 blade scalpel
Large Tegaderm
Biopatch
Catheter

Preparation and Preprocedure Evaluation

The site and choice of catheter depends on the clinical scenario. The subclavian or internal jugular veins are typically preferred because of lower infection rates and thrombosis, but a femoral CVC is appropriate in many situations. For certain procedures or when large volume resuscitation is required, a large bore 8.5 french (2.8 mm) introducer (Cordis) (Fig. 6.7) may be required. When central access is required to give specific medications or provide central venous pressure monitoring, a multilumen CVC (Fig. 6.8) may be more appropriate. (It is important to note that a multilumen CVC is typically inferior to large bore peripheral IV access for rapid volume resuscitation due to the resistance to flow caused by the longer catheter length.) Informed consent should be obtained and the benefits and risks explained. In emergent settings, if the patient or a next of kin is unable to provide timely consent, implied consent may be necessary.

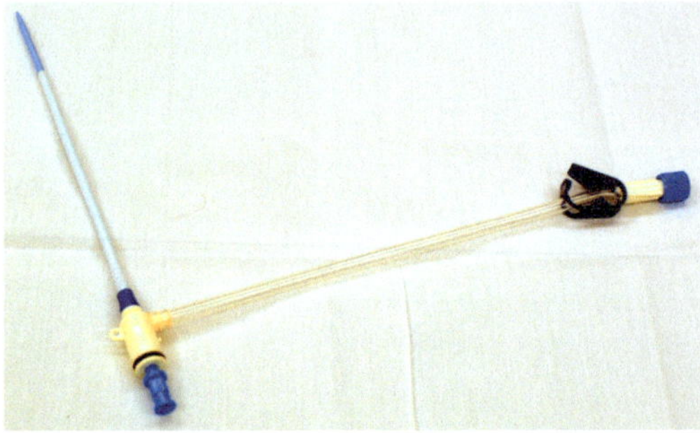

Fig. 6.7 Cordis catheter with dilator in place

Prior to setup, anatomic landmarks should be assessed by ultrasound. First note the location of the target vein and its corresponding artery. Veins will appear to have thin walls versus the thicker walled and pulsatile artery. Note that the artery should not be easily compressible, while the vein should compress with gentle probe pressure. The use of color Doppler may also demonstrate the pulsatile flow of the artery and the steady flow of the vein. Scan up and down to visualize the course of the vein, while also taking note of surrounding structures. It is important to identify surrounding vessels, nerves, lymphatics, or evidence of lung tissue as these structures should be avoided while placing the line.

There are two ways that ultrasound can be utilized to guide the placement of CVCs. The *static approach* describes when ultrasound is used to confirm the location of the target vein and its trajectory and to assess the surrounding anatomy, but is not used during the procedure itself. The

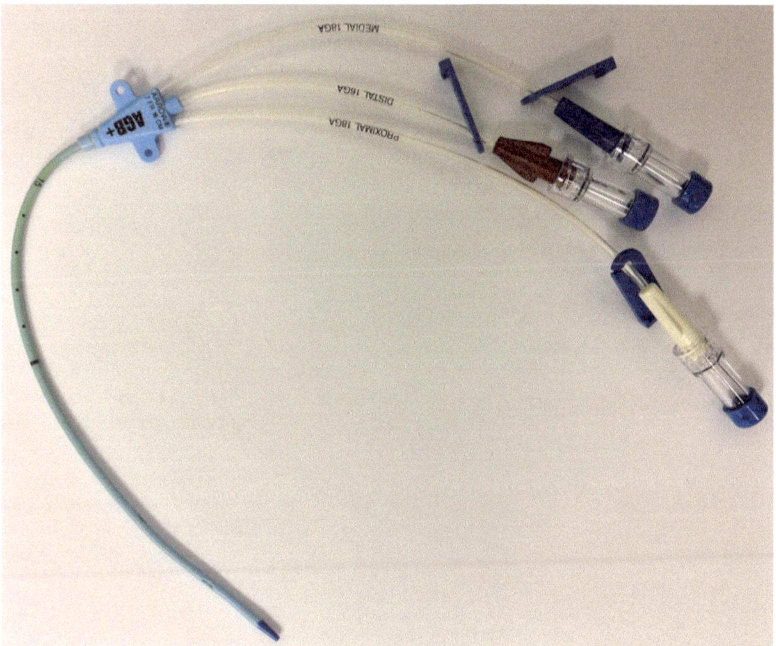

Fig. 6.8 Triple lumen catheter

site of needle insertion over the vein must be marked on the skin prior to sterilization. The *dynamic approach* is when ultrasound is used to provide real-time visualization during needle insertion and help guide needle advancement into the target vessel. It has been found that the static approach has superior first-attempt success rates than the landmark technique (also known as the "blind" technique) alone. It can be done quickly if the practitioner is unable to place the line with the ultrasound probe remaining stable or if a sterile cover is not available. However, the same study found the *dynamic* approach to be superior to both *static* and landmark techniques [4]. The *dynamic* approach is strongly recommended as there is potential for the alignment and orientation of vessels to change with movement (particularly for the internal jugular vein with head and neck movements).

After scanning the vessel, the room should be set up appropriately with ultrasound machine and equipment in locations that permit the operator to easily access equipment and visualize the screen. The patient should be prepared and draped in normal sterile fashion. Clean the patient's skin with chlorhexidine gluconate or a comparable antiseptic solution. The operator should gown and then drape the patient. It is important to have an assistant to aid the operator in handling equipment and the ultrasound probe.

When using a dynamic approach, the ultrasound probe must be placed in a sterile sleeve. A sheath of at least 6 feet in length is important to cover enough cable length to avoid contaminating the sterile field with uncovered cable. However, some radiology procedural sterile sheaths can be so long as to be unmanageable when it comes to dressing a standard ultrasound transducer. Sterile ultrasound sleeves are typically packaged with sterile ultrasound gel. A copious amount of gel should be placed directly in the sleeve prior to inserting the probe to ensure that the entire footprint of the ultrasound probe is covered. The ultrasound probe can then be lowered into the sleeve by the assistant (Fig. 6.9). Rubber bands provided are used to keep the sterile sleeve in place. When applying the rubber band, try to make sure there is a layer of gel in between the transducer footprint and the sterile sleeve free of air bubbles.

In the event that an assistant is not available, a single-operator technique can be used to cover the probe. The probe should be placed in a holder on the ultrasound cart, and gel should be applied prior to the operator gowning. After the operator

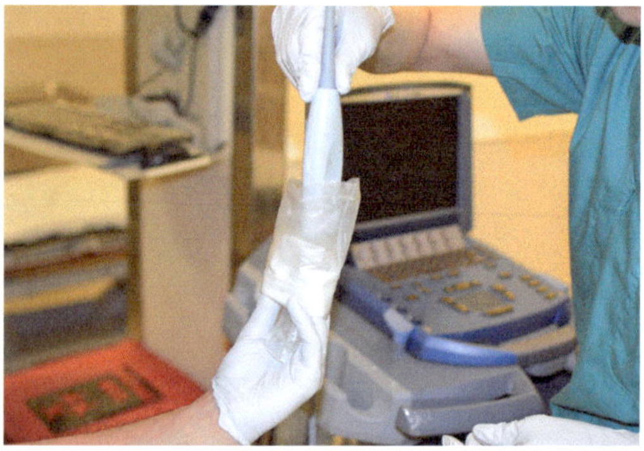

Fig. 6.9 Lowering the probe into the sleeve when an assistant is present

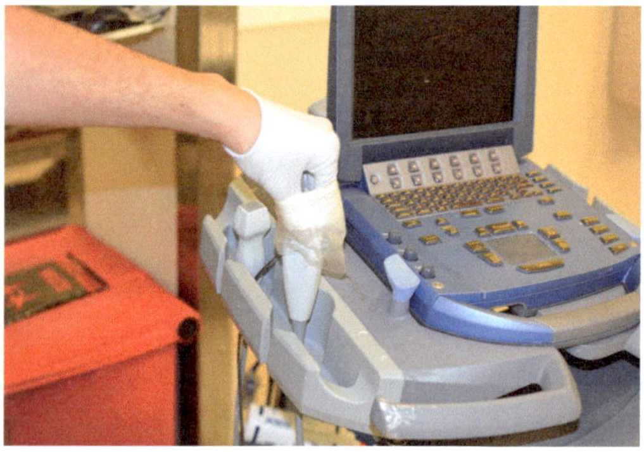

Fig. 6.10 The single operator with a sterile glove can invert the end of the probe cover and grasp the probe

has put on sterile gloves and gown, the operator will place his hand inside the sterile ultrasound cover sleeve and grasp the nonsterile probe as demonstrated in Fig. 6.10. The operator can then grab the corner of the sleeve and pull the cover over the probe and cord as shown in Fig. 6.11.

All equipment should be inventoried and inspected prior to starting the procedure. When using a multilumen CVC, the lumens should be instilled with normal saline to assess for integrity and/or malfunction.

Procedure

The previously determined site of needle entry should be anesthetized using local anesthesia. Always make sure to aspirate prior to instilling the lidocaine to ensure the needle is not inside a

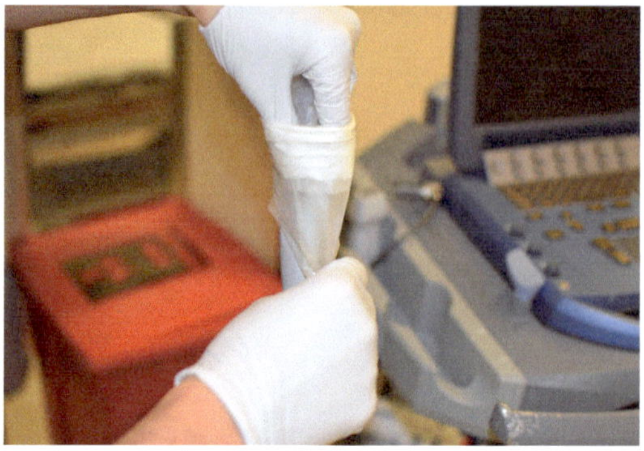

Fig. 6.11 The practitioner then grabs the bottom of the probe cover and pulls it down over the cord

Table 6.1 Advantages and disadvantages of the in-plane, out-of-plane, and oblique needle visualization techniques for dynamic ultrasound-guided central venous catheter placement

	Advantages	Disadvantages
In-plane	Constant needle tip and vessel visualization without any need to move the probe	Potential for cylinder tangential effect May be difficult to keep the vessel and needle within the plane of the beam Cannot see adjacent structures
Out-of-plane	Able to simultaneously view the vessel, and surrounding structures	The probe must be moved with the needle tip to keep it in view Loss of needle tip visualization can result in complications
Oblique	Hybrid approach allowing partial view of vessel and surrounding anatomy with constant needle visualization	May be conceptually more difficult Potential for needle to travel out of plane

vessel. The dynamic approach for ultrasound guidance can be performed using three different needle visualization techniques: in-plane, out-of-plane, and oblique (Table 6.1).

Out-of-Plane Approach

In the out-of-plane approach, the ultrasound beam is insinuated perpendicular to the target

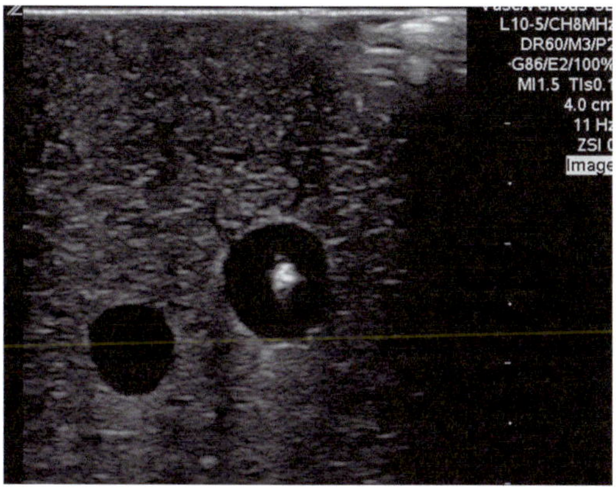

Fig. 6.12 Echogenic needle tip is visualized inside a vein in out-of-plane approach (known as the "target sign")

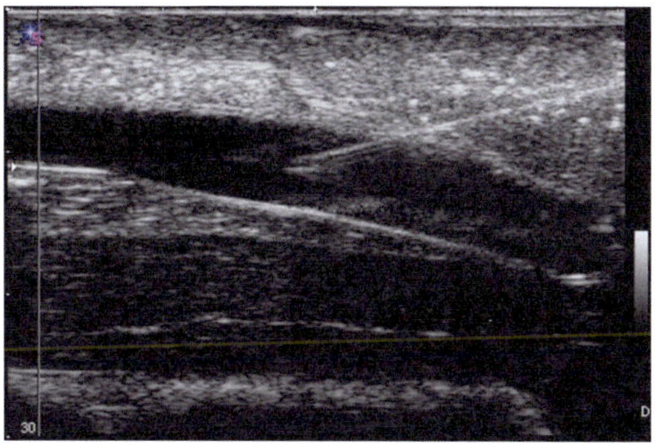

Fig. 6.13 In-plane approach with needle inside the target vessel

vessel causing it to appear as a circle. Once the needle is inserted through the skin, the practitioner should translate the ultrasound probe both proximally and distally to identify the location of the needle tip. The needle tip is seen as a bright, hyperechoic dot with reverberation artifact (Fig. 6.12). Because the needle will also be perpendicular to the ultrasound beam, or "out-of-plane," the practitioner must actively translate the ultrasound probe as the needle is advanced to maintain constant needle tip visualization. If the needle tip is not adequately visualized, the operator can move the needle side to side to create a jiggling effect of the needle tip to aid in its identification. The needle should be slowly advanced toward the vessel while relocating the tip after each manipulation until the needle tip indents and punctures the anterior wall of the target vein. Once the needle tip is properly positioned within the vein, it should appear as a target sign. Again, the ultrasound probe should be moved distally to ensure that the needle does not pass through the back wall of the vein. Once you see the "target sign" fan the probe distally the "target sign" should disappear, and when you fan the probe back proximally the "target sign" should reappear. This indicates the needle tip is in the vessel and is known as the "vanishing target sign" [5].

An advantage of the out-of-plane approach is it allows for simultaneous visualization of the vessel and surrounding structures (artery, nerves, etc.). A common drawback is for the operator to mistake the shaft of the needle for the needle tip, which can result in advancing the needle too far and potentially puncturing the posterior wall of the vein or other nearby structures.

In-Plane Technique

In the in-plane approach, the beam is parallel to the long axis of the target vessel causing the vessel to appear as a rectangle on the screen. The needle is inserted and advanced toward the vessel in this same plane (also known as an "in-plane" approach). The benefit of the "in-plane" technique is the operator does not need to move the probe as the needle is advanced; the needle tip will always be visible so long as the needle remains in the plane of the beam. This minimizes the chances of advancing the needle tip past the posterior wall of the target vessel. Figure 6.13 shows an example of a needle in the vessel in long axis. A disadvantage of the in-plane approach is it requires that the sonographer be able to maintain alignment of the vessel and needle in the beam of the ultrasound probe, which may be difficult in some patients. If the operator swings the syringe either left or right, the needle may move out of plane and become only partially visualized. If the operator accidentally translates or fans the probe, the beam will go from cutting through the main sagittal portion of the vessel to a parasagittal portion which may prevent successful cannulation. This latter issue is often termed the cylinder tangential effect.

Oblique Approach

The oblique approach is a hybrid of the long-axis and short-axis approaches. Starting with an out-of-plane approach, the ultrasound probe is rotated so the vein is visualized midway between its short and long axis. With this technique, the needle is advanced in plane with the ultrasound probe. This allows for both visualization of the full length of the needle and assessment of anatomy around the vein (Fig. 6.14) [6, 7].

One alternate technique is to use the out-of-plane approach when puncturing the skin to make sure the needle enters directly above the vessel and then switches to an in-plane approach to visualize advancement of the needle. Alternatively, the oblique view may be utilized. Upon successful needle placement into the vessel, blood should be able to be aspirated in the syringe. At this point, the syringe can be removed, and dark, nonpulsatile blood should flow out of the needle. The guidewire should be inserted into the needle and advanced into the vein. Ultrasound can be used to visualize the guidewire as it is inserted into the vein (Fig. 6.15).

Guidewires typically have 5 cm hash markings to let the operator know how much guidewire has been inserted. The operator should not insert more than 10–15 cm of guidewire. If ectopy is noted on cardiac monitoring, the guidewire should be pulled back. The operator should never let go of the guidewire as the negative pressure generated by a deep inspiration can cause catheter embolization. A small incision should be made adjacent to the needle just large enough to pass the dilator. The needle can be removed and the dilator inserted while always maintaining control of the guidewire. After the skin and tissue are dilated, the catheter can then be thread over the guidewire using the Seldinger technique. Feed the wire back through the catheter until it comes out at the back end of the catheter (typically the brown port of a triple lumen). Grab the wire coming out at the back end of the catheter, and then advance the catheter into the vein. At this point, the guidewire should be completely removed, and blood should be withdrawn from

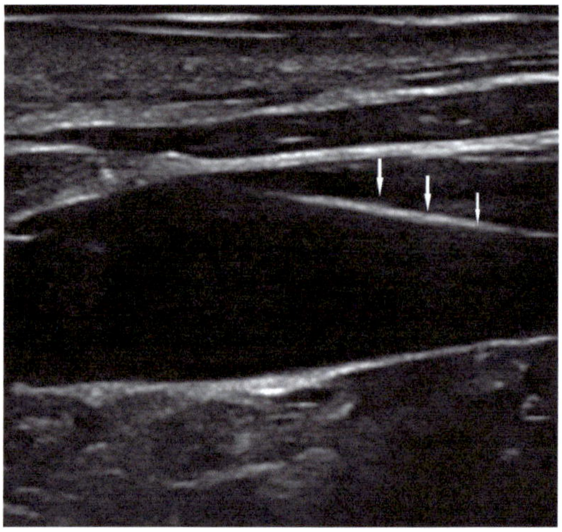

Fig. 6.15 The guidewire (arrows) is visualized inside the vessel in the in-plane approach. (Courtesy of Srikar Adhikari, MD)

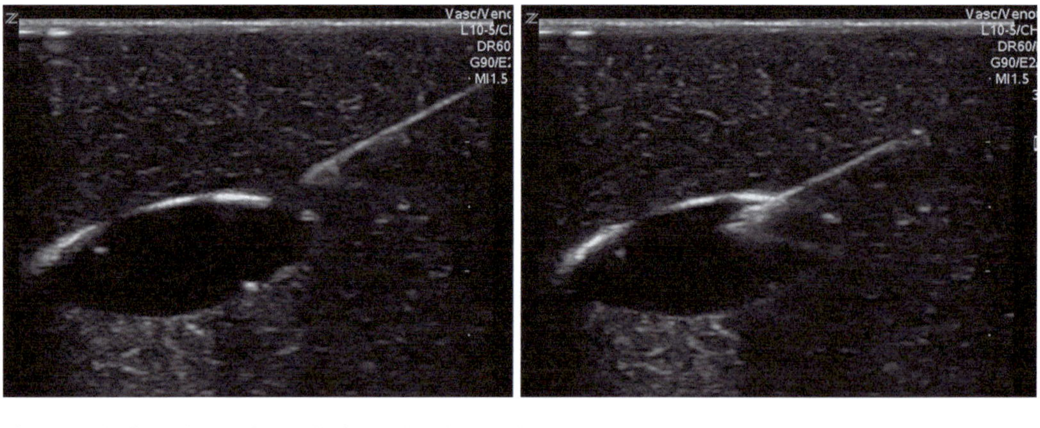

Fig. 6.14 Oblique view as the needle is entering the vessel

the ports. The amount of catheter to be inserted into the patient depends on the location (right internal jugular, 14 cm; left internal jugular or right subclavian, 16 cm; left subclavian, 18 cm). Test each line using the normal saline in the syringe you have prepped making sure that each port is free of any air bubbles prior to flushing. A biopatch should be placed at the skin around the CVC. The CVC should be secured using sutures or specially made clips. The site should finally be cleaned and covered with a Tegaderm™.

When placing a Cordis, the dilator is already within the CVC (Fig. 6.7). Once the blade is used to make an incision in the skin and the needle is removed with the guidewire in place in the vessel, place the Cordis over the guidewire, and push the catheter into place making sure to keep the wire in your hands at all times. Remove the dilator with the wire and place the tubing to the end of the Cordis and flush the line. The line will similarly be sewn into place and covered with a large Tegaderm™.

Internal Jugular Vein Cannulation

Ultrasound-guided internal jugular vein catheterization is often the first choice for many practitioners due to its relative ease of access with ultrasound compared to the subclavian vein, physician familiarity, and a lower rate of catheter-related infections when compared to femoral lines [8]. Accessing the internal jugular vein may be difficult in patients that are unable to lay flat and severely dehydrated (resulting in collapse of the IJ) or who have neck trauma resulting in the need for a cervical collar. Potential complications associated with placement of an internal jugular venous catheter include pneumothorax, bleeding, hematoma formation, arterial cannulation, and laceration of the thoracic duct (left side cannulation) [6]. Ultrasound guidance can decrease the risk of these complications.

When prepping for internal jugular cannulation, the patient should be placed in Trendelenburg position (head of bed down) with the patient's head slightly rotated away from the procedural site (Fig. 6.16). With the practitioner standing at the patient's head, the ultrasound should be positioned next to the patient with the screen in line with the practitioner. The right internal jugular is preferred as it provides a straight course to the superior vena cava. As with the landmark technique, locate the anterior triangle of the neck with the two bellies of the sternocleidomastoid muscle and the clavicle as the inferior portion of the triangle (Fig. 6.17). When scanning this region, the internal jugular vein

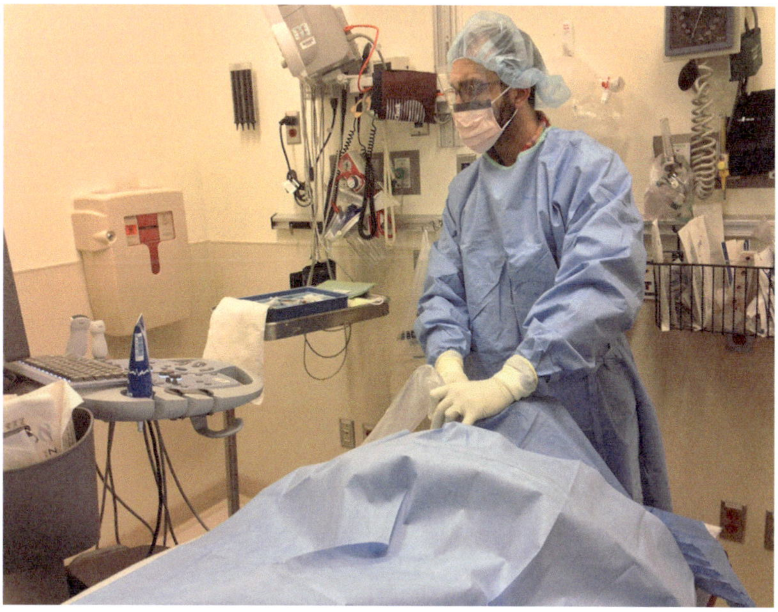

Fig. 6.16 Optimal placement of the ultrasound machine allows both the procedure site and the screen to be easily visualized

can be visualized lateral and superficial to the carotid artery (Fig. 6.18). Figures 6.19 and 6.20 illustrate needle puncturing internal jugular vein in in-plane and out-of-plane approaches. It is important to note that rotating the patient's head may cause the carotid artery to be displaced posterior to the internal jugular vein, increasing the potential for inadvertent arterial puncture. The internal jugular vein should be imaged along its course to assess for its relative position to the carotid artery, vessel depth, and site of maximal diameter. After the catheter is secured, a chest x-ray should be obtained to assess placement. The tip of the line should terminate within the superior vena cava or just above the cavoatrial junction.

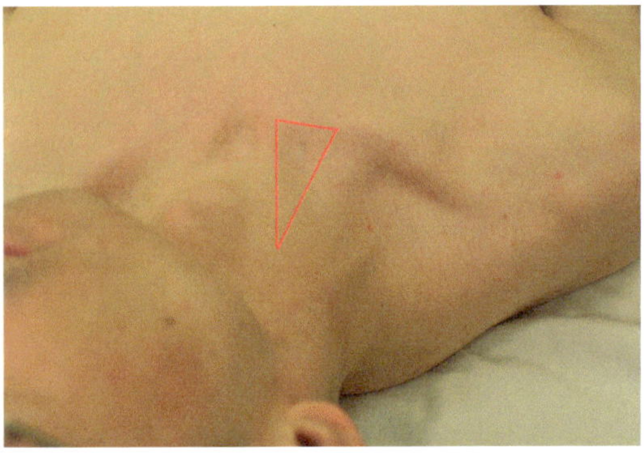

Fig. 6.17 The internal jugular typically is found inside the anterior triangle of the neck, which is defined by the clavicle at the lower border and the two heads of the sternocleidomastoid muscle

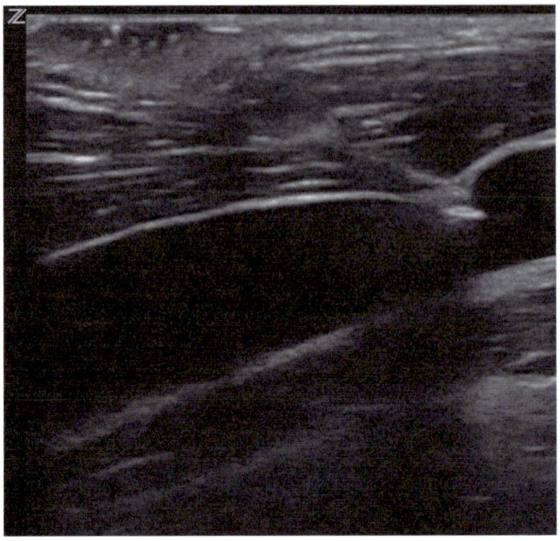

Fig. 6.19 Needle puncturing internal jugular vein in in-plane approach. (Courtesy of Srikar Adhikari, MD)

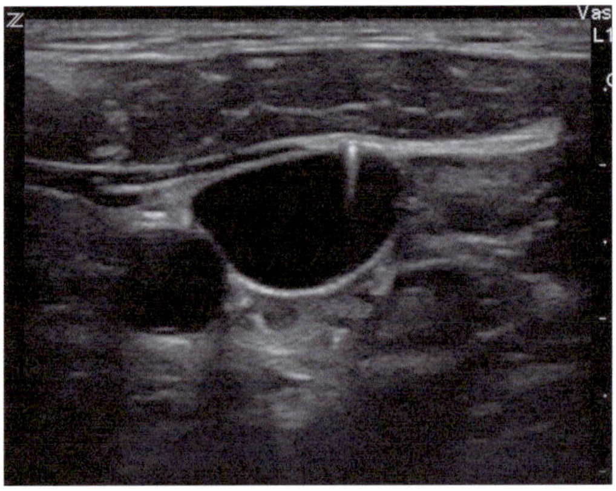

Fig. 6.20 Needle puncturing internal jugular vein in out-of-plane approach. (Courtesy of Srikar Adhikari, MD)

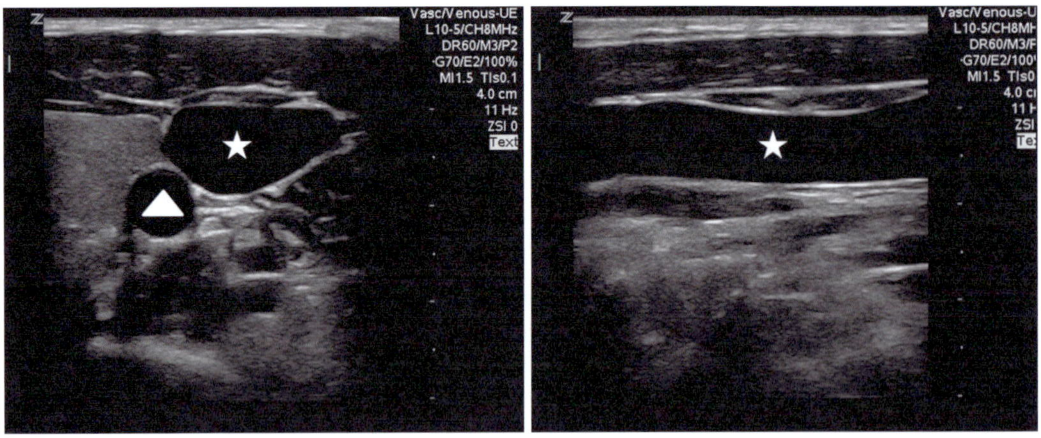

Fig. 6.18 Internal jugular vein (star) and carotid artery (triangle) in short axis (left) and in long axis (right)

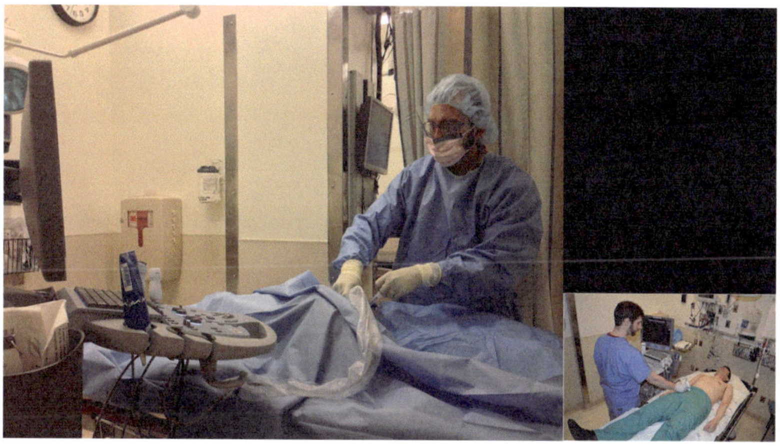

Fig. 6.21 Ultrasound machine positioning for femoral line placement allowing the screen to be in line with the operator

Common Femoral Vein Cannulation

The common femoral vein (CFV) is another option for central venous access, although it has been shown to have higher rates of catheter-related infections than both the internal jugular and subclavian vein. These lines are often placed as temporary central access in emergency situations as they can be placed while the patient is being intubated and during chest compressions or procedures to the chest including thoracentesis or thoracotomy.

The CFV is optimally visualized when the leg is abducted and externally rotated (frog leg position). The operator should be positioned on the side of cannulation with the ultrasound screen in line with the practitioner (Fig. 6.21). The CFV is found just below the inguinal ligament where it travels medial to the common femoral artery and femoral nerve. It is important to make sure the femoral artery is not overlying the femoral vein prior to attempting cannulation (Fig. 6.22).

The line should be placed as noted above. Successful catheter placement can be confirmed with ultrasound by visualizing the catheter within the femoral vein and seeing that the catheter flushes and draws venous blood.

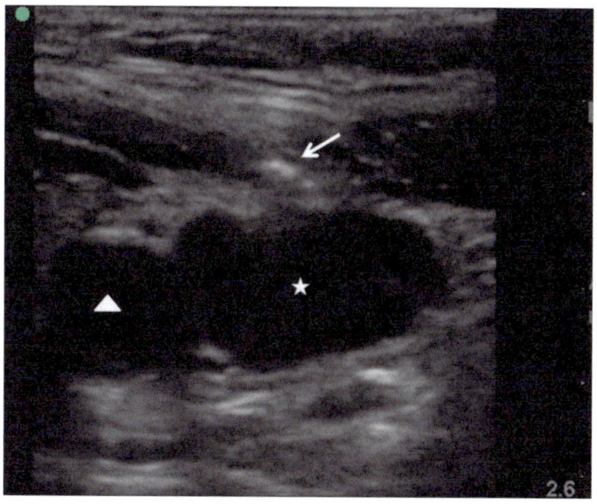

Fig. 6.22 Femoral vein (star) in short axis is distal to the inguinal ligament, the femoral artery (triangle) is seen lateral to the vein, above the vein is a needle approaching the vein, and it is marked by the arrow

Subclavian and Axillary Vein Cannulation

Since 2011, the CDC has recommended that a subclavian or axillary line should be placed over an internal jugular or femoral line to reduce the risk of infection when placing a nontunneled catheter [9]. The lower infection risk of subclavian and axillary venous catheters is sometimes offset by the high risk of pneumothorax – a complication often associated with physician inexperience [6]. Ultrasound guidance can be used to help avoid this risk.

The axillary vein arises from the brachial vein in the axilla and travels across the chest toward the first rib where it becomes the subclavian vein. The axillary vein can be cannulated under ultrasound guidance using the infraclavicular approach. The subclavian vein can be cannulated under ultrasound guidance using the supraclavicular approach. For both approaches, the patient should be placed in Trendelenburg position to minimize the risk of air embolism.

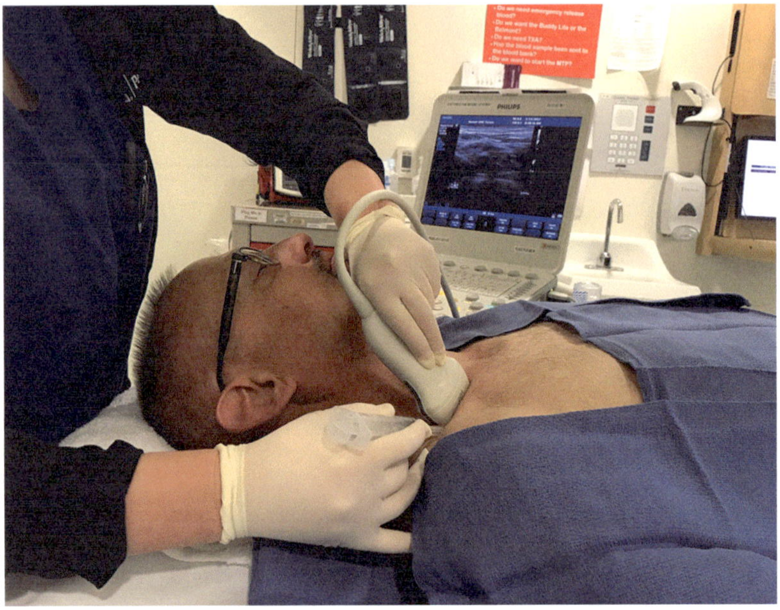

Fig. 6.23 Supraclavicular approach for subclavian vein cannulation using a linear probe

For the supraclavicular approach, the operator should stand at the patient's head with the ultrasound next to the patient and the screen of the ultrasound in line with the practitioner. The linear probe can be used for this approach (Fig. 6.23); however, an endocavitary probe may provide better access to this region given its small footprint (Fig. 6.24). To identify the subclavian vein, first locate the internal jugular vein and track it proximally. The subclavian vein will be seen uniting with the internal jugular vein in the supraclavicular fossa (Figs. 6.25 and 6.26). The vessel can be cannulated using an in-plane technique. If available substitute a neonatal-type, high-frequency micro-convex array probe for the endocavitary probe as it will be easier to wield when attempting vascular access while still providing good access to this site.

For the infraclavicular approach, the practitioner usually stands on the patient's side with the ultrasound machine near the patient's head. Sonographic visualization of the axillary vein is improved when the patient's arm is abducted and externally rotated. The axillary vein can be visualized by placing the transducer on the lateral position of the chest wall (Fig. 6.27). The axillary vein can be followed as it travels inferior to the deltopectoral groove of the clavicle and becomes the subclavian vein as it crosses the first rib (Fig. 6.28). You may be able to see lung sliding

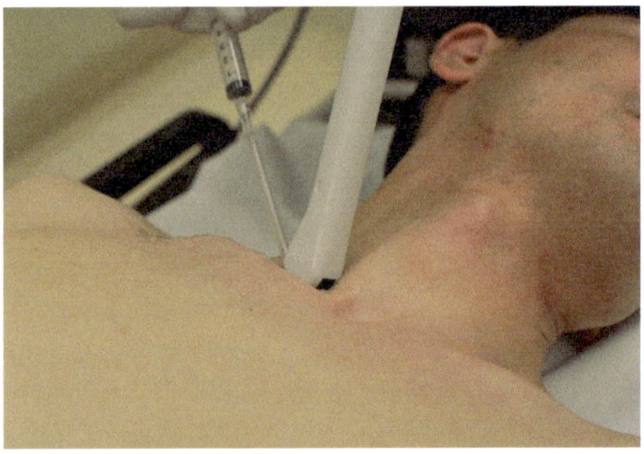

Fig. 6.24 Supraclavicular assessment of the subclavian vein using endocavitary probe

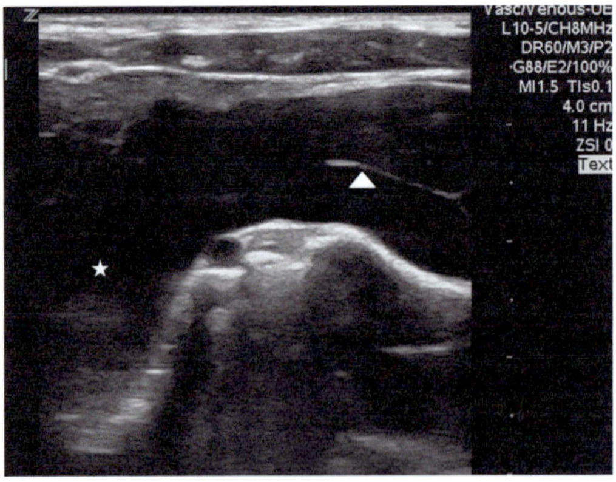

Fig. 6.25 With the linear probe, the subclavian vein is seen (triangle) joining the internal jugular vein (star); a valve is seen in the subclavian vein

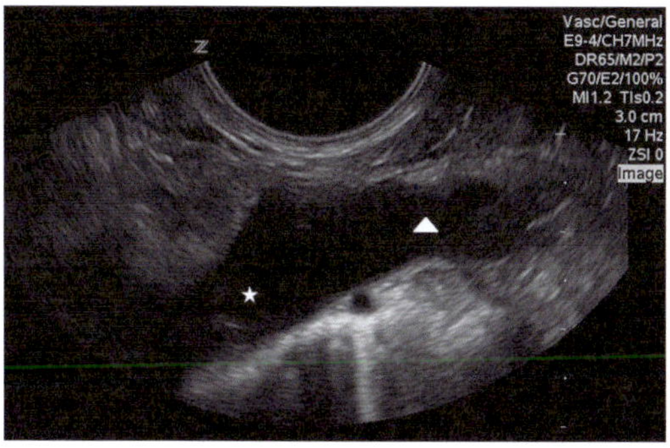

Fig. 6.26 The confluence of the subclavian vein (triangle) and the internal jugular vein (star) is seen with the endocavitary probe

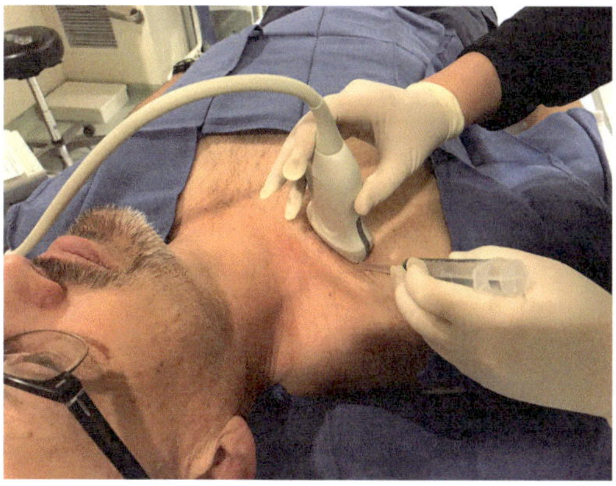

Fig. 6.27 Infraclavicular approach for the assessment of axillary vein

deep to the axillary vein. The axillary vein can be cannulated using either an in-plane or out-of-plane approach as previously described.

An axillary CVC is more easily placed with ultrasound guidance than a subclavian CVC since the clavicle does not obscure the vessel. It has also been demonstrated that the axillary vein tracts away from both its corresponding artery and the rib cage as it courses distally, suggesting less risk of arterial puncture and pneumothorax [10].

Confirming Placement

X-ray has previously been the study of choice to assess for proper placement of upper extremity CVCs. The catheter should be seen coursing along the path of the vein with its tip terminating near the superior vena cava/right atrial junction. A large downside to x-ray confirmation is the time and resources it requires to obtain the image and process it for review. Alternatively, bedside ultrasound can be used to rapidly assess for proper catheter placement using agitated saline. Agitated saline can be made at the bedside with two 5 ml syringes and a three-way stopcock. One syringe should be filled with normal saline and the other empty. Place the two syringes on the stopcock, and close the third end so that the

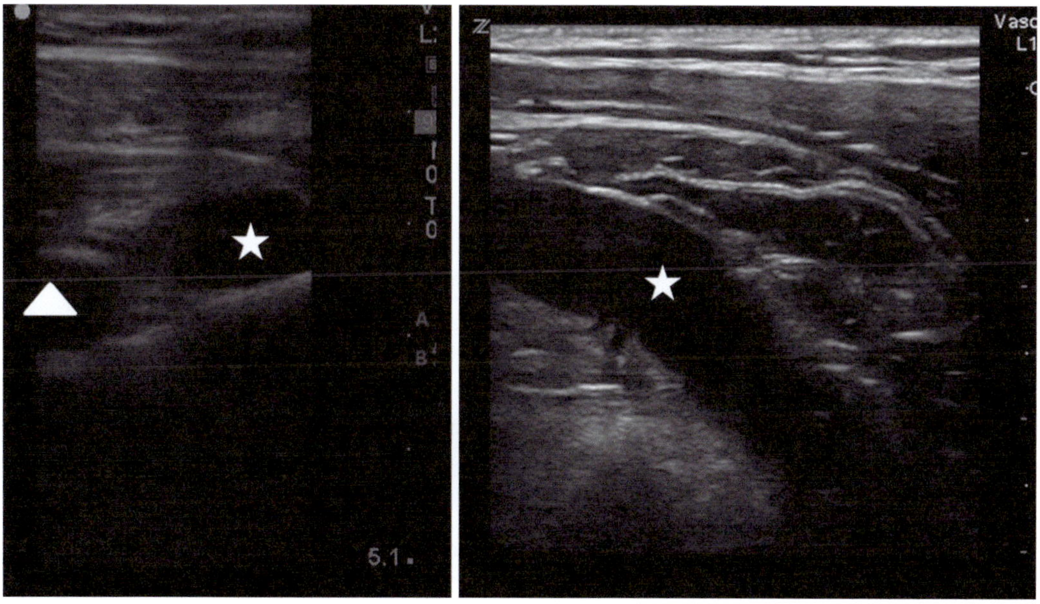

Fig. 6.28 The axillary vein (star) and artery (triangle) in short axis (left image) and the axillary vein (star) long axis (right image)

syringes are flowing into one another. "Agitate" the saline by quickly moving the saline between the two syringes. Once this is complete (10–30 seconds of agitation) (Fig. 6.29), instill the saline into the central line while using ultrasound to visualize the right atrium and ventricle. If the catheter is correctly placed, agitated normal saline bubbles (Fig. 6.30) will be seen within the right atrium and right ventricle [11]. Subclavian CVC placement sometimes results in cannulation of the ipsilateral internal jugular vein. A technique to detect this complication is to flush normal saline into the CVC while placing the palm of your hand on the patient's neck. If a thrill is palpated when fluid is instilled, the line should be reattempted [12].

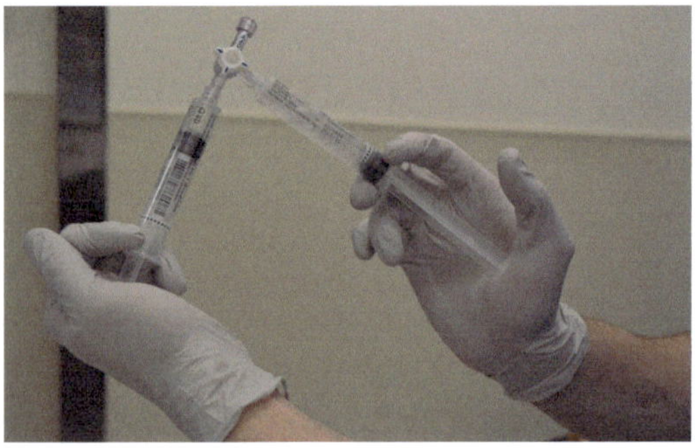

Fig. 6.29 Agitated saline is made by rapidly shifting saline between two syringes via a three-way stopcock

Complications

Pneumothoraces

This is a risk when placing subclavian and internal jugular CVCs. Ultrasound can evaluate for a pneumothorax after line placement more quickly and accurately than portable chest x-ray [13]. With the patient lying supine, the linear probe is placed in the midclavicular line with the probe marker toward the patient's head. The pleural line can be identified as a hyperechoic line between the inferior aspects of the ribs (Fig. 6.31). As the patient breaths, the sonographer should note sliding or "shimmering" of the lung pleura. In the case of a pneumothorax, this will be absent. Occasionally, comet tails may be seen which is an indication of normal lung tissue and rules out a pneumothorax in this region. The sonographer should scan between multiple rib spaces to ensure that the patient does not have a small or focal pneumothorax. Use of M-mode may also help the sonographer. In the event of a pneumothorax and absent lung sliding, there will be no motion detected, and the "barcode" sign (Fig. 6.32) will be seen. Alternatively, when lung sliding is present, one will see the "seashore" sign (Fig. 6.33) [11].

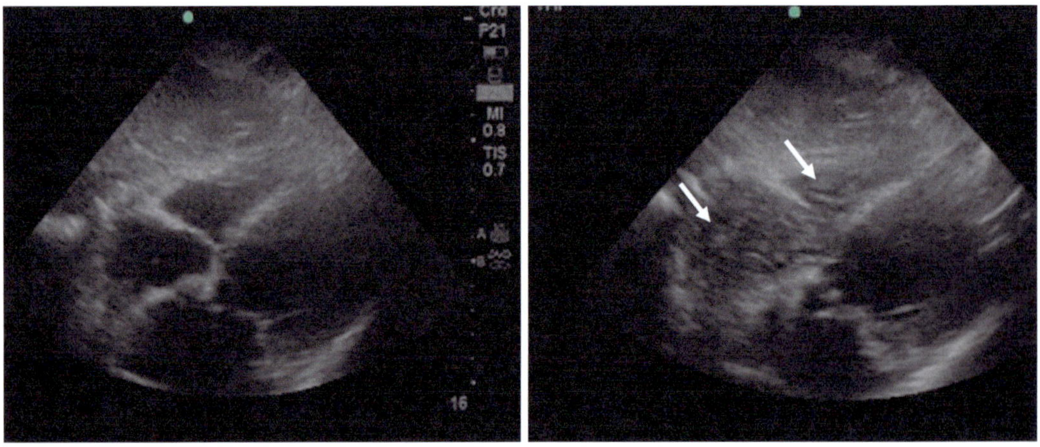

Fig. 6.30 Before (left) and after (right) agitated saline is flushed through a CVC. The right atrium and ventricle fill with the hyperechoic microbubbles of the agitated saline (arrows)

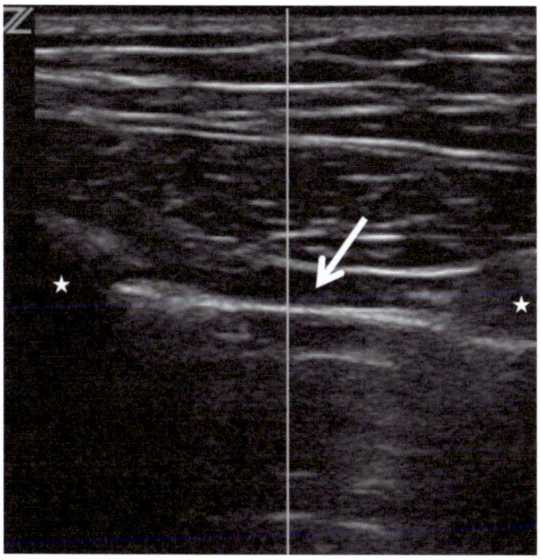

Fig. 6.31 Hyperechoic pleural line of lung between two ribs (starred)

Infections

Nontunneled CVCs are at the highest risk for central line-associated bloodstream infections (CLABSI) with femoral lines yielding the highest infection rate. Intrinsic or non-modifiable risk factors for infection are patient age, underlying disease or conditions, and patient gender (increased risk in males and the elderly). Extrinsic or modifiable risk factors include prolonged hospitalization before CVC insertion, multiple CVCs, parenteral nutrition, femoral or internal jugular access site, heavy microbial colonization at insertion site, multilumen CVCs, lack of maximal sterile barriers for CVC insertion, and CVC insertion in an intensive care unit or emergency department [14]. Using ultrasound guidance for CVC insertions helps

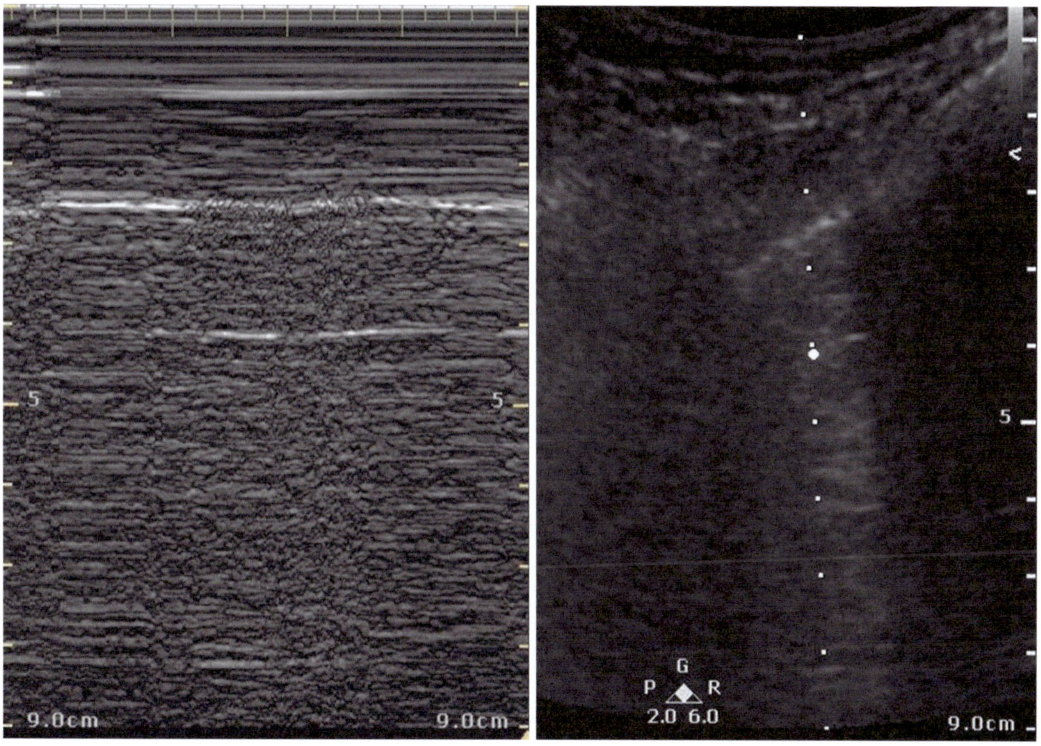

Fig. 6.32 "Seashore sign" seen in M-mode indicating normal lung sliding

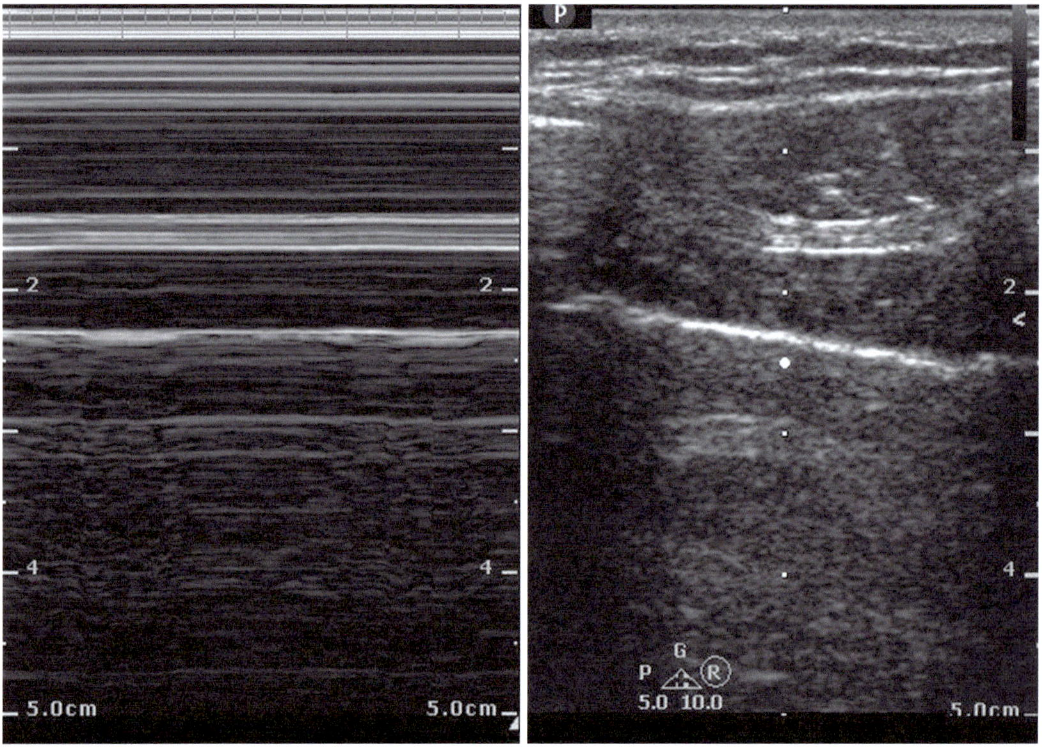

Fig. 6.33 "Barcode sign" which denotes no lung sliding, concerning for a pneumothorax

decrease the risk of associated infections by decreasing the number of cannulation attempts. Adherence to full barrier precaution technique throughout the procedure is also vital in reducing infection rates. Additionally, the continued need for central access should be frequently reassessed to minimize the duration that CVCs are in place.

Other Complications

Other potential complications of CVC placement include arterial puncture, hematoma formation, arteriovenous fistula formation, intraluminal dissection, venous air embolism, retroperitoneal bleeding, pseudoaneurysm, a lost wire which may cause an atrial wall rupture, thrombus formation, nerve injury, anaphylaxis from an antibiotic impregnated catheter, thoracic duct injury (with left-sided cannulation), or catheter malposition [6].

Pearls and Pitfalls

- A common pitfall in the out-of-plane approach is to mistake the shaft of the needle for the tip resulting in advancing the needle too far which can lead to posterior wall, artery, or lung perforation.
- When using the out-of-plane approach, the transducer must be constantly repositioned to maintain visualization of the needle tip. Slightly jiggling the needle can also help localize the tip.
- Taking time to set up the room appropriately making both CVC materials and ultrasound

equipment easily accessible will improve overall success of the procedure.

- Visualize the target vessel in both the long and short axis prior to starting the procedure to ensure there is no variant anatomy or barriers to line placement (clot, stenosis).
- A useful approach is to start in the out-of-plane approach to make sure the needle entry is directly over the vessel and then switch to an in-plane approach to advance the needle into the vein.
- Consider the subclavian or axillary vein when the internal jugular vein is completely collapsed due to dehydration as there is a high likelihood of posterior wall puncture.
- Use of ultrasound for subclavian cannulation is associated with better outcomes and, in at least one study, a zero incidence of pneumothorax [17].

Key Points

- Ultrasound guidance improves success and reduces the risk of complications when placing CVCs.
- Ultrasound can be used for placement of internal jugular, subclavian/axillary, and femoral lines.

Integration into Clinical Practice

Ultrasound decreases complications and improves success when placing CVCs. Ultrasound guidance for internal jugular cannulation is recommended by multiple organizations. Ultrasound guidance should be routinely used for CVC placement to enhance patient safety. Use of ultrasound guidance is considered as standard of practice in current clinical practice.

Evidence

- 2015 Cochrane review on ultrasonography for internal jugular line placement found that use of ultrasound when compared to the landmark technique reduced arterial punctures, number of attempts, and time to successful cannulation [1].
- 2013 meta-analysis found decreased risks of cannulation failure, arterial puncture, hematoma, and hemothorax in adult patients for which ultrasound guidance was used for CVC placement [15].
- First-pass success is significantly increased by use of ultrasound guidance in internal jugular vein cannulation [16].

References

1. Brass P, Hellmich M, Kolodziej L, Schick G, Smith AF. Ultrasound guidance versus anatomical landmarks for internal jugular vein catheterization. Cochrane Database Syst Rev. 2015;1:CD006962.
2. Brass P, Hellmich M, Kolodziej L, Schick G, Smith AF. Ultrasound guidance versus anatomical landmarks for subclavian or femoral vein catheterization. Cochrane Database Syst Rev. 2015;1:CD011447.
3. Shekelle P, Dallas P. Use of real-time ultrasound guidance during central line insertion: brief update review. In: Agency For Health Research and Quality (US), editor. The New England Journal of Medicine: AHRQ; Boston, MA 2013. p. 172–7.
4. Milling TJ Jr, Rose J, Briggs WM, Birkhahn R, Gaeta TJ, Bove JJ, et al. Randomized, controlled clinical trial of point-of-care limited ultrasonography assistance of central venous cannulation: the Third Sonography Outcomes Assessment Program (SOAP-3) Trial. Crit Care Med. 2005;33(8):1764–9.
5. Thomas S, Moore CL. The vanishing target sign: confirmation of intraluminal needle position for ultrasound guided vascular access. Acad Emerg Med. 2013;20(10):e17–8.
6. Troianos CA, Hartman GS, Glas KE, Skubas NJ, Eberhardt RT, Walker JD, et al. Guidelines for performing ultrasound guided vascular cannulation: recommendations of the American Society of Echocardiography and the Society of Cardiovascular Anesthesiologists. J Am Soc Echocardiogr. 2011;24(12):1291–318.
7. Phelan M, Hagerty D. The oblique view: an alternative approach for ultrasound-guided central line placement. J Emerg Med. Elsevier. 2009;37(4):403–8.

8. McGee DC, Gould MK. Preventing complications of central venous catheterization. N Engl J Med. 2003; 348(12):1123–33.
9. O'Grady NP, Alexander M, Burns LA, Dellinger EP, Garland J, Heard SO, et al. Summary of recommendations: guidelines for the prevention of intravascular catheter-related infections. Clin Infect Dis. 2011;52(9):1087–99.
10. Galloway S, Bodenham A. Ultrasound imaging of the axillary vein—anatomical basis for central venous access. Br J Anaesth. 2003;90(5):589–95.
11. Duran-Gehring PE, Guirgis FW, McKee KC, Goggans S, Tran H, Kalynych CJ, et al. The bubble study: ultrasound confirmation of central venous catheter placement. Am J Emerg Med [Internet]. 2014.; Available from: https://doi.org/10.1016/j.ajem.2014.10.010.
12. Rath GP, Bithal PK, Toshniwal GR, Prabhakar H, Dash HH. Saline flush test for bedside detection of misplaced subclavian vein catheter into ipsilateral internal jugular vein†. Br J Anaesth. 2009; 102(4):499–502.
13. Nagarsheth K, Kurek S. Ultrasound detection of pneumothorax compared with chest X-ray and computed tomography scan. Am Surg. 2011;77(4):480–4.
14. Commission J, Others. Preventing central line--associated bloodstream infections: a global challenge, a global perspective. Oak Brook: Joint Commission Resources; 2012.
15. Wu S-Y, Ling Q, Cao L-H, Wang J, Xu M-X, Zeng W-A. Real-time two-dimensional ultrasound guidance for central venous cannulation: a meta-analysis. Anesthesiology. 2013;118(2):361–75.
16. Augoustides JG, Horak J, Ochroch AE, Vernick WJ, Gambone AJ, Weiner J, et al. A randomized controlled clinical trial of real-time needle-guided ultrasound for internal jugular venous cannulation in a large university anesthesia department. J Cardiothorac Vasc Anesth. 2005;19(3):310–5.
17. Kilbourne MJ, Bochicchio GV, Scalea T, Xiao Y. Avoiding common technical errors in subclavian central venous catheter placement. J Am Coll Surg. 2009;208(1):104–9.

Ultrasound-Guided Ear, Nose, and Throat Procedures

7

Richard Amini and Parisa Javedani

Introduction

Head and neck procedures are routinely performed by healthcare providers in acute care settings. Traditionally, anatomical landmarks are used to determine accurate location and approach when performing these procedures. However, the success and complication rates for landmark-based techniques are quite variable due to anatomical variations. The evaluation of superficial regions of the face and neck is shallow, and as a result, imaging with high-frequency ultrasound probes can provide high-resolution images ideal for the diagnostic workup and procedural guidance. High-resolution ultrasound for evaluation of head and neck soft tissue swelling is far superior to the physical examination and provides a very high sensitivity (96%) and specificity (82%), and cysts as small as 2–3 mm can be identified [1]. More importantly, the use of ultrasound guidance has been demonstrated to improve success rates, minimize inadvertent injury to surrounding tissue, and improve patient experiences.

R. Amini (✉)
University of Arizona, Department of Emergency Medicine, Tucson, AZ, USA
e-mail: ramini@aemrc.arizona.edu

P. Javedani
Colorado Permanente Medical Group, Denver, CO, USA

Advantages of Ultrasound Guidance

The benefit of ultrasound guidance is perhaps most realized when evaluating for and performing needle aspiration of tonsillar and peritonsillar infections. A recent RCT compared anatomical landmark techniques to ultrasound imaging for the diagnosis and drainage of PTAs and found that ultrasound was superior in the following ways: diagnostic accuracy, ultrasound 100% vs. landmark 75%; successful drainage, ultrasound 100% vs. landmark 50%; and consultation of otolaryngology, ultrasound 7% vs. landmark 50% [2]. In small lesions (10–15 mm), landmark guidance in fine needle aspiration leads to 3 times as many failed samples [3]. Ultrasound guidance not only allows the physician to evaluate the relevant anatomy but also allows real-time visualization of the needle as the procedure is performed. A thorough understanding of the basic principles of ultrasound, sonographic anatomy, and manual dexterity skills is essential in the use of ultrasound for procedural guidance.

Head and Neck Cutaneous Abscess Drainage

Anatomy

Anatomy of the head and neck includes an extensive supply of nerves and vasculature. When evaluating for an abscess, a keen eye should be used

S. Adhikari, M. Blaivas (eds.), *The Ultimate Guide to Point-of-Care Ultrasound-Guided Procedures*, https://doi.org/10.1007/978-3-030-28267-7_7

to evaluate for vital anatomical structures before the start of the procedure. For example, in the lateral anterior region of the neck, the carotid artery and internal jugular vein are located below the sternocleidomastoid and should be identified so as not to cause vascular injury during incision and drainage or needle aspiration (Fig. 7.1). Due to the extensive network of neurovascular branches, needle aspiration is the favored technique for a majority of abscesses of the head and neck.

Clinicians must also be familiar with sonographic evaluation of the airway. Air-tissue interface can help the operator identify relevant anatomy. In the mouth, air-tissue interface can be identified as a hyperechoic line which follows the curvature of the tongue (Fig. 7.2a) and as a hyperechoic line between the gum line/teeth and the cheek (Fig. 7.2b). In the neck, the interface is used to identify the trachea (Fig. 7.2c).

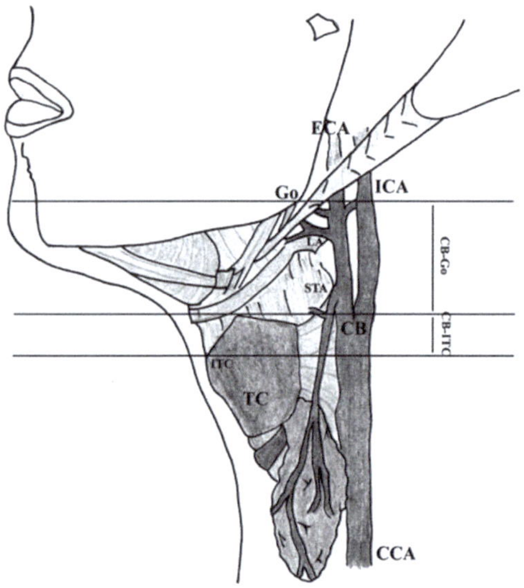

Fig. 7.1 Anatomy of the lateral neck (TC thyroid cartilage, CB carotid bifurcation, CB–Go carotid bifurcation–gonion, CB–ITC carotid bifurcation–isthmus of thyroid cartilage, CCA common carotid artery, ECA external carotid artery, ICA internal carotid artery, STA superior thyroid artery, LA lingual artery). (Reproduced from Topography of carotid bifurcation: considerations for neck examination. Surg Radiol Anat. 2008;30: 383–387-p. 384)

Physical examination findings of head and neck swelling are not reliable, whereas sonographic evaluation purports a sensitivity >90% and specificity >80% [1]. Clinicians performing cutaneous procedures of the head and neck should use ultrasound to increase success rates and minimize complications.

Indications

The vast majority of etiologies behind swelling and/or discomfort of the head or neck include cellulitis, abscess, cyst, lymphadenopathy, or salivary gland swelling (Fig. 7.3). Patients who are found to have edema or swelling should undergo sonographic evaluation for anechoic fluid collections. As mentioned these patients should generally undergo aspiration or incision and drainage.

Contraindications

Head and neck infections (dental infections, facial infections, peritonsillar abscess, etc.) can create direct or indirect airway compression. As a result, the patient's airway should be assessed prior to starting the procedure. Patients in whom airway obstruction or airway compromise is deemed a risk factor should not undergo bedside drainage, and surgical consultation should be considered.

Equipment/Probe Selection

As with evaluation of most superficial structures, the high-frequency (15–6 MHz) linear array probe should be used. Color Doppler can help evaluate for hyperemia and aid in the identification of surrounding neurovascular structures. Lidocaine with or without epinephrine should be readily available. Chlorhexidine, a sterile probe cover, and #11 blade scalpel or 18 or 20 gauge needle attached to a 10 mL syringe should also be available (Fig. 7.4).

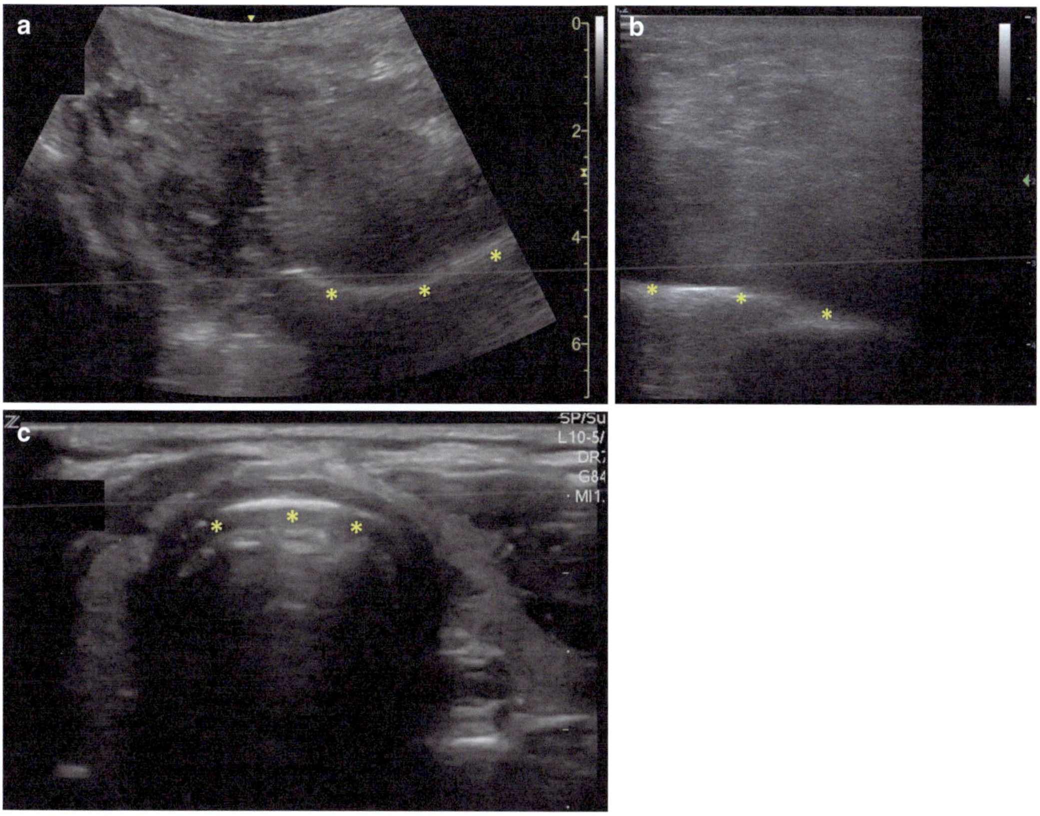

Fig. 7.2 Mucosa and air interface. (**a**) Transcervical imaging of the oropharynx demonstrates the tongue and soft palate interface (asterisks). (**b**) Soft tissue imaging of the face demonstrates the cheek and gingiva interface (asterisks). (**c**) Airway imaging. The trachea is identified as a result of the mucosa-air interface in a supine patient. In all three images, the hyperechoic line between surfaces is accentuated by trapped air

Preparation/Preprocedural Evaluation

For cutaneous procedures of the head and neck, the gurney should be at a height comfortable for the physician. The patient's head should be comfortably turned to the contralateral side, and the neck should be extended to maximize access to the affected area. Topical anesthetic, such as lidocaine-epinephrine-tetracaine gel, can be used over the affected area to minimize discomfort. In certain scenarios, clinicians may choose to provide anxiolysis with benzodiazepines or systemic pain control with a short-acting narcotic. Prior to the procedure, depth of the abscess cavity from the surface of the skin, size of the abscess, and surrounding structures should be evaluated using ultrasound. Color Doppler should be used to identify adjacent vessels which should be avoided during the procedure.

Procedure

The linear array transducer should be used to scan the area in question in both the sagittal and transverse planes; whenever possible, the patient's contralateral side should be imaged for comparison. An anechoic fluid collection with echoic contents often with posterior acoustic enhancement is concerning for abscess. This should be distinguished from cellulitis, which can have a cobblestone appearance without fluid collections

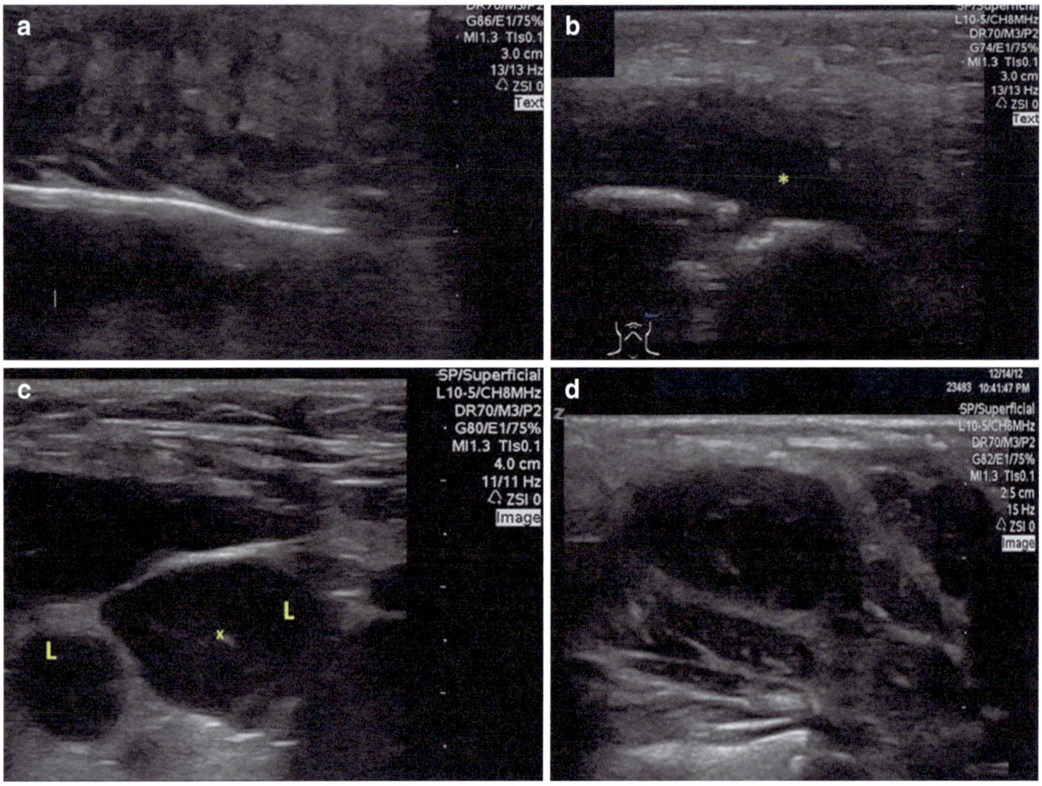

Fig. 7.3 (**a**) Soft tissue swelling of the face with cobblestone appearance consistent with cellulitis. (**b**) Anechoic fluid collection from periapical dental abscess (asterisk). (**c**) Lymphadenitis (L) with echogenic hilum (x). (**d**) Salivary gland inflammation

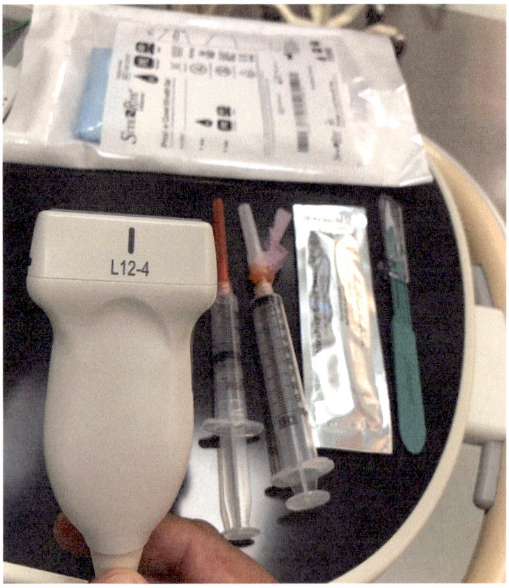

Fig. 7.4 Linear array transducer and other equipment for incision and drainage

(Figs. 7.5 and 7.6). The physician should gently compress the affected area for squish sign, and color Doppler flow can be used to confirm the lack of vascularity within the cavity (Fig. 7.7). If a fluid collection is located, the boundaries, depth from the skin surface, and estimated size of the cavity should be noted. The relevant adjacent anatomy should be evaluated; and the physician should be mindful of the underlying structures in the neck which include the thyroid, parathyroid, trachea, and vasculature. When draining an abscess of the face, care must be taken to avoid the facial nerve and branches of the trigeminal nerve. When draining abscesses of the neck, care must be taken not to injure the underlying neurovascular structures, and special care must also be taken to remain superficial to the platysma.

Once the abscess and relevant anatomy have been visualized and imaged in at least two planes, the affected area can be anesthetized. The cutane-

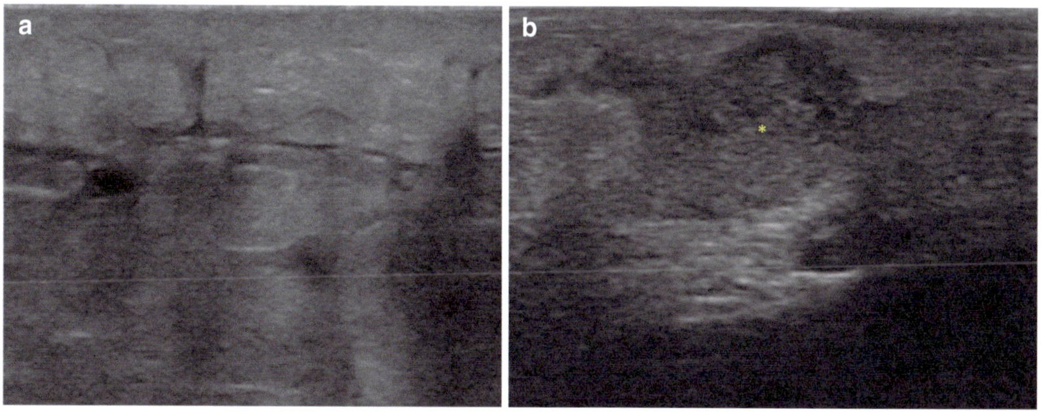

Fig. 7.5 (**a**) Soft tissue swelling with presence of cobblestone appearance consistent with cellulitis. (**b**) Soft tissue swelling with anechoic fluid collection (asterisk) suggesting abscess

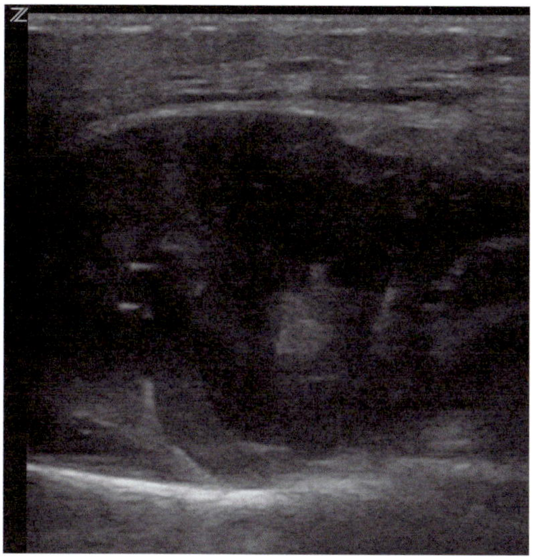

Fig. 7.6 B-mode image of anechoic facial abscess with posterior acoustic enhancement

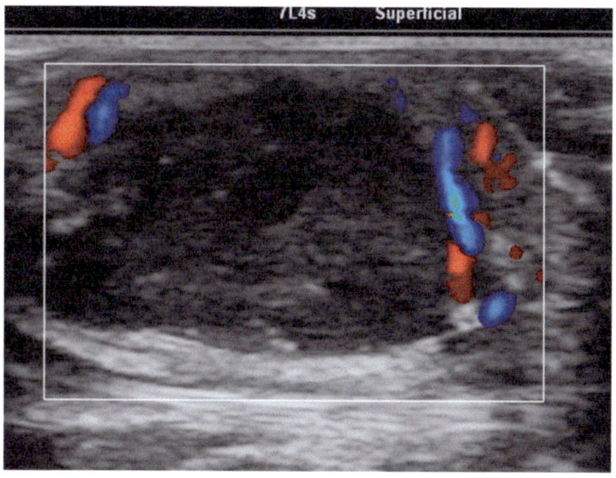

Fig. 7.7 On color Doppler, no flow noted within the abscess cavity; however, hyperemia is seen surrounding the abscess cavity

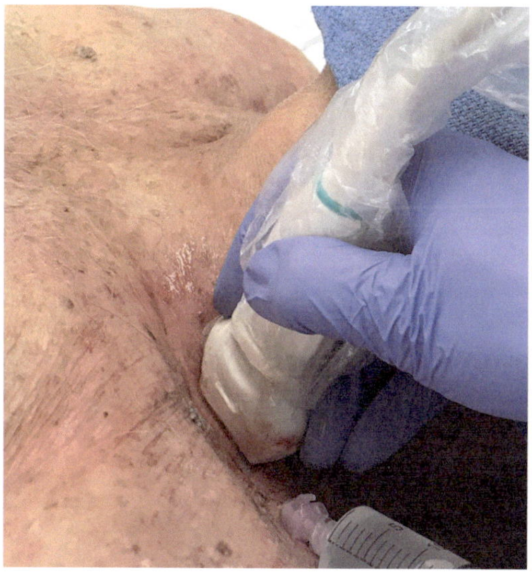

Fig. 7.8 Needle aspiration using in-plane approach

ous area should be cleansed with chlorhexidine. The probe should be covered with a tegaderm, and gel should be placed on top of the probe. Using an 18 or 20 gauge needle attached to a 10 mL syringe, advance the needle tip under ultrasound guidance using an in-plane approach (Fig. 7.8). If necessary, make a small incision using a #11 blade scalpel, and use blunt dissection to break up loculated fluid collections (Fig. 7.9a, b). Extensive abscesses may require irrigation with normal saline to aid in breakdown of loculations. Ultrasound should be used after drainage is complete to verify complete evacuation of the abscess cavity (Fig. 7.10).

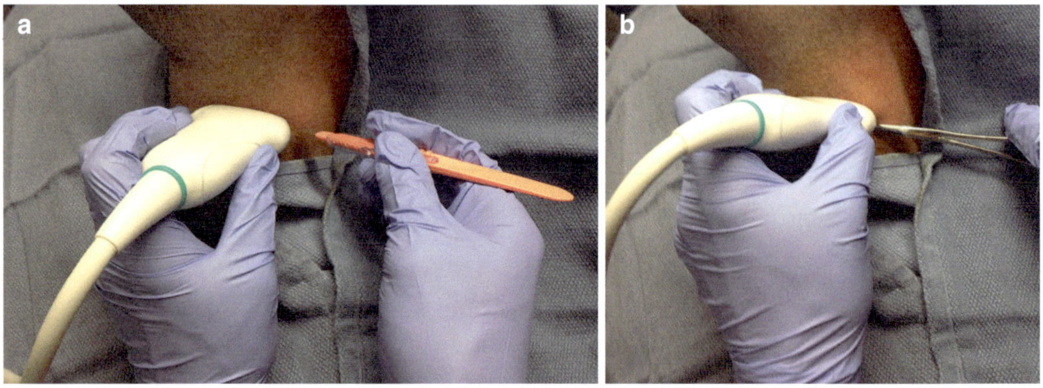

Fig. 7.9 Ultrasound-guided incision and drainage. (**a**) Probe positioning for incision. (**b**) Probe positioning for drainage

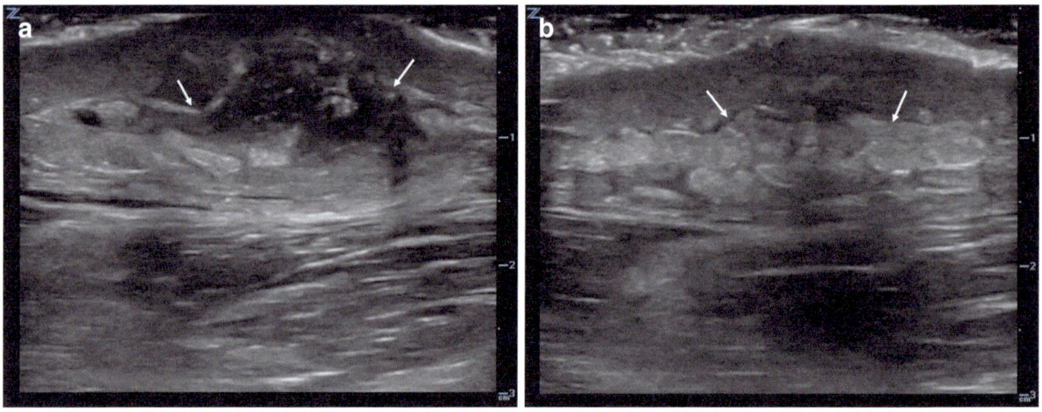

Fig. 7.10 (**a**) Anechoic abscess cavity (arrows) prior to incision and drainage. (**b**) Post incision and drainage image confirming abscess evacuation, collapsed abscess cavity (arrows)

Complications

Injury to the surrounding neurovascular structures is a complication associated with head and neck cutaneous procedures. Additionally, lymph nodes may be difficult to distinguish from an abscess. Color Doppler can aid in the identification of vascular structures and lymph nodes. In addition, ultrasound should be used to verify complete evacuation of the abscess cavity. A partially drained abscess may result in the need for further intervention in the future.

Pearls/Pitfalls

1. Injury to surrounding neurovascular structures can be avoided by utilizing color Doppler during the initial evaluation and performing the procedure under ultrasound guidance.
2. Purulent material in the abscess cavity may appear isoechoic. For this reason, any findings should be compared to the contralateral side, color Doppler can be used to demonstrate hyperemic glands or nodes, and compression can help demonstrate abscess content motion.
3. The use of 18 gauge needles is preferred as purulent material may be difficult to aspirate through smaller caliber needles.
4. If purulent material is too viscous to aspirate, a #11 blade scalpel can be used to create a small puncture sufficient to allow for drainage.
5. Use gray-scale imaging and color Doppler imaging to evaluate for necrotic lymph nodes and glands.
6. In-plane approach is recommended while performing needle aspiration.

Integration into Clinical Practice

Physical examination of cutaneous swelling of the head and neck has poor diagnostic utility, whereas ultrasound has a sensitivity >90%. Ultrasound-guided incision and drainage of head and neck abscesses can provide definitive treatment. Furthermore, ultrasound-guided drainage can help prevent the occurrence of common complications, including injury to the surrounding neurovascular structures.

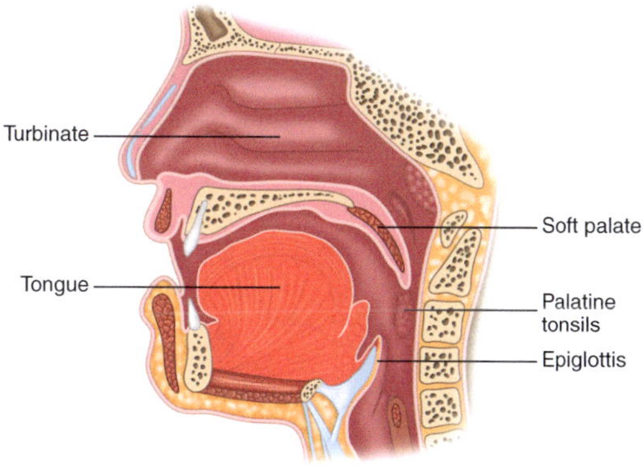

Fig. 7.11 Anatomy of the pharynx and tonsillar tissue

Evidence

High-resolution ultrasound provides a very high sensitivity (96%) and specificity (82%) for identification of purulent collections in evaluation of head and neck swelling [1]. Ultrasound-guided fine needle aspiration has a sensitivity of 89–98% and specificity of 95–98% in the differentiation of neck masses [4]. Yusa et al. described the utility of ultrasound guidance for draining deep face and neck abscesses. In addition, ultrasound guidance has been shown to be helpful in the drainage of submasseteric space abscess and needle aspiration of lateral masticator space [5, 6].

> **Key Points**
> - Ultrasound-guided aspiration of cutaneous swelling of the head and neck will increase success rates, decrease complications, and as a result improve patient care and experience.
> - Hand dexterity and sonographic needle guidance skills are required and can easily be cultivated with practice.

Peritonsillar Abscess Drainage

Anatomy

The throat is divided into three parts: the nasopharynx, oropharynx, and hypopharynx. The nasopharynx includes the nasal cavity and soft palate, the oropharynx includes the posterior mouth down to the superior edge of the epiglottis, and the hypopharynx includes the epiglottis to the cricoid cartilage (Fig. 7.11). Found in the oropharynx, the palatine tonsils are defined anteriorly by the tonsillar pillar and the glosopalatine muscles and posteriorly by the tonsillar pillar and the pharyngopalatine muscle. The palatine tonsil itself is located between the palatoglossal and palatopharyngeal arch. Each tonsil has a number of ingrowths known as tonsillar crypts. During an infection, the peritonsillar space evolves into peritonsillar cellulitis. Peritonsillar abscesses form when the surrounding infection spreads into the tonsillar capsule. In addition to the evaluation of palatine tonsils, clinicians should be familiar with sonographic anatomy of the tongue, soft palate, and carotid artery.

Indications

Patients will often present with any or all of the following: trismus, odynophagia, "hot potato" voice, edema and erythema of the surrounding peritonsillar tissue, cervical lymphadenopathy, limitation of neck movements, torticollis, tonsillitis, tonsillar displacement, and uvula deviation away from the affected side [7, 8]. Intraoral ultrasound can help identify PTA versus peritonsillar cellulitis (PTC) (Fig. 7.12).

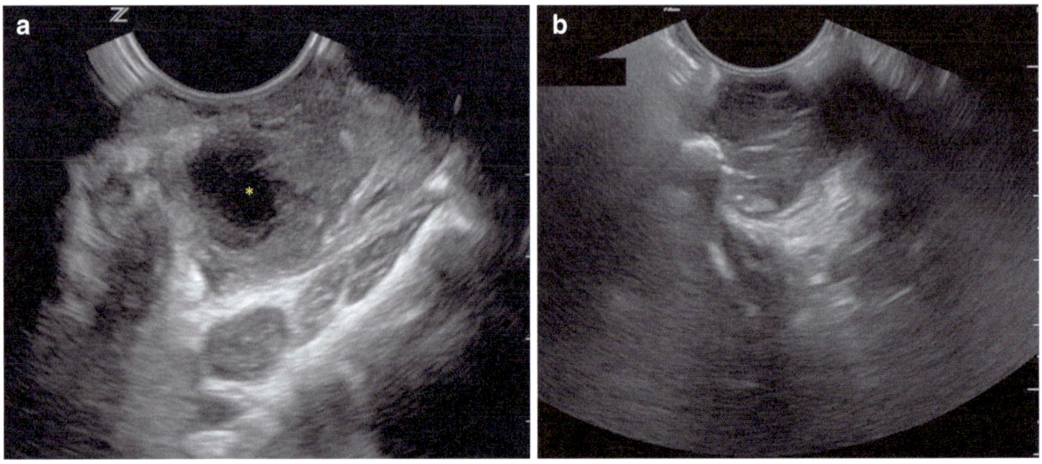

Fig. 7.12 Ultrasound imaging of the peritonsillar space is essential to differential tonsillar swelling with abscess. (**a**) B-mode showing peritonsillar abscess (asterisk). (**b**) Tonsillar swelling consistent with peritonsillar cellulitis

Contraindications

If there is concern for possible airway obstruction or patient noncompliance during the procedure, an alternative method of drainage, such as intra-operative drainage under general anesthesia, should be considered.

Equipment/Probe Selection

Although the intraoral approach is the most widely utilized technique for ultrasound-guided PTA drainage, the transcervical approach is a great option for patient with significant trismus which can limit placement of the endocavitary transducer into the oropharynx. When conducting the transoral approach, the high-frequency (12–2.5 MHz) curved array endocavitary probe (Figs. 7.13 and 7.14a) is required for optimal oropharynx imaging. When the transcervical approach is conducted, the low-frequency (5–2 MHz) curved array transducer or a (10–5 MHz) linear transducer is used (Fig. 7.15a).

Preparation/Preprocedural Evaluation

An airway assessment should be performed prior to starting the procedure, and necessary airway equipment should be readily available at the bedside. The patient should be seated upright, with the bed at a height comfortable for the physician performing the procedure. A topical anesthetic spray should be applied to the affected peritonsillar tissue. Five percent lidocaine ointment or 2% lidocaine jelly can be placed on a tongue depressor and given to the patient in the form of a "popsicle" as a useful anesthetic adjunct. Nebulized 4% lidocaine can provide additional analgesia, and systemic analgesia may be necessary. A 2 in. 18 gauge needle or an 18 gauge spinal needle with the plastic sheath attached to a 10 mL or 20 mL syringe should be available at the bedside. One percent lidocaine without epinephrine should be available in the event the patient requires further analgesia prior to starting the procedure.

PTA should be distinguished from PTC, with PTA appearing as an enlarged tonsil with heterogeneous or cystic appearance and PTC appearing as an enlarged tonsil with a homogenous or striated appearance (Fig. 7.12) [9]. A cobblestone appearance typical of cellulitis may be noted in advanced PTC. Measure the depth of the abscess cavity from the mucosal surface, as this will determine the length of needle required. Measure the length and width of the abscess cavity to determine the overall size of the abscess, and estimate the expected amount of fluid to be drained (Figs. 7.8c and 7.9c). Finally, in short or

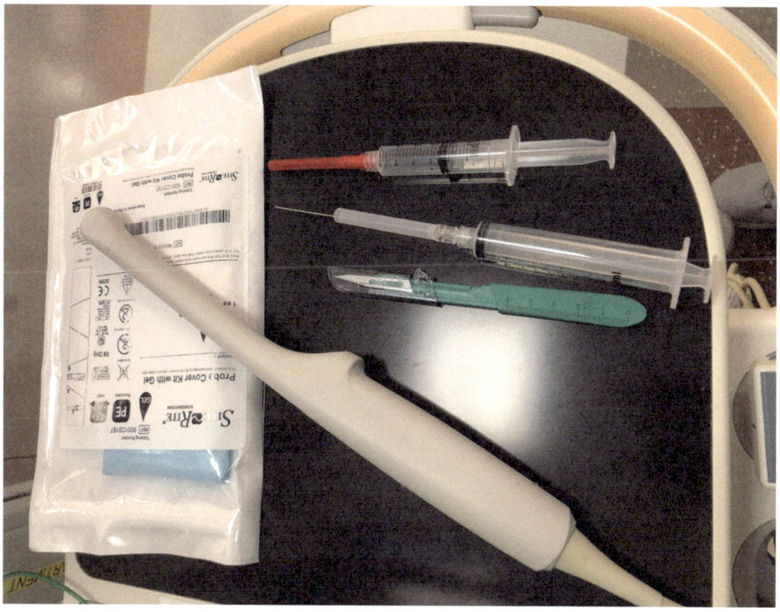

Fig. 7.13 High-frequency endocavitary probe for intraoral approach

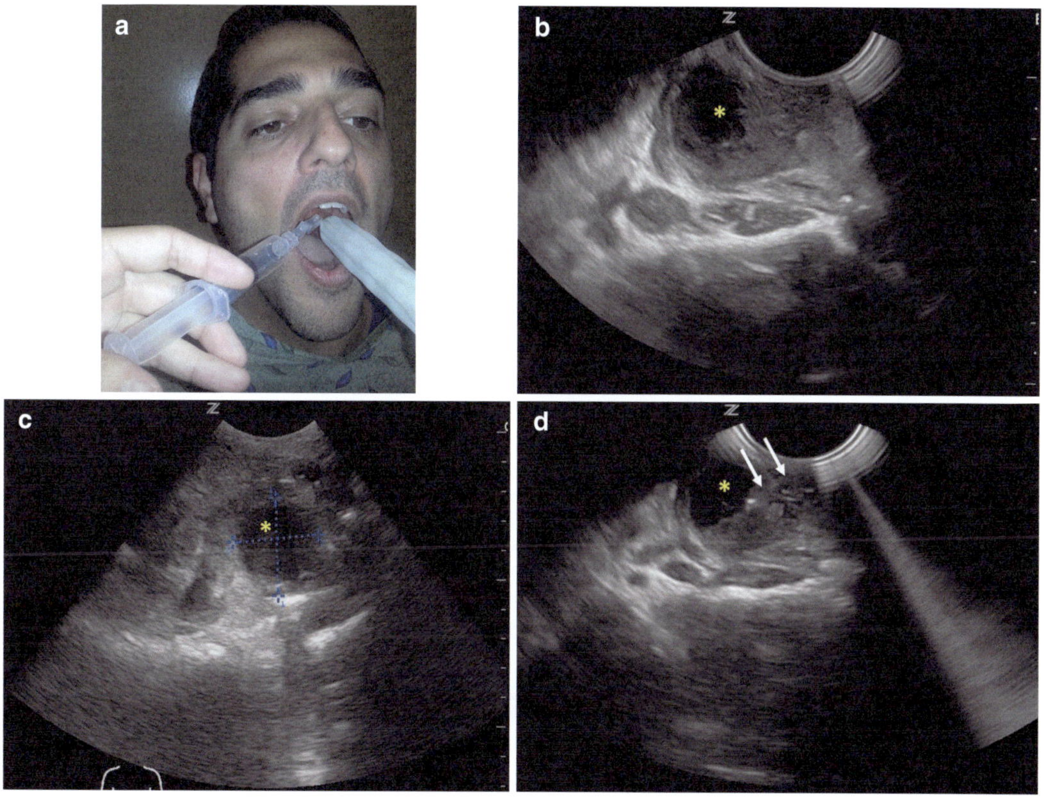

Fig. 7.14 Intraoral approach for PTA aspiration. (**a**) Endocavitary probe and the needle are inserted into the mouth. (**b**) Identification of a PTA with anechoic fluid collection (asterisk). (**c**) Measure the size and depth of the abscess cavity. (**d**) PTA drainage with direct needle visualization (arrows)

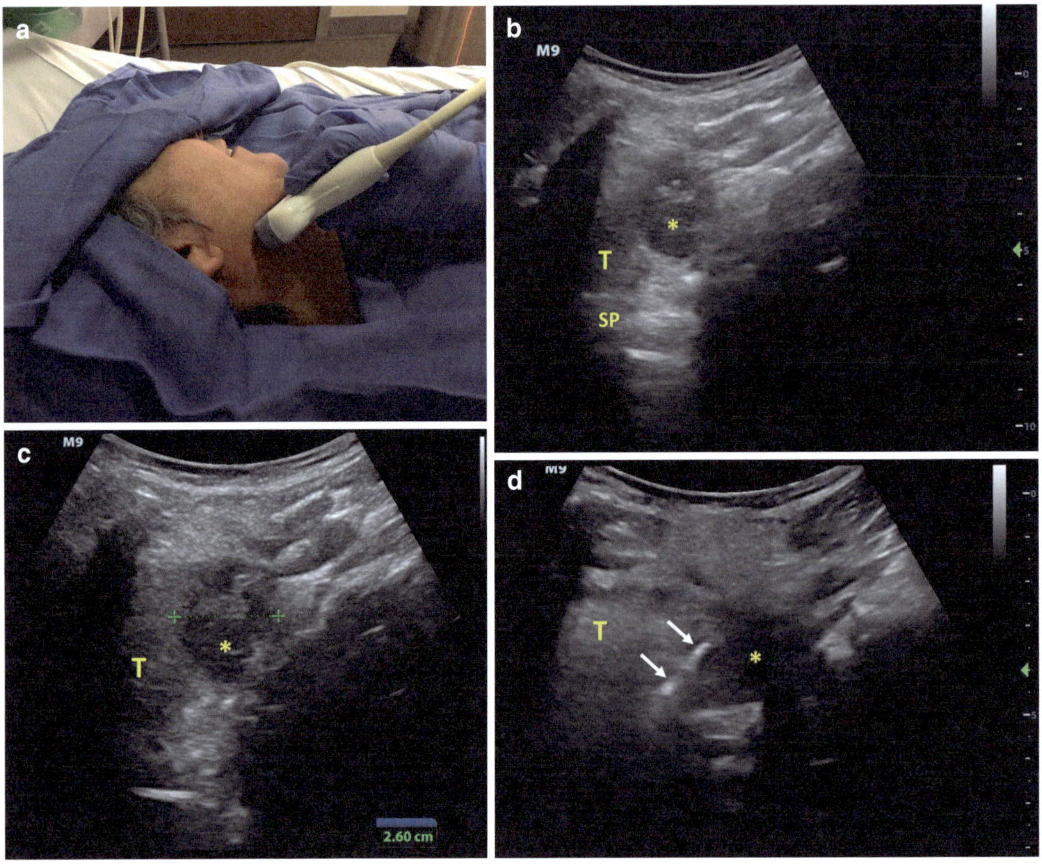

Fig. 7.15 Transcervical approach for PTA aspiration. (**a**) Curved array transducer provides imaging in the submandibular region while the needle is inserted into the mouth. (**b**) Identification of a PTA with isoechoic fluid collection (asterisk) (T-Tonsil, SP-Soft palate). (**c**) Measure the size and depth of the abscess cavity. (**d**) PTA drainage with direct needle visualization (arrows)

transverse axis, determine the relationship of the abscess cavity to the carotid artery. The carotid artery will appear as a small, pulsatile, tubular structure, generally 0.5–2.5 cm posterior to the abscess cavity, and use of a color Doppler can help in its identification (Fig. 7.16). Place a small amount of gel over the transducer, and cover the probe with a sheath or condom. Insert the probe into the pharyngeal region, and scan in both the long and short axis.

Procedure

Intraoral Approach

When performing the intraoral approach to PTA drainage, the endocavitary transducer can be inserted from either the ipsilateral side in line with the mandible or from the contralateral side (Fig. 7.14a). Advance the transducer and image the oropharynx and identify the PTA (Fig. 7.14b). Measure the abscess size and total distance from the carotid artery (Fig. 7.14c). Insert the needle at the middle (in order to align it with the emanating ultrasound beam) of the probe tip, and slowly advance the needle only after the needle tip is visualized on ultrasound. If the needle tip is not identified, the needle should not be advanced further (Figs. 7.14d and 7.17).

Transcervical Approach

When performing the transcervical approach to PTA drainage, the curved array transducer can be used transcutaneously on the ipsilateral side in the

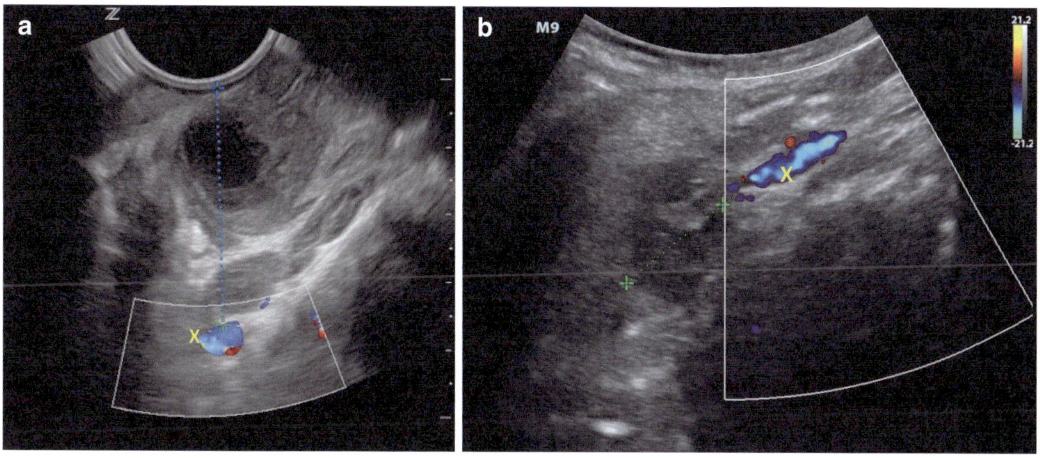

Fig. 7.16 (a) Intraoral ultrasound image of a left PTA fluid collection. The letter (x) marks the carotid artery. (b) Transcervical ultrasound image of a left PTA fluid collection. The letter (x) marks the carotid artery

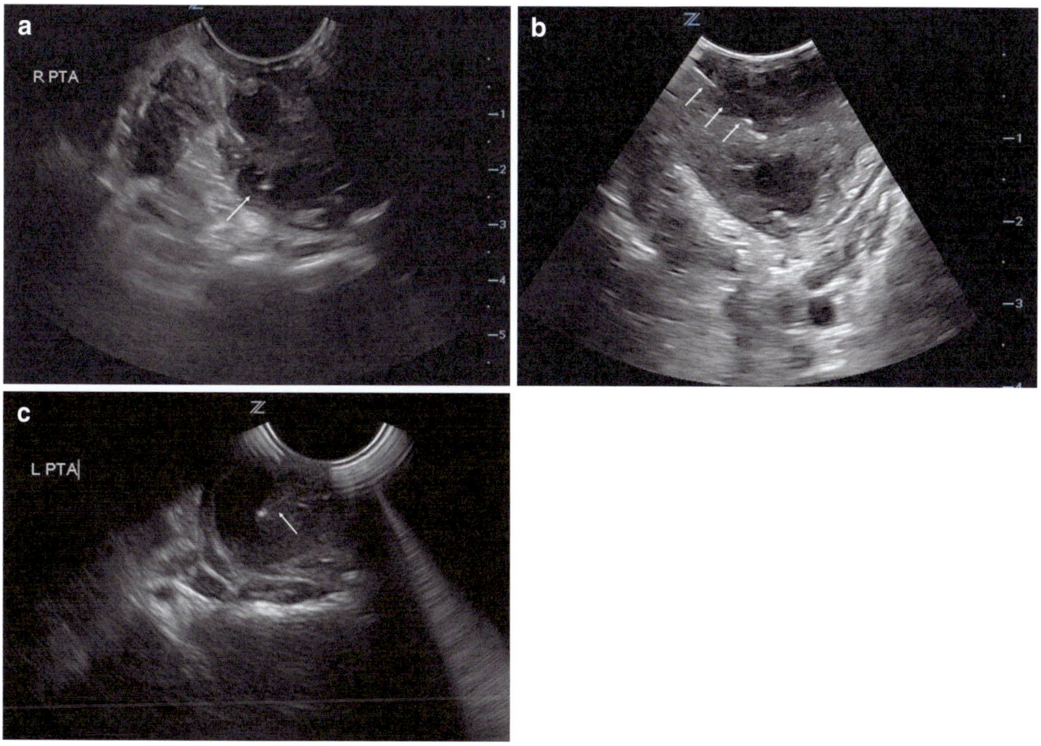

Fig. 7.17 (a) Needle tip (arrow) visualized during real-time ultrasound-guided drainage. (b) Needle shaft and tip (arrows) are seen prior to pentretating abscess cavity. (c) Echogenic needle tip (arrow) in the abscess cavity

submandibular space (Fig. 7.15a). As with the intraoral approach, the operator must first evaluate relevant anatomy and identify the PTA (Fig. 7.15b). Be sure to measure the abscess size and total distance from the carotid artery (Fig. 7.15c). Insert the needle in line with the mandible or from the contralateral side, and slowly advance the needle only after the needle tip is visualized on ultrasound. If the needle tip is not identified, the needle should not be advanced further (Fig. 7.15d).

Whether one chooses to perform the intraoral or the transcervical approach, evaluation for the

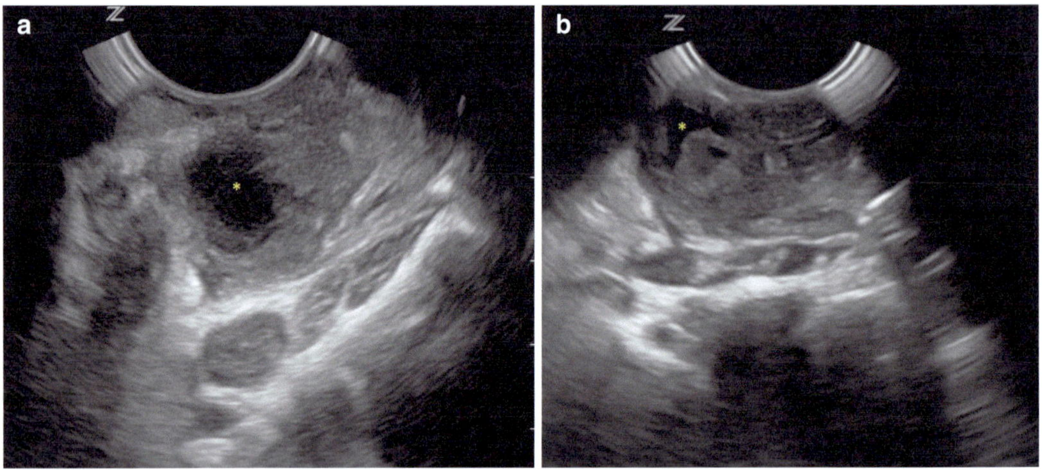

Fig. 7.18 Peritonsillar abscess. (**a**) Prior to drainage, anechoic abscess visualized. (**b**) Post drainage-collapsed abscess cavity is seen

carotid artery using color Doppler is necessary to avoid inadvertent injury. With either approach, a 2 in. 18 gauge needle should be attached to a 10 mL or 20 mL syringe for aspiration. Alternatively, the plastic sheath on an 18 gauge spinal needle can be trimmed to the premeasured depth to prevent injury to the carotid artery. A loculated abscess cavity may require injection with saline to aid in breakdown of loculations and allow for successful needle aspiration. Complete evacuation of the abscess cavity should be confirmed on ultrasound (Fig. 7.18).

Complications

Patient cooperation is key for this procedure to be successful; systemic analgesia and topical analgesia used in combination will help maximize patient cooperation. Using ultrasound to distinguish PTA from PTC prior to the procedure will minimize failures. Inadvertent injury to the carotid artery is a theoretical risk associated with PTA needle aspiration and can be minimized by measuring the distance from the abscess cavity to the vessel.

Pearls/Pitfalls

1. Ultrasound evaluation can help minimize the potential for a dry tap and distinguish between PTA and PTC. Heterogeneous/isoechoic abscesses (those with thick purulent material) can also be mistaken for cellulitis. Compression of the peritonsillar space can create movement within the purulent fluid.
2. The hand-eye coordination and dexterity required for this procedure require practice.
3. Determining the distance of the abscess cavity from the carotid artery can help avoid carotid puncture. Color Doppler can help with visualizing the carotid artery.
4. Measuring the abscess cavity can provide a rough estimate of how much fluid is contained in the abscess cavity.
5. Measure the depth of the abscess cavity so you can choose the appropriate length of needle.
6. Aspiration under real-time ultrasound guidance requires skill and practice. If you lose your needle tip on ultrasound, it is best not to advance any further to avoid inadvertent carotid puncture.
7. A loculated abscess may require saline injection to facilitate adequate drainage.
8. PTA drainage requires a cooperative patient and confident physician. Adequate pain management and light sedation are pivotal to success.
9. Encountering an unusually deep PTA may actually represent a retropharyngeal abscess (RTA). RTA can be drained using the same technique if visualization is adequate. Needle length required can increase up to 4 or 5 inches for RTA drainage.

Integration into Clinical Practice

This procedure should take approximately 20 minutes from start to finish. Routine use of intraoral ultrasound for evaluation of peritonsillar swelling can provide an accurate diagnosis with minimal side effects. If PTA is the underlying etiology, intraoral ultrasound can provide real-time evaluation of the relevant anatomy, thereby minimizing risk of harm in this bedside procedure. Patients found to have no abscess on a prescan or having a dry tap of an "at-risk area" can be brought back in 1 or 2 days for a rescan. Some will be noted to have developed a clear abscess in that time, and an aspiration can be performed at that time.

Evidence

Prior studies have demonstrated the superiority of ultrasound-guided needle aspiration over the traditional landmark approach [2, 7, 10]. A recent RCT compared anatomical landmark techniques to ultrasound imaging for the diagnosis and drainage of PTAs and found that ultrasound was superior in the following ways: diagnostic accuracy, ultrasound 100% vs. landmark 75%; successful drainage, ultrasound 100% vs. landmark 50%; and consultation of otolaryngology, ultrasound 7% vs. landmark 50% [2]. Literature for transcervical evaluation of PTA is limited; however, a recent study noted the sensitivity to be 80% and the specificity to be 93% [11].

Key Points

- Ultrasound-guided PTA needle aspiration requires practice, but real-time use of intraoral ultrasound can aid in visualization of relevant anatomy and minimize potential complications.
- Needle guidance for PTA drainage increases procedural success and minimizes consultation of otolaryngology colleagues.
- Transoral approach is diagnostically more accurate than the transcervical approach; however, transcervical approach can be useful for needle guidance in patients with severe trismus.

Suppurative Lymph Node Aspiration

When conducting procedures of the head and neck, it is imperative that clinicians understand the variable appearance of lymph nodes. Lymph nodes tend to be oval and smooth bordered and have an echogenic central hilum (Fig. 7.19). During infections, they may become reactive and will demonstrate increased blood flow in color Doppler mode (Fig. 7.20a, b). When lymph nodes succumb to infections, necrosis can occur. Intranodal necrosis may appear as a cystic area (cystic necrosis) within the lymph node or as a hyperechoic area within the lymph node (coagulation necrosis), but both are pathologic (Figs. 7.20c, 7.21 and 7.22). Lymph nodes round in shape with peripheral flow are considered abnormal (Figs. 7.23 and 7.24). Finally, a suppurative lymphadenitis will present with ultrasound findings similar to an abscess (Fig. 7.20d) [12]. A clinician may need to perform a needle aspiration or needle biopsy of this structure. Topical anesthetic, such as lidocaine-epinephrine-tetracaine gel, can be used over the affected area to minimize discomfort. Chlorhexidine, a tegaderm, and a 21 or 22 gauge needle are attached to a 10 mL syringe. Ultrasound guidance should direct the needle for biopsy or aspi-

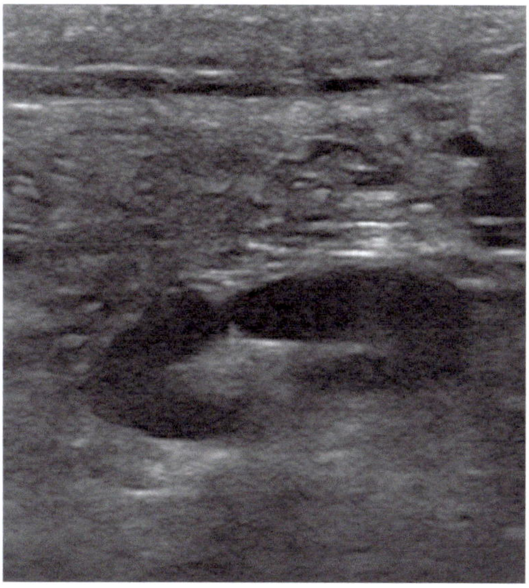

Fig. 7.19 Normal oval lymph node echogenic central hilum

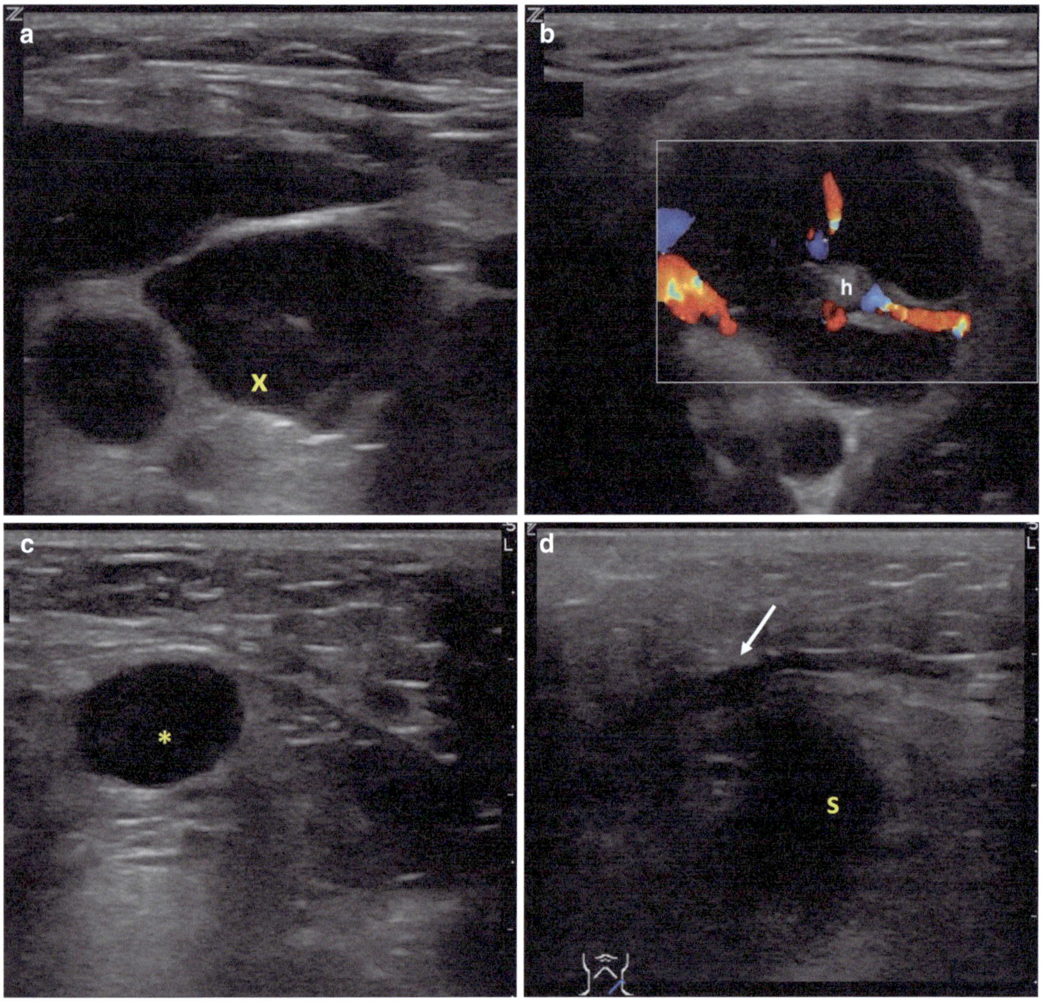

Fig. 7.20 Lymph node evaluation. (**a**) Normal lymph node with echogenic central hilum (x). (**b**) Enlarged reactive lymph node with color Doppler imaging demonstrating increased hilar flow (h-hilum). (**c**) Round lymph node with anechoic center (asterisk) similar in appearance to a cyst. (**d**) Necrotic and suppurative lymph node (s) with surrounding fluid collection

ration, and the clinician should advance the needle into the region of interest using in-plane approach. Ultrasound-guided fine needle aspiration has a sensitivity of 89–98% and specificity of 95–98% for successful FNA. The use of ultrasound in FNA has reduced negative FNA rates from 15% to <2% [4].

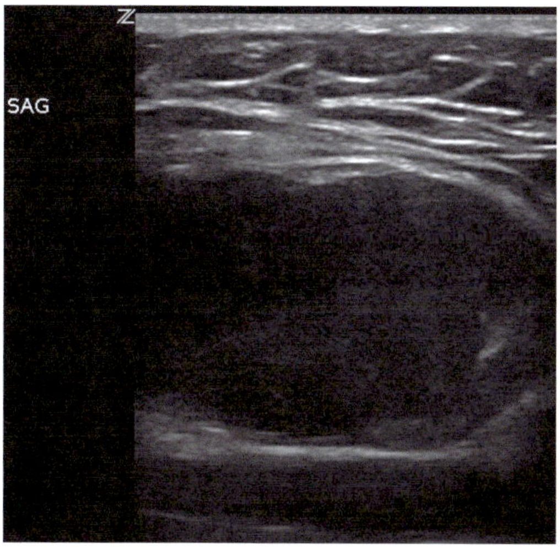

Fig. 7.21 Intranodal coagulation necrosis with echogenic debris

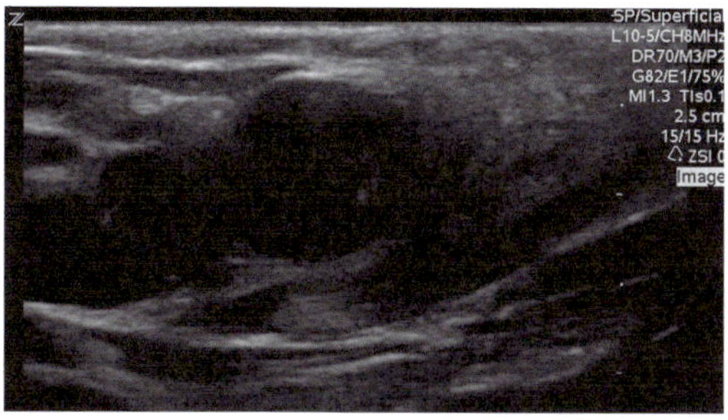

Fig. 7.22 Abnormal shape with intranodal cystic necrosis and loss of echogenic hilum

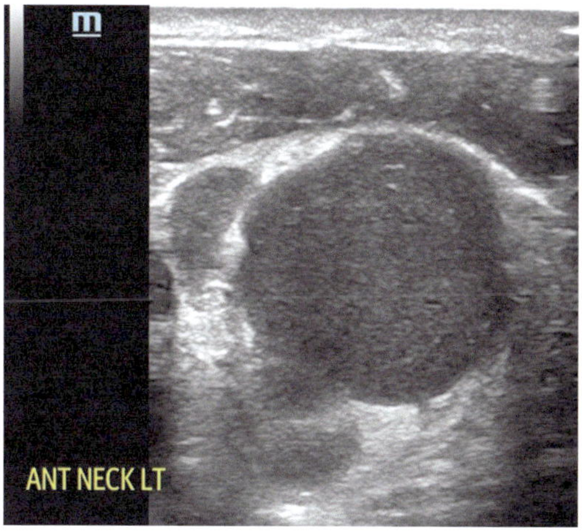

Fig. 7.23 Abnormal shape (round) and loss of normal echotexture

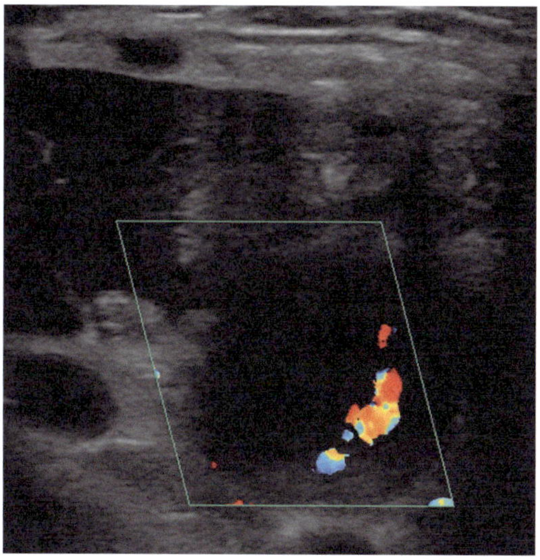

Fig. 7.24 Peripheral flow noted in this necrotic lymph node

References

1. Mallorie CN, Jones SD, Drage NA, Shepherd J. The reliability of high resolution ultrasound in the identification of pus collections in head and neck swellings. Int J Oral Maxillofac Surg. 2012;41(2):252–5.
2. Costantino TG, Satz WA, Dehnkamp W, Goett H. Randomized trial comparing intraoral ultrasound to landmark-based needle aspiration in patients with suspected peritonsillar abscess. Acad Emerg Med. 2012;19(6):626–31.
3. Cesur M, Corapcioglu D, Bulut S, et al. Comparison of palpation-guided fine-needle aspiration biopsy to ultrasound-guided fine-needle aspiration biopsy in the evaluation of thyroid nodules. Thyroid. 2006;16(6):555–61.
4. Ying M, Bhatia KS, Lee YP, Yuen HY, Ahuja AT. Review of ultrasonography of malignant neck nodes: greyscale, Doppler, contrast enhancement and elastography. Cancer Imaging. 2013;13(4):658–69.
5. Sivarajasingam V, Sharma V, Crean SJ, Shepherd JP. Ultrasound-guided needle aspiration of lateral masticator space abscess. Oral Surg Oral Med Oral Pathol Oral Radiol Endod. 1999;88(5):616–9.
6. Yusa H, Yoshida H, Ueno E, Onizawa K, Yanagawa T. Ultrasound-guided surgical drainage of face and neck abscesses. Int J Oral Maxillofac Surg. 2002;31(3):327–9.
7. Lyon M, Blaivas M. Intraoral ultrasound in the diagnosis and treatment of suspected peritonsillar abscess in the emergency department. Acad Emerg Med. 2005;12(1):85–8.
8. Grisaru-Soen G, Komisar O, Aizenstein O, Soudack M, Schwartz D, Paret G. Retropharyngeal and parapharyngeal abscess in children--epidemiology, clinical features and treatment. Int J Pediatr Otorhinolaryngol. 2010;74(9):1016–20.
9. Buckley AR, Moss EH, Blokmanis A. Diagnosis of peritonsillar abscess: value of intraoral sonography. AJR Am J Roentgenol. 1994;162(4):961–4.
10. Blaivas M, Theodoro D, Duggal S. Ultrasound-guided drainage of peritonsillar abscess by the emergency physician. Am J Emerg Med. 2003;21(2):155–8.
11. Araujo Filho BC, Sakae FA, Sennes LU, Imamura R, de Menezes MR. Intraoral and transcutaneous cervical ultrasound in the differential diagnosis of peritonsillar cellulitis and abscesses. Braz J Otorhinolaryngol. 2006;72(3):377–81.
12. Reshma VJ, Shihab Anwar A, Abdulla Mufeed V, Johnson K. Characterization of cervicofacial lymphnodes – a clinical and ultrasonographic study. J Clin Diagn Res. 2014;8(8):ZC25–8.

Ultrasound-Guided Musculoskeletal Procedures

8

Bret Nelson, Joshua Guttman, and David Spinner

Introduction

Musculoskeletal (MSK) procedures are performed by physicians from multiple specialities, including emergency medicine, physiatry, orthopedic surgery, sports medicine, internal medicine, and family medicine. Procedures vary widely by practice environment and include treatment of chronic ailments such as calcific tendinosis to acute injuries like fractures requiring reduction. Traditionally, these procedures were performed via landmark guidance and at times need to be repeated if not successful. The addition of ultrasound to the standard procedure allows the clinician to visualize anatomic areas of interest, increasing the probability of success. In this chapter, we describe the use of ultrasound in assisting commonly performed MSK procedures.

B. Nelson (✉)
Department of Emergency Medicine, Mount Sinai Hospital, New York, NY, USA
e-mail: bret.nelson@mssm.edu

J. Guttman
Department of Emergency Medicine, Emory University Hospital, Atlanta, GA, USA

D. Spinner
Department of Rehabiliation Medicine, Mount Sinai Hospital, New York, NY, USA

Advantages of Ultrasound Guidance

The main advantage of ultrasound guidance is it allows for direct visualization of both the structure of interest and the needle, if used. In procedures involving aspiration or injection, both the target structure and the needle can be seen in real time, allowing the clinician to adjust needle direction or position to reach the area of interest. Thus, directly visualizing the needle and surrounding anatomy increases the success rate of the procedure.

During procedures, such as joint or fracture reductions, imaging to confirm success may be performed immediately, obviating the need to transport the patient to the radiology suite for confirmation. Most importantly, if procedural sedation is used and the procedure is unsuccessful, another attempt may be performed immediately while the patient is still sedated. This means less risk of multiple procedural sedations, decreased pain, less frustration for both the patient and provider, and decreased length of stay.

Equipment and Probe Selection

Ultrasound equipment required for all MSK procedures discussed in this chapter is reviewed here. MSK ultrasound procedures may be performed with any available point-of-care

S. Adhikari, M. Blaivas (eds.), *The Ultimate Guide to Point-of-Care Ultrasound-Guided Procedures*, https://doi.org/10.1007/978-3-030-28267-7_8

ultrasound machine. Some machines have musculoskeletal presets (such as "MSK," "superficial," or "small parts"); however, this is not required. The clinician can adjust the frequency, depth, gain, and focus appropriately to optimize the scan.

Most MSK procedures are performed using a high-frequency (7.5 MHz or more), linear array probe, as this probe creates the highest-resolution images. In some procedures, such as hip arthrocentesis in an adult, the high-frequency probe does not give adequate depth to allow visualization of the target of interest. In those cases, the clinician can either decrease the frequency on the probe or switch to a lower-frequency probe, such as the curvilinear probe typically used for visualization of abdominal structures. Additionally, in more muscular or obese patients, the curvilinear probe may be needed to provide the extra depth to visualize the target.

Bursal Aspiration and Injection

Bursae may become inflamed due to infection, or aseptic causes, such as trauma; overuse; connective tissue disorders, such as rheumatoid arthritis or systemic lupus erythematosus; uremia; or gout and pseudogout. Ultrasound can be used to assist in the diagnosis of bursitis by confirming the anatomic location of pain and tenderness. In addition, ultrasound can guide needle placement for aspiration of bursa contents for fluid analysis or injection of anesthetic or anti-inflammatory agents.

Anatomy

Bursae are in general located adjacent to the joints and serve to cushion and remove friction between the joints, tendons, and bones. They are lined by synovial membrane and are filled with viscous fluid which should appear anechoic on ultrasound. There are several commonly encountered bursae in acute care.

Shoulder The subacromial-subdeltoid bursa lies above the intertubercular groove of the humerus, deep to the deltoid muscle (Fig. 8.1). It reduces friction between the rotator cuff, the coracoacromial arch, and the deltoid muscle.

Hip The trochanteric bursa (also referred to as the subgluteus maximus bursa) is located lateral

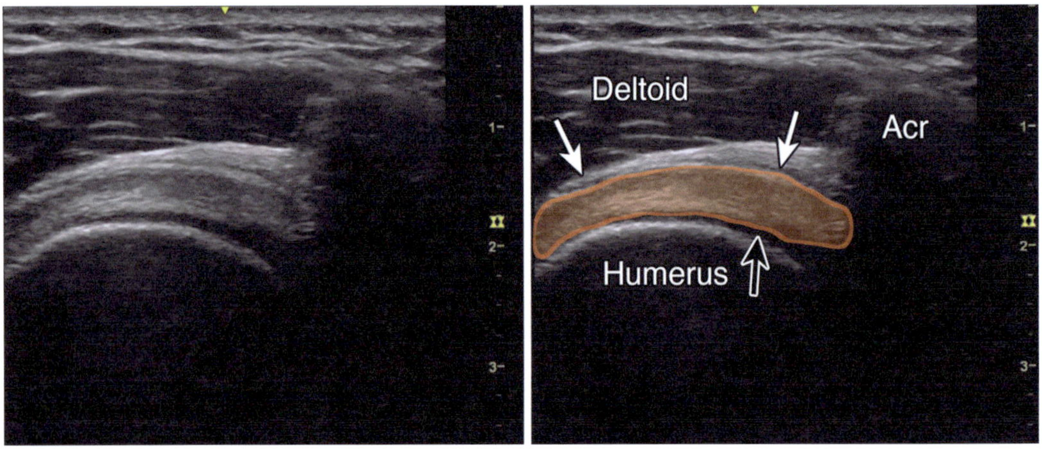

Fig. 8.1 Subacromial subdeltoid bursa (bounded by arrows) in coronal plane. The humerus, deltoid muscle, and acromion (Acr) are visible as well

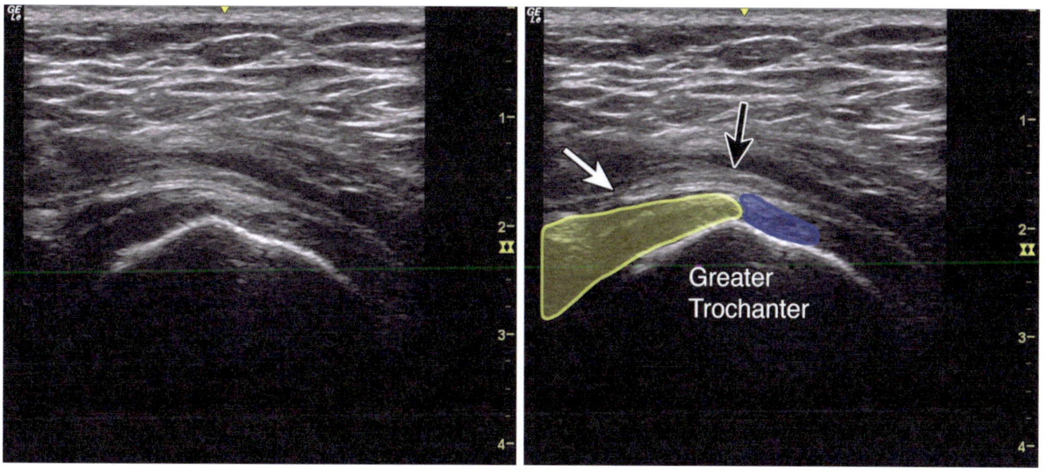

Fig. 8.2 Subgluteus maximus bursa (trochanteric bursa) indicated by white arrow. Purple indicates gluteus minimus attaching to anterior facet. Orange indicates gluteus medius attaching to lateral facet. Black arrow indicates iliotibial tract

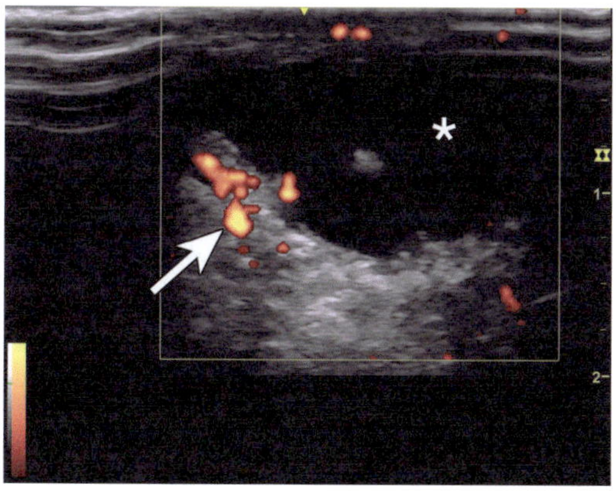

Fig. 8.3 Inflamed olecranon bursa (∗); color power Doppler demonstrates surrounding hyperemia

to the proximal femur, between the insertion of the gluteus medius and gluteus minimus muscles into the greater trochanter of the femur (Fig. 8.2).

Elbow The olecranon bursa is located over the extensor surface of the proximal ulna and extending over the tip of the bony olecranon process itself (Fig. 8.3).

Indications

- Aspiration of fluid from an inflamed bursa for analysis
- Injection if anti-inflammatory medications into the bursa

Contraindications

- Cellulitis overlying the needle entry site (relative contraindication)

Preparation

Equipment setup for bursa aspiration is the same as standard landmark-guided approaches. When ultrasound is used, a sterile ultrasound sheath (probe cover) and sterile gel should be used.

Procedure

1. Patient positioning is the same as landmark-guided approaches.
2. Longitudinal and transverse views of the bursa should be obtained sonographically to

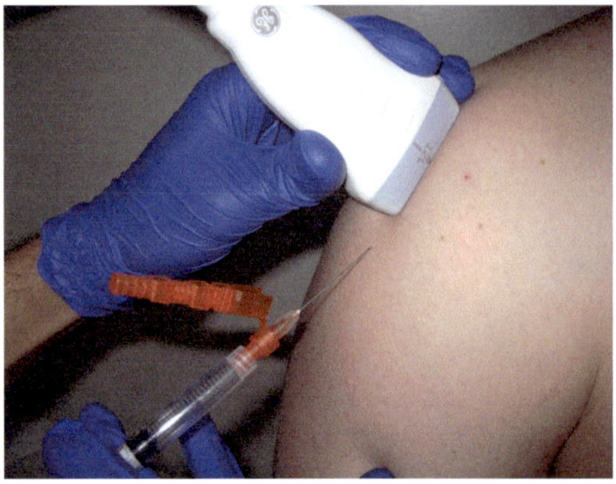

Fig. 8.4 Setup for subacromial subdeltoid bursa aspiration or injection

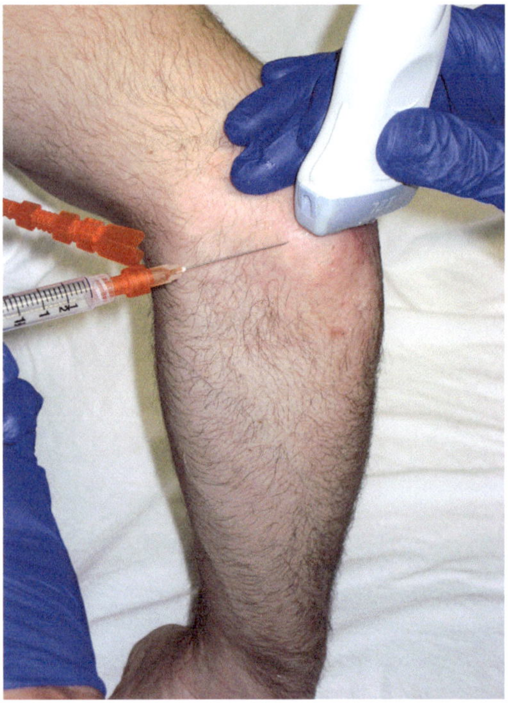

Fig. 8.5 Setup for olecranon bursa aspiration or injection

confirm the location of the bursa and that hypoechoic fluid exists within it (Figs. 8.4 and 8.5).

3. An in-plane needle visualization approach can be used to visualize the needle path from the skin to the bursa, as well as fluid injection if that is performed (Figs. 8.6, 8.7, and 8.8).

Complications

- Infection
- Bleeding
- Hematoma
- Injury to neurovascular structures

Pearls

- For olecranon bursa aspiration, elbow flexion can put some pressure on the bursa which aids drainage.
- The subacromial, subdeltoid bursa should be examined through a range of shoulder abduction to highlight its position.
- Hip rotation can make subgluteus maximus bursitis more evident.

Pitfalls

- The olecranon bursa is a frequent site of septic bursitis; confirm a sterile (aseptic) bursitis prior to steroid injection.

Integration into Clinical Practice

Ultrasound can be used to confirm the location and appearance of the bursa in cases of suspected bursitis. Then under appropriate sterile real-time guidance, a needle can be directed into the bursa for fluid analysis or injection.

Evidence

A review of studies comparing the two approaches found subacromial-subdeltoid bursa injection was 63% successful in cases where palpation was used; ultrasound guidance increased the success rate to 100% [1].

A recent Cochrane review of 290 patients in five studies found that image guidance provided no outcome benefit (pain, function, or adverse events) for patients compared to blind glucocorticoid injection for shoulder pain. Thus, the authors

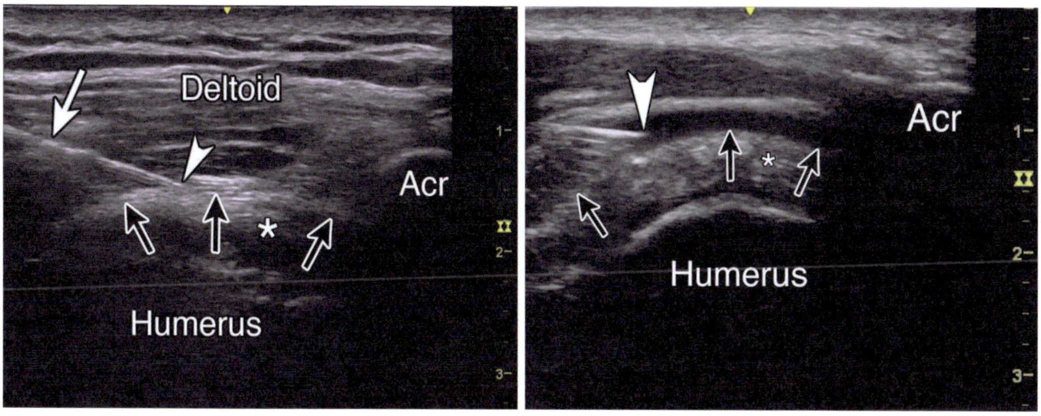

Fig. 8.6 Sonographic guidance of subacromial subdeltoid needle bursa aspiration or injection. In the left image, white arrow highlights needle position, white arrowhead (needle tip), black arrows (bursa) and supraspinatus tendon (asterisk). In the right image, anechoic anti-inflammatory bursal injection (black arrows) is visible along with the needle tip (white arrowhead) and supraspinatus tendon (asterisk) (Acr-acromion)

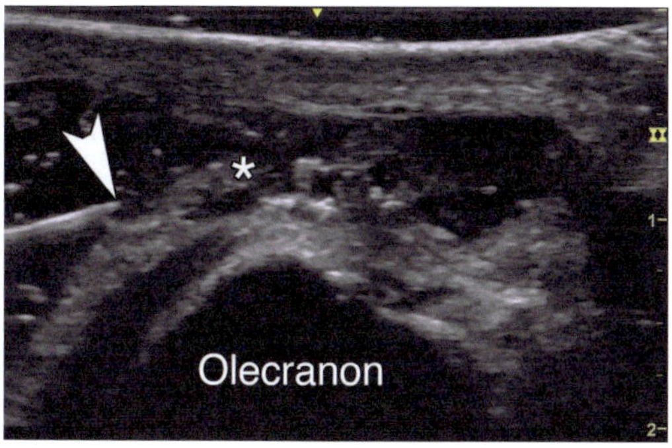

Fig. 8.7 Sonographic guidance of needle into the olecranon bursa (asterisk). Arrowhead is needle tip

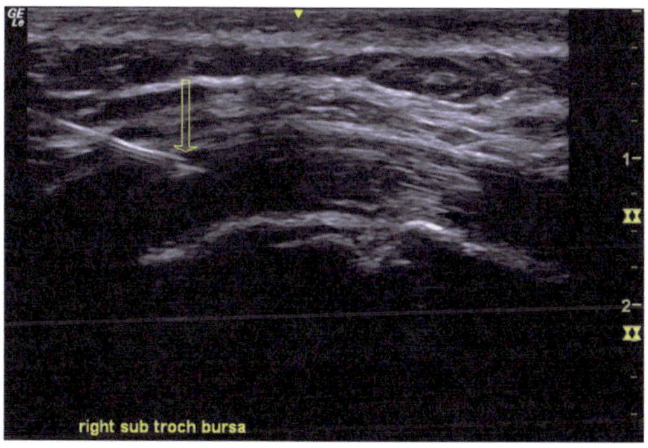

Fig. 8.8 Injection into the trochanteric bursa. The needle tip path is marked by the arrow, and anechoic anti-inflammatory injection is visible

concluded that despite the fact that ultrasound may improve accuracy of injection into the shoulder, there was no added outcome benefit to ultrasound use [2].

Key Point

- Examine bursae through the joint's full range of motion.

Arthrocentesis and Joint Injection

Arthrocentesis is commonly performed for diagnostic and therapeutic indications in multiple joints throughout the body. The procedure has traditionally been landmark guided, but there is a range of difficulty in accessing certain joints, and patient body habitus or acute discomfort may make the procedure more challenging. Thus, ultrasound can be used to confirm an effusion is present and to guide needle placement into the synovial joint for fluid aspiration or injection of analgesic or anti-inflammatory medications.

Anatomy

The sonographic appearance of a joint space is comprised of bright, hyperechoic cartilage and bony interfaces creating a "seagull sign" (Fig. 8.9). Depending on the joint and pathology, tendon origins and insertions may be visible, and anechoic or hypoechoic synovial fluid may be visible.

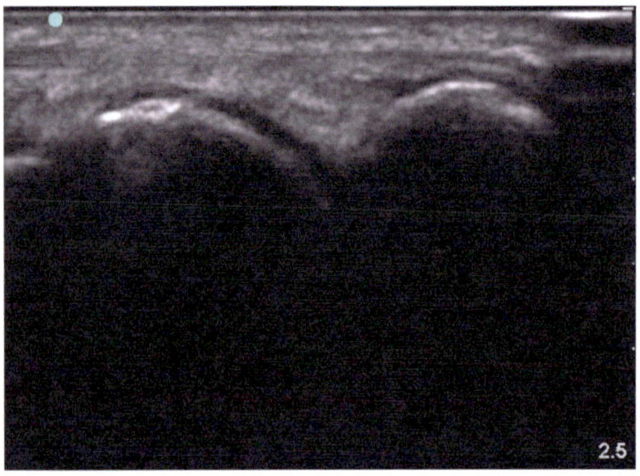

Fig. 8.9 The "seagull sign" created by two adjacent cartilage interfaces curving in toward each other and suggesting a seagull's wings

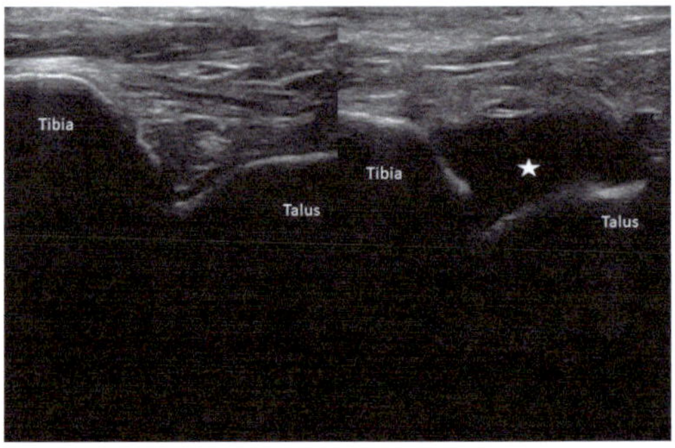

Fig. 8.11 Normal ankle joint (left), including the distal tibia and talus. Effusion (star) on the right

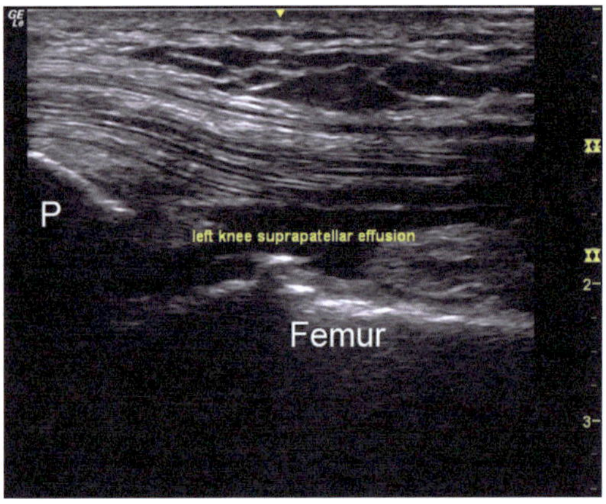

Fig. 8.10 Knee joint – the distal femur, patella, and effusion are visible

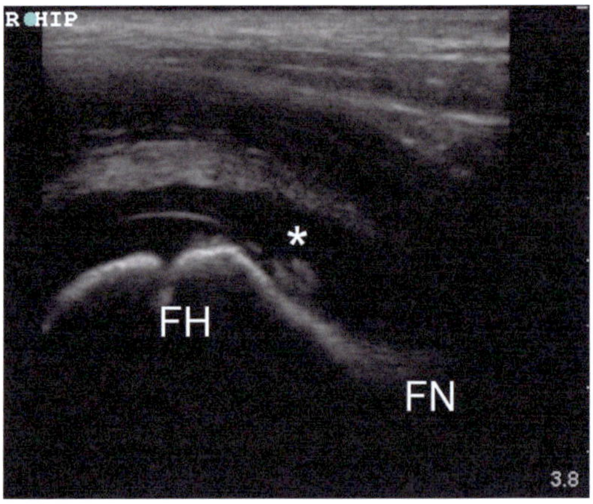

Fig. 8.12 Hip effusion (*), with underlying femoral head (FH) and femoral neck (FN)

Knee The distal femur, proximal tibia, and patella are often easily visualized sonographically, though not always in the same view (Fig. 8.10). The patellar tendon will be visible as well and can serve as a landmark for underlying effusion.

Ankle Following the distal tibia distally, the joint space with the talus will become visible (Fig. 8.11).

Hip With the probe orientated obliquely along the anterior hip along the axis of the femoral neck, the acetabulum, femoral neck, and femoral head will be visible (Fig. 8.12).

MTP joint The joint space between the metatarsal and proximal phalanxes is readily visible; a water bath can be helpful if the structures are too superficial (Fig. 8.13).

Elbow Effusion may be visualized in several locations, including the annular recess, coronoid fossa, or olecranon fossa (Fig. 8.14).

Shoulder The glenohumeral joint may be visualized and from an anterior or posterior approach and several different approaches toward needle guidance have been described. From the anterior

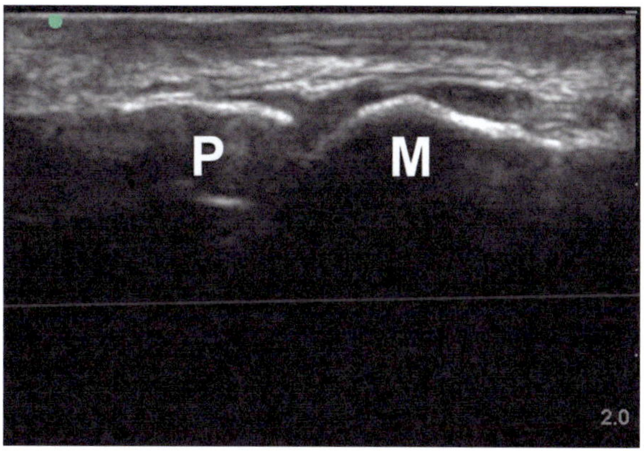

Fig. 8.13 Metatarsal (M)-phalangeal (P) joint

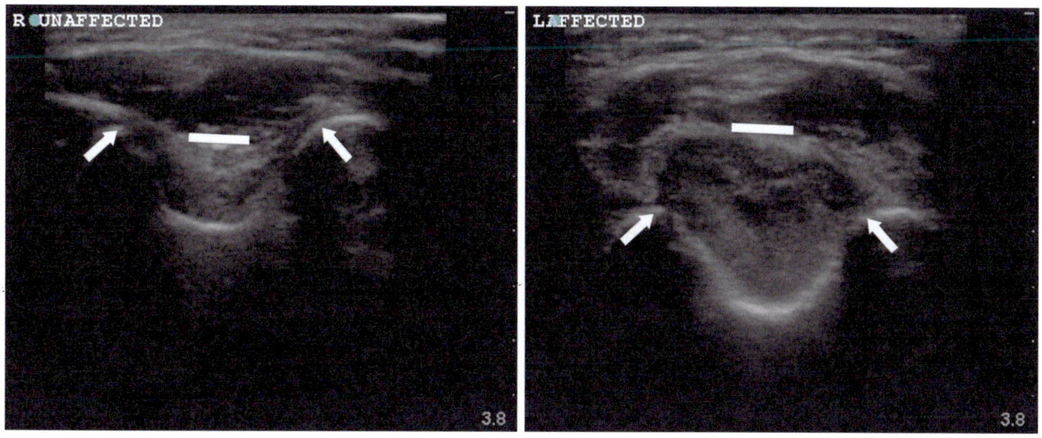

Fig. 8.14 The olecranon fossa (arrows) with joint capsule (horizontal line). Left is normal; capsule does not extend past fossa. On the right, effusion (in this case hematoma) extends past the fossa

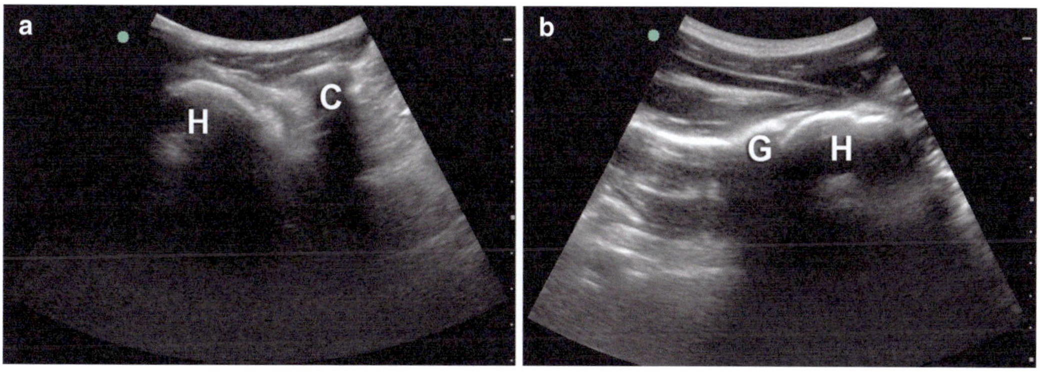

Fig. 8.15 Glenohumeral joint from anterior approach (**a**) Humeral head (H) and coracoid (C) are visible. Posterior approach (**b**) demonstrating the glenoid (G) and humeral head (H)

approach, the humeral head is visible deep and lateral to the coracoid process. From the posterior approach, the glenoid fossa is visible medial to the humeral head (Fig. 8.15).

AC joint The acromioclavicular joint is very superficial, located at the lateral edge of the clavicle (Fig. 8.16).

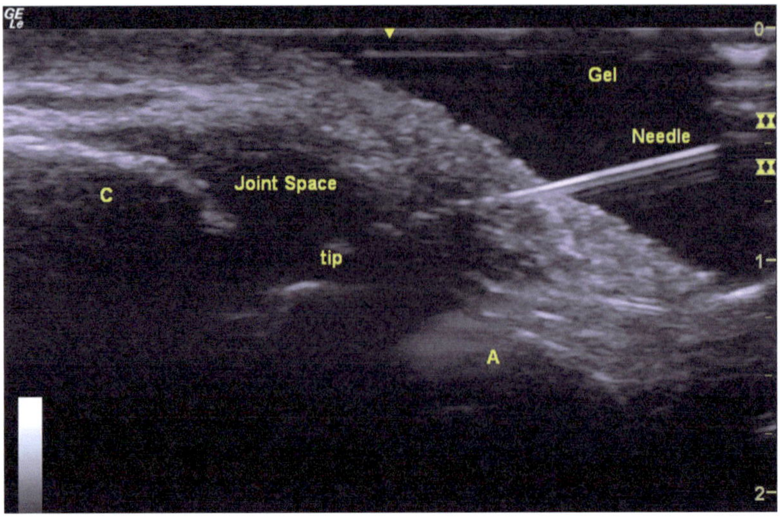

Fig. 8.16 Acromion (A)-clavicular (C) joint, demonstrating needle guidance for injection

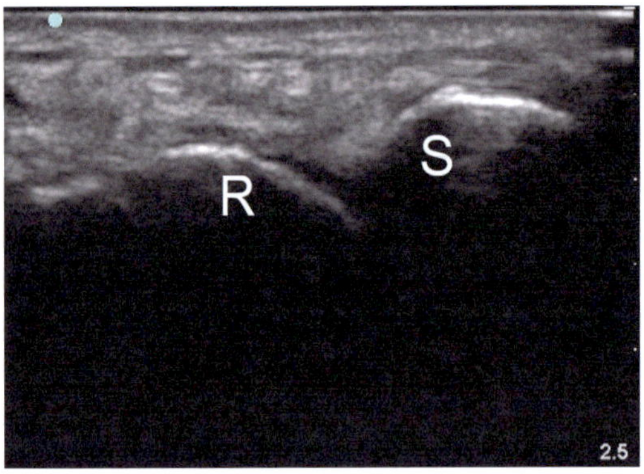

Fig. 8.17 Joint space between the radius (R) and scaphoid (S)

Wrist Following the distal radius to its distal edge, the radiocarpal joint will become visible (Fig. 8.17).

Indications

- Fluid analysis for diagnostic evaluation of a new effusion
- Evaluation of possible septic joint
- Aspiration of fluid to relieve pain and pressure of an effusion or fluid collection
- Injection of anesthetic or anti-inflammatory medication

Contraindications

- Cellulitis overlying the needle entry site (relative contraindication)
- Mass or vessel overlying the needle entry site

Preparation

Standard preparation for arthrocentesis should be maintained, including creating a sterile prep site and assembling appropriate anesthesia, syringes, needles, drapes, and other equipment. In order to visualize needle entry in real time, a sterile probe sheath and sterile gel should be used.

Procedure

1. The ultrasound probe should be placed over the joint of interest, and the typical appearance of a joint space should be confirmed.
2. The presence of joint effusion should be confirmed by noting an anechoic space without Doppler flow above the joint cartilage.
3. At this point, the needle should be directed in the plane of the ultrasound beam toward the joint space. The needle progress may be observed in real time until joint fluid is aspirated.

4. In some cases, ultrasound may be used to confirm the presence and location of joint fluid, at which point the proper location and trajectory of needle placement will be noted but performed without direct ultrasound visualization. This technique is more feasible for larger joints where the procedure itself is less challenging and there is less benefit to holding the ultrasound probe for the duration of the procedure.

Complications

- Infection
- Bleeding
- Hematoma
- Injury to nerves, vessels, and tendons

Pearls

- Joint effusion may be hypoechoic instead of anechoic in the presence of debris, immune reaction, infection, or other causes.
- Joint effusions should compress under probe pressure.

Pitfalls

- It is quite feasible to perform a sterile joint aspiration using real-time ultrasound guidance. Do not let the introduction of the ultrasound probe alter the sterility of the procedure.

Integration into Clinical Practice

Ultrasound can rapidly confirm the presence of joint effusion prior to considering arthrocentesis or joint injection. Local anatomy can be assessed, including the presence of any vessels, nerves, or other structures to be avoided with your needle.

Evidence

Glenohumeral joint and knee joint injection were each 79% successful with landmark technique; ultrasound guidance increased success to 95% for the shoulder and 99% for the knee [1]. An emergency department-based study of ultrasound-guided knee arthrocentesis demonstrated the technique had equal success compared with a landmark-based approach. However, ultrasound guidance yielded less pain for patients and shorter procedure time and was less technically difficult for emergency providers [3].

Key Points

- Ultrasound may be especially useful in confirming effusions in smaller or deeper joints.
- Sonographic guidance for needle approach can assist in avoiding vessels, nerves, and other sensitive structures en route to the effusion.

Fracture Reduction

Distal radius fractures are one of the most commonly encountered fractures in both the adult and pediatric population. Ultrasound has been shown to be accurate compared to radiography for detecting distal radius fractures. Ultrasound can show the amount of fracture displacement and can also be used to determine adequate reduction. Traditionally, adequacy of reduction is assessed blindly. Once the clinician determines that reduction is successful, the wrist is splinted, and the patient is sent for post-reduction x-rays. If the alignment is inadequate, then the splint must be removed and a second reduction attempt performed. This may include additional procedural sedation and increases the patient's length of stay. Some settings have access to fluoroscopy, where reduction can be assessed immediately at the bedside. While fluoroscopy is accurate, purchase and maintenance of the machine add additional costs. It also adds radiation, a concern especially in pediatric patients. Ultrasound has advantages over both these techniques, allowing real-time objective assessment of fracture reduction similar to fluoroscopy, without the additional cost and radiation.

While ultrasound can theoretically be used to reduce any fracture, it has been most extensively described in distal radius fractures, and therefore this section will focus specifically on distal radius fractures. In particular, it will focus only on the use of ultrasound to guide the procedure, as the reduction technique is described in other procedural texts.

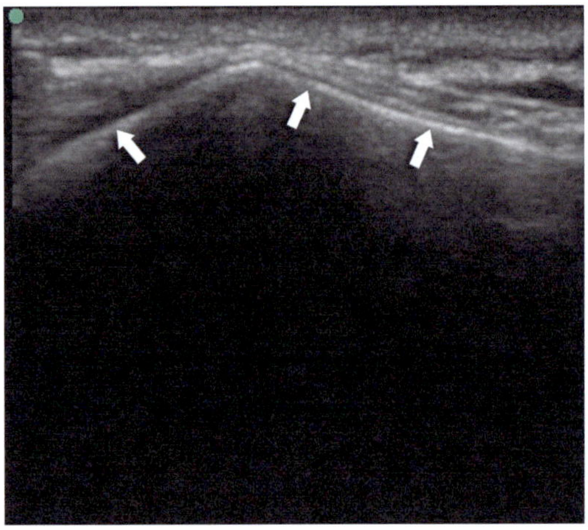

Fig. 8.18 Normal radius, shown in longitudinal plane. Arrows highlight bright echogenic bony cortex

Anatomy

Distal radius fractures can be easily visualized on ultrasound. The radius has the appearance of a linear bright hyperechoic line with shadow in the far field when viewed in longitudinal plane (Fig. 8.18). The radiocarpal joint and lunate can be seen at the distal end of the radius. The radius can also be scanned in short axis and can be followed distally to the joint line. The long-axis view is the highest yield when assessing for fractures.

A fracture is diagnosed by visualizing a disruption of the radial bony cortex. The amount of displacement can be estimated by noting the distance between the proximal and distal bony fragments (Fig. 8.19). Angulation of the bone may also be noted. Associated hematoma can be seen.

Indications

- Any fracture that may be clearly visualized on ultrasound, most commonly distal radius, with or without associated ulnar fractures

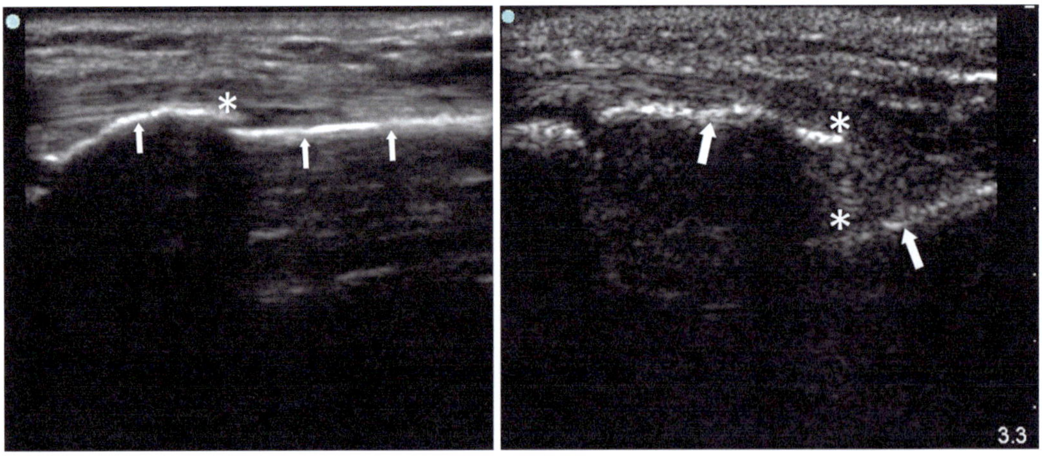

Fig. 8.19 Minimally displaced fracture (left) and significantly displaced fracture (right). Arrows highlight the cortex; asterisks denote fracture site

Contraindications

- Open fracture, such that the ultrasound gel would come into contact with tissue

Preparation

The fracture should first be interrogated with ultrasound. Multiple orthogonal views should be used, similar to the orthogonal views taken with x-ray. The following three images should be taken in long axis (Fig. 8.20):

(a) Posteroanterior view from the dorsal surface
(b) Anteroposterior view from the volar surface
(c) Lateral view

Additionally, a transverse view (d) may be helpful. Typically, the dorsal surface views will be the most helpful, as distal radius fractures tend to have dorsal displacement. It should be noted which views identify the fracture and any displacement. An image of the fracture should be saved prior to reduction for documentation. Enough towels should be available to wipe the ultrasound gel off the patient in between reduction attempts.

Procedure

1. Reduction should proceed in the usual manner.
2. Once adequate reduction is felt to be achieved, the ultrasound should be used to evaluate the fracture in multiple planes, taking into account the views taken prior to reduction.
3. If there is still fracture displacement noted on the ultrasound, then a second reduction attempt should be performed.
4. Steps 2 and 3 should be repeated as often as necessary until adequate reduction is achieved,

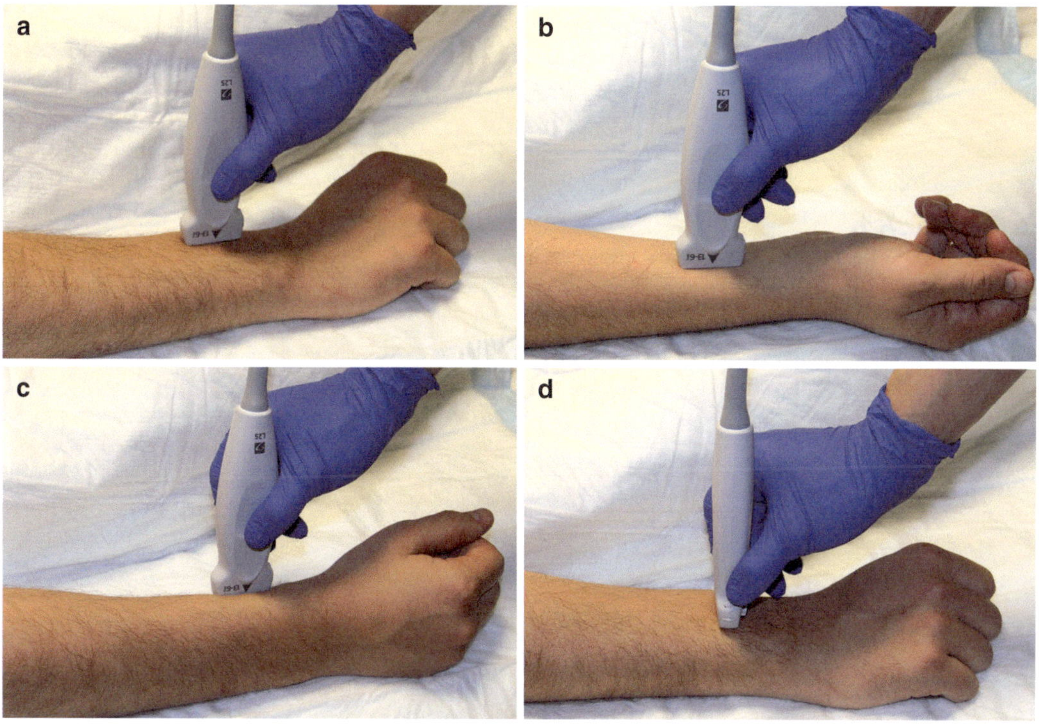

Fig. 8.20 Positioning of the ultrasound probe to obtain orthogonal views of the fracture site. Longitudinal dorsal surface (**a**), volar surface (**b**), lateral (**c**) and transverse (**d**) views

or it is determined that closed reduction will not be successful.
5. Once reduction is achieved, the patient should be splinted and sent for post-reduction x-rays.

Fracture reduction is achieved when the two ends of the fractured cortices are aligned, with minimal to no displacement or angulation of the bone. The fracture should be looked at in AP, lateral, and short-axis planes to confirm adequate reduction.

Complications

- Bleeding
- Hematoma
- Injury to neurovascular structures
- Injury to ligaments and tendons

Pearls

- If the initial reduction attempt is unsuccessful, then use ultrasound to determine what further manipulations are required. For example, if there is persistent dorsal displacement, then further reduction efforts can focus on correcting the dorsal displacement.
- If performing the reduction, have an assistant assigned to the ultrasound. Fracture visualization can be easily taught, and the clinician does not need to spend extra time placing ultrasound gel and wiping it off.

Pitfalls

- Not looking at orthogonal planes. Displacement can be in dorsal, volar, or lateral planes, therefore confirming reduction in multiple planes prior to splinting.

Integration into Clinical Practice

Ultrasound can be incorporated into any fracture reduction being done in the emergency department (ED). While it is has been best studied in distal radius and ulnar fractures, it has the potential to assist any fracture reduction, by identifying adequate alignment on any fracture that can be visualized with ultrasound. It has similar advantages both in the operating room and in the ED and has been used in both scenarios. If a reduction is being done in the ED or intensive care unit (ICU) by an orthopedic surgeon, the emergency physician or intensivist can assist by employing ultrasound to assess for adequacy of reduction.

Evidence

Bedside ultrasound has been shown to be accurate in detecting long bone fractures. Detection of distal radius fractures has a sensitivity of 96–100% and a specificity of 93–100% [4]. In studies on adult patients with distal radius fractures, ultrasound performed similarly to fluoroscopy and showed better alignment as compared to blind reduction [5, 6]. In one study, there was a reduced need for operative fixation in the ultrasound group [6]. In pediatrics forearm fracture reductions, success rate with the use of ultrasound was found to be 92% [7]. When ultrasound was compared to fluoroscopy for adequacy of reduction, ultrasound had a specificity of 98%. Therefore, ultrasound was accurate in ruling in an adequate reduction. However, in that same study, ultrasound did not perform as well when looking for inadequate reduction (sensitivity 50%), whereby reduction was deemed to be unacceptable by ultrasound, but acceptable by fluoroscopy [8]. Overall, the literature supports the use of ultrasound in assessing the adequate reduction, but it still needs to be confirmed by post-reduction x-rays.

Key Points
- Ultrasound is accurate in identifying long bone fractures and is most useful when guiding distal radius and ulnar fractures.
- Ultrasound can be employed multiple times during a reduction to assess the adequacy, but should be performed prior

to splinting, to assess the adequacy of reduction.

- Orthogonal views should always be obtained.
- Reduction should be confirmed with post-reduction x-rays.

Hematoma Block

A hematoma block is the injection of local anesthetic at the site of the hematoma overlying a fracture, in order to induce anesthesia for reduction, or for pain control. It is traditionally done without the use of imaging. The clinician palpates the site of the fracture, introduces the needle into the area that he or she palpates the fracture, and attempts to aspirate blood from the hematoma to confirm proper needle placement. If the hematoma is not aspirated, the clinician must reorient the needle or restart the procedure, increasing both length of the procedure and patient discomfort. Additionally, in comminuted fractures and in patients with a large body habitus, the fracture site may be difficult to palpated, decreasing the effectiveness of a hematoma block. Ultrasound mitigates these factors by easily visualizing the site of fracture and allowing accurate injection of anesthetic. While it has not been studied, clinical practice usage strongly suggests that ultrasound use would increase the effectiveness, as the needle can be guided onto the fracture site, as opposed to just entering the hematoma.

Anatomy

A hematoma block may be performed at any anatomic area with a fracture. It is employed most commonly in distal radius fractures, but has been described in other fractures as well.

Indications

- Any accessible fracture site easily visualized with ultrasound

Contraindications

- Visualized vasculature impeding needle access to the fracture site
- Skin and soft tissue infection overlying the needle entry site
- Neurovascular compromise requiring emergent fracture reduction
- Allergy to local anesthesia

Preparation/Pre-procedural Evaluation

In planning the procedure, clinician should survey the fracture site and hematoma with ultrasound in both the longitudinal and transverse planes, or long and short axis, to locate the site of fracture and evaluate for any surrounding vasculature (Fig. 8.19). Should there be significant vasculature or the fracture site is not well visualized, then the procedure should not be performed. If the fracture site is deemed accessible by ultrasound, then the clinician should be in preparation. The ultrasound machine should be placed on the opposite end of the patient, in a position that allows the clinician to visualize the screen without rotating his or her head (Fig. 8.21). The depth and gain should be adjusted a priori, based

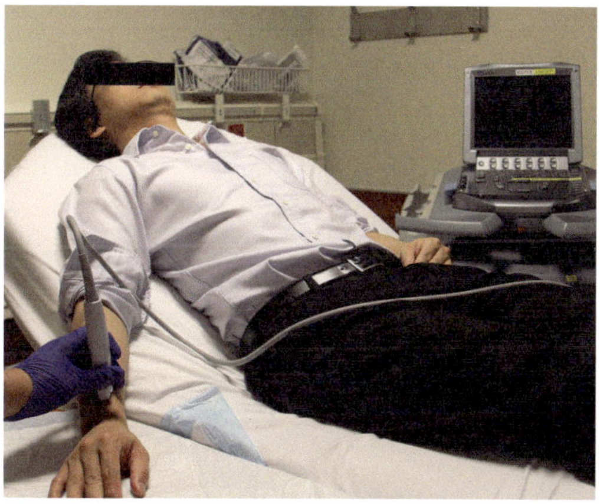

Fig. 8.21 Proper positioning of the clinician relative to the patient and ultrasound machine. Note that the clinician can view the ultrasound machine and perform the procedure without rotating his or her head or body

on the anatomic survey. During the ultrasound survey, the clinician should determine whether the needle will enter the skin at the proximal or distal end of ultrasound probe. This should take into account both the handedness of the provider and the anatomy surrounding the fracture. The clinician should assess for an unobstructed needle path.

The extremity should be placed in a position that maximizes procedural success while minimizing patient discomfort. The ideal position allows the clinician to steady the nondominant hand holding the ultrasound probe to maintain stability, while allowing for ease of proper needle placement with the dominant hand (Fig. 8.22). Much of this determination will need to be individualized, taking into account the patient's mobility, other associated injuries, and location of the fracture. The following suggestions are general guidance for specific anatomic locations. For radius, ulnar, and hand fractures, the extremity can be placed on a flat surface, such as a tray table, when possible. For humeral shaft fractures, the patient can be rolled onto their other shoulder, with the humerus lying flat on the patient's thorax and the ultrasound placed on the lateral humerus (Fig. 8.23). For humeral head fractures, the patient should be seated if possible, or sheets can be placed behind the patient to allow access to the posterior shoulder (Fig. 8.24). For femur fractures, the patient should remain supine and will unlikely tolerate any movement. For tibia fractures, the leg can be externally rotated, and, for fibula fractures, the leg can be internally rotated, if tolerated by the patient.

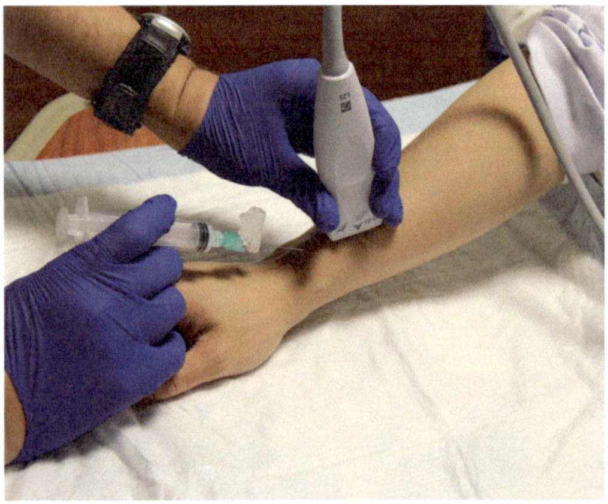

Fig. 8.22 Proper positioning of the ultrasound probe on the patient in preparation for the procedure

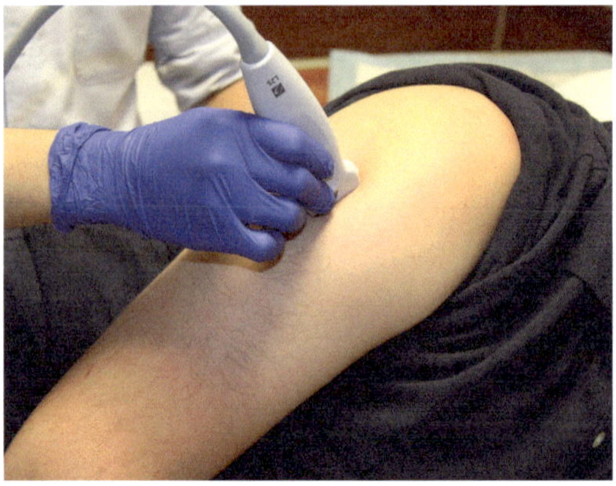

Fig. 8.23 Patient position and probe placement for the evaluation of humeral shaft fractures (probe held along long axis of the bone)

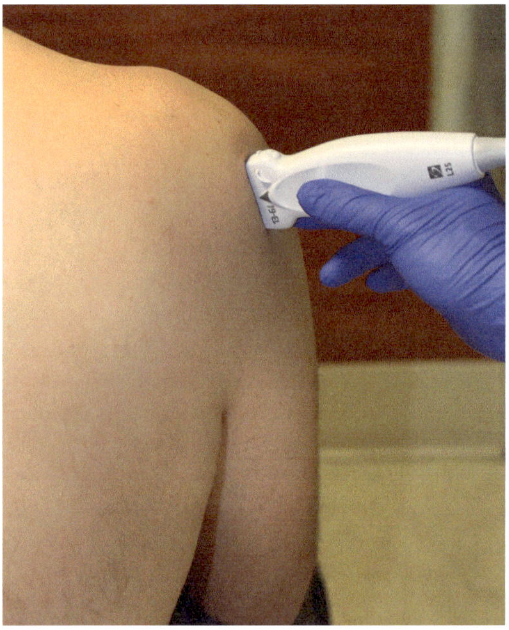

Fig. 8.24 Patient position and probe placement for the evaluation of humeral head fractures (probe held along long axis of the bone)

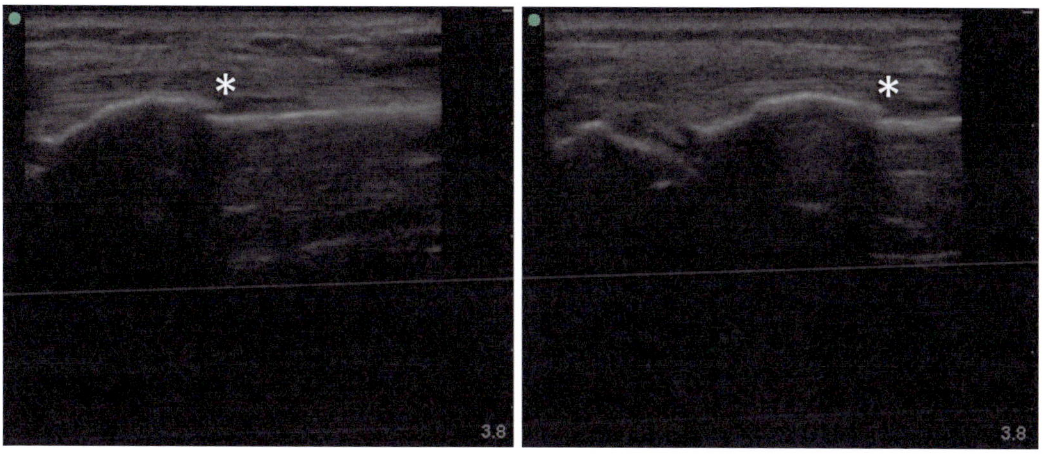

Fig. 8.25 Ultrasound image of a distal radius fracture (left), and probe adjustment to bring the fracture site (∗) closer to the end of the screen (right). This facilitates performance of the procedure by minimizing the distance the needle needs to travel

Equipment

- Sterile drape/towels and gloves
- Chlorhexidine or povidone-iodine antiseptic solution
- Needle of adequate depth (1.5-inch 20–22-gauge needle for superficial bones, a 18–22-inch spinal needle for deeper bones)
- 10–12-cc syringe
- 10 cc of local anesthetic: Lidocaine 1–2% or bupivacaine 0.25–0.5%, with our without epinephrine
- Sterile ultrasound probe cover (commercial cover or tegaderm)
- Sterile ultrasound gel
- A dressing such as an adhesive bandage or gauze

Lastly, as in all other procedures, the clinician should adjust the height of the bed to allow for minimal bending and maximum provider comfort during the procedure. The clinician may choose to sit if space allows.

Procedure

1. Prepare and drape the area in the usual aseptic fashion to maintain maximum sterility.
2. Place the antiseptic cover on the ultrasound probe in the usual fashion and place sterile ultrasound gel on the probe.
3. Place the ultrasound probe over the underlying fracture in longitudinal plane, so the bone is seen in long axis, as a linear hyperechoic line. By convention, the probe marker should be pointed proximally.
4. The probe may then be moved slightly proximally or distally, so that the fracture site is closer to the needle entry site, to minimize the distance needed for the needle to traverse to reach the target (Fig. 8.25).
5. Once the ultrasound probe is placed at its proper location and the target is visualized, the needle can be inserted. It should be inserted in-plane with the probe, in the center of the probe. Some ultrasound probes have markers indicating the center of the probe (Fig. 8.26).
6. The needle should then be guided to the fracture site with direct visualization on the ultrasound screen (Fig. 8.27). The needle depth can be adjusted as needed.
7. Once the needle is visualized and confirmed to be at the fracture site, the clinician injects 10 ml of local anesthetic. The anesthetic can be visualized as anechoic fluid at the site of injection (Fig. 8.28).

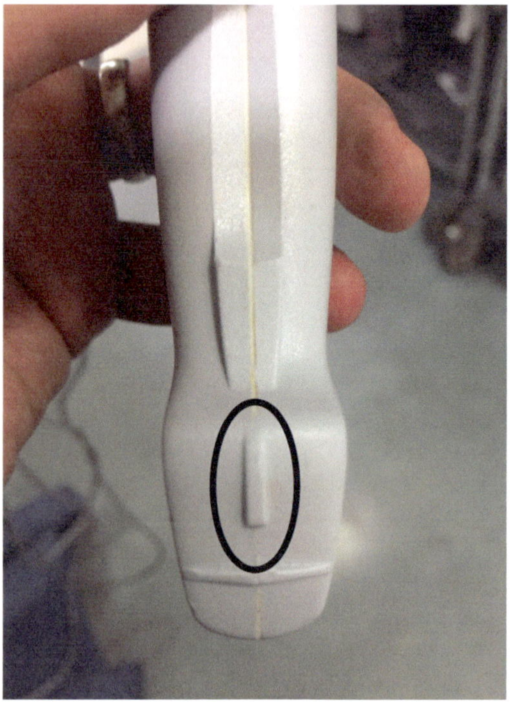

Fig. 8.26 Probe with a marker showing the center of the probe. The needle should be inserted under this marker, to ensure the needle is in the center of the screen

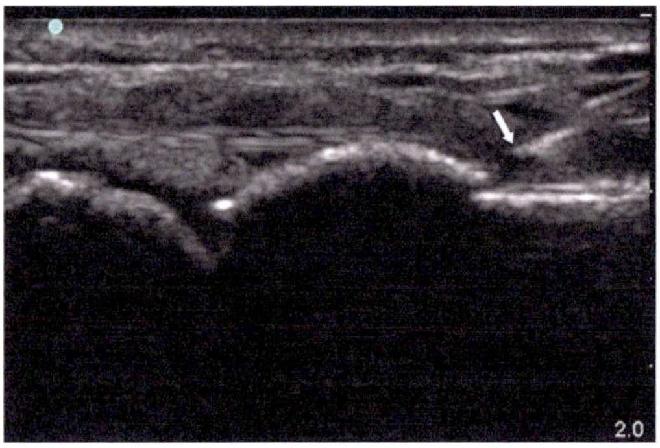

Fig. 8.27 Ultrasound image showing the needle in-plane. The needle (arrow is tip) is followed until it is seen entering the fracture site

8. Once the anesthetic has been injected, the needle is withdrawn, and a dressing is placed on the insertion site. The needle should be disposed of in an appropriate sharp container.

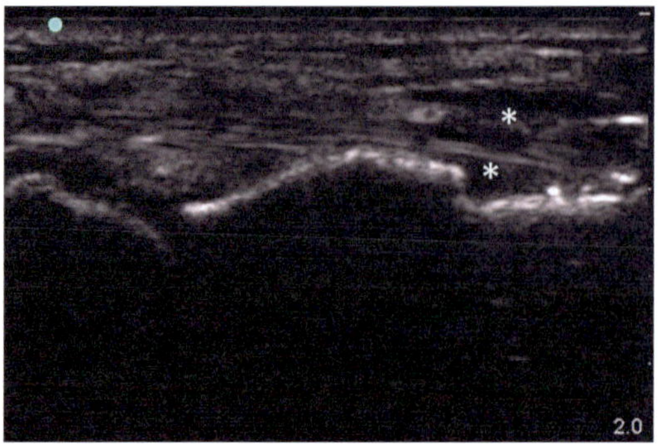

Fig. 8.28 Ultrasound image of the fracture site, after anesthetic has been injected. Note the appearance of anechoic fluid (*)

Complications

There are few complications noted with this procedure. Pain associated with needle insertion can be minimized by creating a wheal of anesthetic at the skin surface prior to needle insertion, as well as injecting anesthetic during needle insertion to anesthetize the soft tissue. If this is to be performed, extra anesthetic should be prepared as to have an adequate volume to inject at the fracture site.

It is also possible to inject local anesthesia into the vasculature, inducing local anesthesia toxicity. This complication can be virtually eliminated if the needle and tip are visualized during the entire procedure and do not enter any visualized vasculature. If the needle tip is lost, the clinician should stop moving the needle and locate the needle tip. If the needle tip still cannot be identified, then the needle should be withdrawn and the procedure restarted. Additionally, the clinician can aspirate prior to injecting local anesthetic to assure that he or she is not injecting into a vessel. Note that a small amount of blood will often be aspirated from the hematoma.

Pearls

- Map the entire procedure prior to sterile preparation of the area. This will give the procedure the maximal chance of success.

- Err on the side of having a longer, rather than shorter, needle. If a needle is too short, then it will not reach the target prior to hubbing at the skin. The distance from the skin surface to the fracture site can be measured on the ultrasound screen, to assure adequate length.

Pitfalls

- Not visualizing the needle throughout the procedure. If during the procedure, the needle is lost, then the probe can be slid from side to side while maintaining the long axis, to find the needle. Alternatively, the clinician can rock the probe, changing the angle of insonation and allowing better needle visualizing.
- Assuming that if no blood is aspirated at the fracture site, the needle is not in the right position. Aspiration may not always reveal blood. The key is to visualize the needle tip directly at the fracture site.

Integration into Clinical Practice

Hematoma blocks can be easily incorporated into clinical practice. They are easy to learn and may be performed rapidly. Hematoma blocks can be considered for all fracture patients, but are most useful in patients who are at high risk of complications associated with procedural sedation, such as the elderly and those with pre-existing lung disease. Placement of a successful hematoma block allows for more rapid discharge from the ED, the reduction to be done in a non-monitored setting, and spares the patient the side effects of procedural sedation. Even in patients not undergoing fracture reduction, a hematoma block can relieve the pain associated with an acute fracture, increasing patient comfort and satisfaction. Additionally, in teaching institutions, a hematoma block is ideal for junior trainees. Because the patient is not undergoing procedural sedation, the clinician may feel more comfortable allowing the trainee more time to perform a successful reduction, while not worrying about prolonged procedural sedation time.

Evidence

There is a single randomized control trial assessing the effectiveness of ultrasound-guided hematoma blocks [9]. One hundred forty ED patients with distal radius fractures were randomized to either an ultrasound-guided hematoma block or procedural sedation. The authors found similar pain scores and patient satisfaction, with lower complications and a shorter length of stay with the hematoma block. There are several case reports, which include hematoma blocks for humerus, sternum, and femoral neck fractures [10–12].

Key Points

- An ultrasound-guided hematoma block should be considered in all patients with an acute fracture, whether or not reduction is planned.
- Map out the procedure before proceeding; visualize the fracture on ultrasound and determine the appropriate site for needle entry.
- Visualize the needle tip at all times, injecting when the needle tip reaches the fracture site.

Joint Reduction

Although joint dislocations are often clinically obvious, there are cases where radiologic evaluation is often employed to confirm the diagnosis or rule out complications of the injury. X-rays are typically used after reduction attempts to confirm success and occasionally during the procedure when placement is in doubt. Ultrasound can assist joint reductions in real time to confirm anatomy and has several advantages over x-rays. The ultrasound can be performed at the point of care, while the patient remains in the procedure area. Thus, there is less risk of the patient requiring re-sedation after an initial unsuccessful reduction. Sonographic assessment can be made as many times as needed during the procedure without concern for radiation or increased costs. Finally, ultrasound can assess dynamic, moving anatomy, such as the appearance of a bone or joint through a range of motion. Although bedside fluoroscopy boasts several similar advantages of ultrasound over x-rays performed in the radiology department, that procedure still emits ionizing radiation to the patient (and operator) and cannot visualize soft tissues such as muscles, joint effusions, or tendons as well. Although some case reports describe several different types of joint reductions which may be assisted with ultrasound, this section will focus on anterior shoulder dislocations due to the relative frequency of this pathology, since it has been described most frequently in the literature.

Anatomy

Ultrasound may be used to evaluate the position and relationship between the glenoid fossa and humeral head. With an anterior dislocation, the humeral head is displaced inferiorly (below the glenoid). With a curvilinear transducer placed in a transverse orientation just below the scapular spine, the glenoid fossa and humeral head should be visible (Fig. 8.29). In a normal shoulder, the humeral head articulates with the glenoid fossa, and this can be visualized through a range of internal and external shoulder rotation. In the setting of anterior dislocation, the humeral head will be visualized anterior to the glenoid fossa.

Indications

- Suspected shoulder dislocation

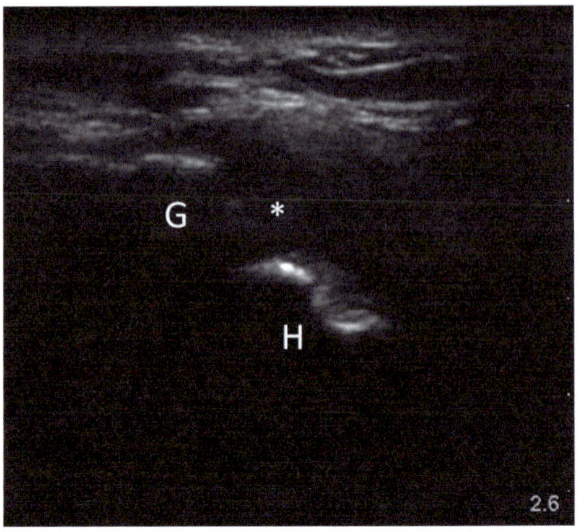

Fig. 8.29 With the transducer placed in a transverse orientation just below the scapular spine, the glenoid fossa (G) and humeral head (H) should be visible. In this case, the anterior (deep) displacement of the humeral head and presence of hematoma (∗) are diagnostic of anterior dislocation

Contraindications

- Suspected open fracture

Preparation

Either a low-frequency curvilinear transducer or a higher-frequency linear array probe may be used. Gel is required; beyond that, the reduction procedure itself will require standard equipment for the reduction approach chosen by the operator.

Procedure

1. Place the patient in a position of comfort, typically sitting with their back to the operator.
2. The ultrasound machine should be placed in front of the patient such that the operator, standing behind the patient, can visualize both the shoulder and the ultrasound screen (Fig. 8.30).
3. Place the transducer in a transverse orientation just below the spine of the scapula.

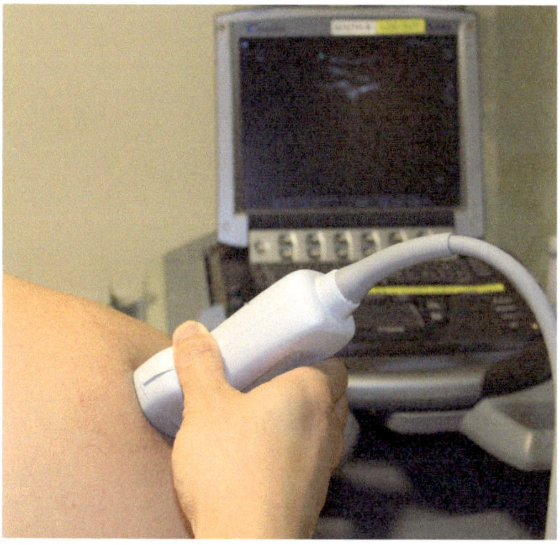

Fig. 8.30 The ultrasound machine should be placed in front of the patient such that the operator, standing behind the patient, can visualize both the shoulder and the ultrasound screen

4. Visualize the glenoid and humeral head to confirm dislocation.
5. Reduction should proceed in the usual manner.
6. Once adequate reduction is felt to be achieved, the ultrasound should be used to evaluate the glenohumeral joint again using the same approach described above. If the shoulder is indeed reduced, the humeral head should be visible within the glenoid fossa through a range of internal and external rotation of the shoulder.

Complications

The use of ultrasound should not itself create a complication, unless the images are misinterpreted. Complications of the shoulder reduction technique itself remain the same.

Pearls

- If the anatomy seems atypical or confusing, assess the unaffected side to establish the pattern of normal for a particular patient.
- Dynamic internal and external rotation can help locate the humeral head and establish the stability of its relationship with the glenoid fossa.
- Although a curvilinear transducer is recommended by many authors, a high-frequency linear transducer may be used in some patients as well.

Pitfalls

- When the transducer angle approaching the glenoid or humeral head is too far from perpendicular, the bony anatomy can appear fuzzy or distorted. Fan through the joint to establish the optimal angle.

Integration into Clinical Practice

Ultrasound can be incorporated prior to or instead of x-ray to confirm a diagnosis of dislocation. It can also be used to anesthetize the joint, using an intraarticular anesthetic injection or nerve block described (in other chapters). Some authors have noted x-rays are not necessary in the evaluation and management of uncomplicated shoulder dislocations. One could interpret this sentiment to imply ultrasound may not be needed either, or that operators who consistently use x-rays could safely use ultrasound instead.

Evidence

A prospective observational study of 73 patients with suspected dislocation demonstrated ultrasound had perfect sensitivity and specificity for the initial diagnosis of dislocation compared to standard 3-view shoulder x-rays [13]. Test characteristics were the same for post-reduction confirmation of proper shoulder joint alignment.

Key Points

- Use contralateral anatomy to confirm pathology.
- Ultrasound is used to confirm anatomy before and after reduction attempts; it is not necessary to visualize the reduction in real time.

Foreign Body Removal

The detection and treatment of soft tissue foreign bodies is a clinical challenge and represents an area of medicolegal risk for acute care providers in many practice settings. Pain, tenderness, redness, and swelling may be indicators of infection, foreign body, abscess, or all three. Ultrasound can be used to distinguish these entities and may provide insight where physical examination and conventional x-ray fall are equivocal.

Anatomy

In normal soft tissue, the layers of the skin, subcutaneous fat, fascia, and bone are all readily visible (Fig. 8.31). Foreign bodies will have a variety of appearances based on their anatomic location, depth, size, and density. Metallic foreign bodies will often demonstrate reverberation artifact, causing bright echogenic lines to appear on the ultrasound screen distal to the foreign body (Fig. 8.32). Foreign bodies made of wood, plastic, and other materials with densities different than the surrounding tissue will shadow if they are large enough.

Indications

- Any suspected foreign body

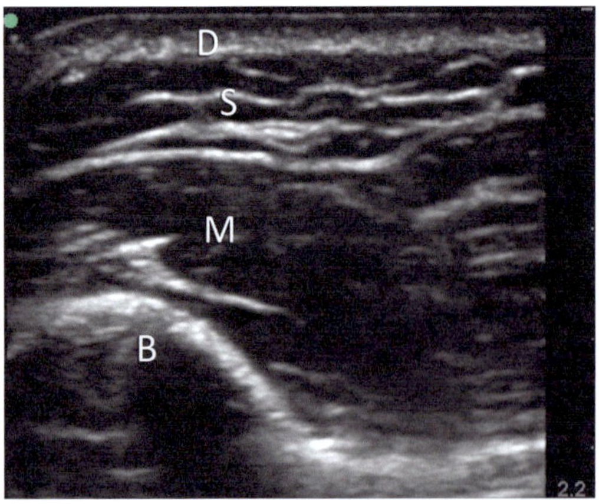

Fig. 8.31 Sonographic appearance of normal soft tissue demonstrating layers of the dermis (D), subcutaneous fat (S), muscle (M), and bone (B)

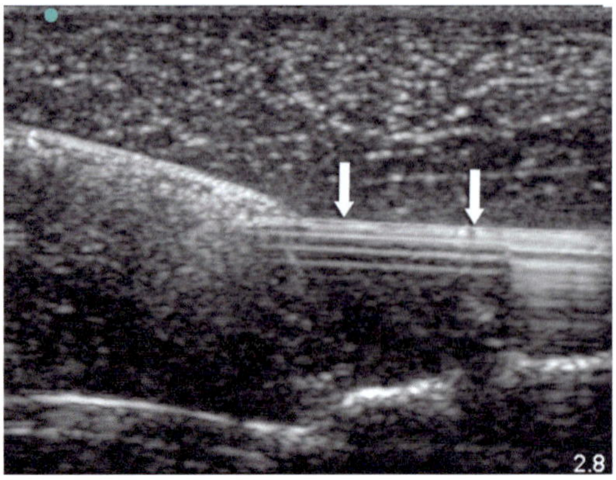

Fig. 8.32 Metallic foreign bodies will often demonstrate reverberation artifact, causing bright echogenic lines to appear on the ultrasound screen distal to the foreign body. In this case, multiple linear parallel lines originate from a needle beneath the skin surface (arrows)

Contraindications

- In the setting of an open or grossly contaminated wound, care should be taken to ensure the transducer is covered in a sterile sheath, and sterile gel is used to make contact with the skin or soft tissues.

Preparation

A high-frequency linear probe will best image superficial foreign bodies. A small-gauge needle and syringe are necessary for infiltration of local anesthetic. Alligator forceps, scalpel, tissue hooks, and other instruments may be necessary based on the preferred method of foreign body removal.

Procedure

1. Slowly scan over the area of suspected foreign body in two orthogonal planes.
2. Once the foreign body is detected, its depth, size, and orientation should be assessed.
3. Once localized, the area surrounding the foreign body may be anesthetized by directing an anesthetic-filled syringe with needle toward the foreign body. This is accomplished under direct

ultrasound visualization, typically with the needle in the plane of the ultrasound beam. Injecting small amounts of local anesthetic against the foreign body will "hydro-dissect" the foreign body away from the surrounding tissue, numbing the area and often improving sonographic visualization. In some areas of the body, a nerve block could be considered instead of or in addition to the local infiltration.

4. After anesthesia, there are several approaches to removing the foreign body. The choice will depend on a number of factors including the composition, position, and size of the foreign body, operator experience, patient comfort, availability of specialty consultants, etc.
   (a) Direct a needle to the foreign body, and dissect down through the tissue using the needle as a guide. This open technique is most helpful in the setting of foreign bodies which are large, near other sensitive structures, or composed of pieces. It can also be used in concert with a specialist consultant accustomed to open dissection – you localize, they dissect.
   (b) Insert a small alligator forceps in the plane of the ultrasound beam, and grasp the foreign body, removing it along the path of insertion (Fig. 8.33). This technique is best suited to smaller, more linear foreign bodies which are unlikely to break apart.

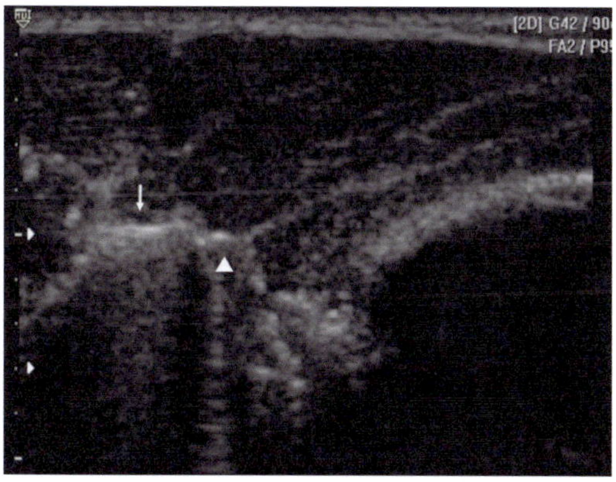

Fig. 8.33 BB pellet (arrowhead) removal with an alligator forceps (arrow) under ultrasound guidance. (Courtesy of Michael Blaivas, MD)

Complications

The visualization of foreign bodies using ultrasound should not in itself create a complication unless misdiagnosis occurs. Complications of foreign body removal include bleeding, infection, damage to nearby structures, and other standard reported complications.

Pearls

- Have a high index of suspicion when patients report a foreign body sensation, and use their self-reported location as your starting point when scanning.
- When a foreign body is not visualized, ensure you are using the highest-frequency setting on your transducer.
- Consider a standoff pad or water bath if structures are too superficial.
- Look for acoustic shadowing – sometimes the shadow cast is more apparent than the object casting the shadow.

Pitfalls

- Small (less than a few mm) foreign bodies will be difficult to visualize on ultrasound because they will not cast a shadow.
- Foreign bodies with tissue-like density are also challenging since no contrast will be visible between the echogenicity of the foreign body and surrounding tissue.

Integration into Clinical Practice

Consider using ultrasound prior to, or instead of, radiography to detect foreign bodies. Ultrasound may be especially useful in the setting of a small number of foreign bodies and those which are radiolucent such as wood or plastic.

Evidence

Several studies describe the rather heterogeneous experience of ultrasound guidance for foreign body removal. In one center, 95 foreign bodies of varying composition (glass, metal, vegetable, plastic, and stone) were removed from 62 patients under constant ultrasound guidance [14]. In this series, the authors guided a scalpel from the skin to the foreign body under ultrasound guidance, then passed a forceps along that tract to grasp, and removed the foreign body. Another study reports 252 (88% of a possible 287) successful foreign body retrievals under constant ultrasound guidance, with 15 unsuccessful extractions and 12 which were not attempted due to local anatomy or the composition of the foreign body [15].

Key Points

- Ultrasound is accurate in identifying foreign bodies, even some that may be radiolucent.
- Use ultrasound to identify the position and location of the foreign body, but also nearby sensitive vascular or nervous structures.

Intraosseous Access Placement

Intraosseus needle insertion is increasingly being used for critical vascular access with the advent of rapid, drill-based delivery systems. It is recommended by ACLS and PALS guidelines for critical patients in whom rapid intravenous access cannot be obtained. Traditionally, intraosseus needle placement is confirmed by aspiration of the bone marrow, firm needle position, and infusion of fluid without pressure. However, these do not necessarily confirm the needle has not penetrated the deep cortex into the soft tissue behind the bone, and extravasation of infused fluid is a potential risk. Recently, reports of ultrasound use to confirm intraosseus placement and proper function lend an additional tool to help confirm proper placement.

Anatomy

Several sites are commonly used for intraosseus placement. In young children, the proximal tibia is recommended. In adults and older children, the distal tibia, proximal humerus, malleoli, or sternum may be used. Sonographically, bony cortex will be readily visible as a bright echogenic line deep to the skin and soft tissue.

Indications

- Intraosseus vascular access is recommended for critically ill patients in whom rapid vascular access cannot be obtained.

Contraindications

- Fracture of the target bone
- Cellulitis over insertion site

Preparation

A high-frequency linear probe is needed to confirm placement of the intraosseus needle. Standard equipment should be assembled for the intraosseus needle insertion itself.

Procedure

1. Intraosseus needle placement should proceed in accordance with manufacturer's instructions.
2. Place a high-frequency linear probe near to insertion site in the transverse and longitudinal planes.
3. While visualizing the cortex near the needle insertion site, activate the color or power Doppler function, and place the Doppler box beneath the cortex. Flush the needle with saline, and assess for color flow within the cortex (Fig. 8.34).

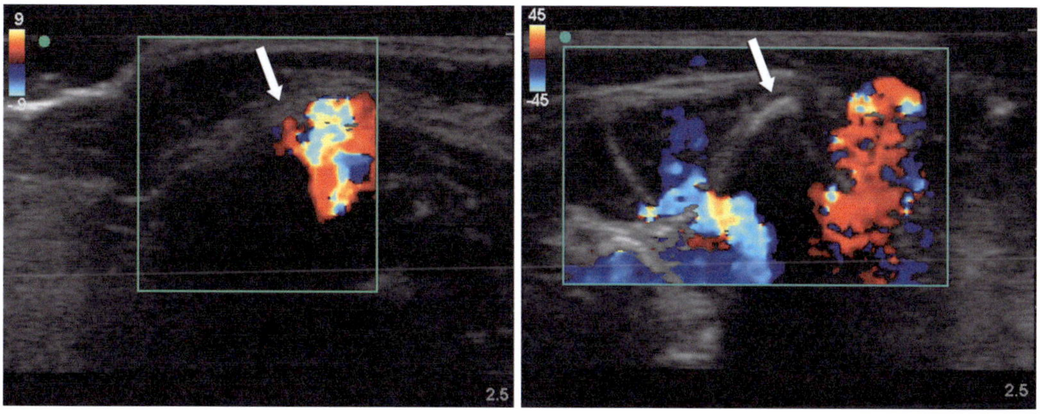

Fig. 8.34 Intraosseus (left) and extraosseus (right) flow of a saline flush through the needle. Bony cortex is white arrow. (Courtesy of Jim Tsung MD, MPH)

Complications

Ultrasound confirmation of intraosseus placement should not introduce any new complications beyond the procedure itself, unless images are misinterpreted.

Pearls

- Power Doppler is more sensitive to low-flow Color Doppler and should therefore give a more reliable signal in intraosseus infusions.
- Imaging the bony cortex in the transverse plane may facilitate sampling closer to the point of needle entry and ensure the proper bone is being imaged.

Pitfalls

- Intraosseus needles can become dislodged, especially during patient transport. Consider reimaging if the line no longer flushes easily or if displacement is suspected.

Integration into Clinical Practice

Ultrasound confirmation should be attempted immediately after intraosseus needle insertion, as the first flush is pushed through the device. Thus, the procedure should not take longer than the needle insertion itself.

Evidence

Several case series have demonstrated the efficacy of ultrasound confirmation of intraosseus needle placement. In the most recent, ultrasound properly identified abnormal, extraosseus flow in all misplaced needles and intraosseus flow in all properly positioned needles ($n = 6$) [16].

> **Key Point**
> - Ultrasound confirmation of flow with saline flush may increase the accuracy of assessing proper needle placement in critically ill patients.

References

1. Daley E, Bajaj S, Bisson L, et al. Improving injection accuracy of the elbow, knee, and shoulder: does injection site and imaging make a difference? A systemic review. Am J Sports Med. 2011;39:656–62.
2. Bloom JE, Rischin A, Johnston RV, Buchbinder R. Image-guided versus blind glucocorticoid injection for shoulder pain. Cochrane Database Syst Rev. 2012;(8):CD009147.
3. Wiler JL, Costantino TG, Filippone L, Satz W. Comparison of ultrasound-guided and standard land-

mark techniques for knee arthrocentesis. J Emerg Med. 2010;39:76–82.
4. Kozaci N, Ay MO, Akcimen M, et al. Evaluation of the effectiveness of bedside point-of-care ultrasound in the diagnosis and management of distal radius fractures. Am J Emerg Med. 2015;33(1):67–71.
5. Kodama N, Takemura Y, Ueba H, Imai S, Matsusue Y. Ultrasound-assisted closed reduction of distal radius fractures. J Hand Surg Am. 2014;39(7):1287–94.
6. Ang SH, Lee SW, Lam KY. Ultrasound-guided reduction of distal radius fractures. Am J Emerg Med. 2010;28(9):1002–8.
7. Barata I, Spencer R, Suppiah A, Raio C, Ward MF, Sama A. Emergency ultrasound in the detection of pediatric long-bone fractures. Pediatr Emerg Care. 2012;28(11):1154–7.
8. Dubrovsky AS, Kempinska A, Bank I, Mok E. Accuracy of ultrasonography for determining successful realignment of pediatric forearm fractures. Ann Emerg Med. 2015;65(3):260–5.
9. Fathi M, Moezzi M, Abbasi S, Farsi D, Zare MA, Hafezimoghadam P. Ultrasound-guided hematoma block in distal radial fracture reduction: a randomised clinical trial. Emerg Med J. 2015;32(6):474–7.
10. Lovallo E, Mantuani D, Nagdev A. Novel use of ultrasound in the ED: ultrasound-guided hematoma block of a proximal humeral fracture. Am J Emerg Med. 2015;33(1):130 e131–2.
11. Wilson SR, Price DD, Penner E. Pain control for sternal fracture using an ultrasound-guided hematoma block. J Emerg Med. 2010;38(3):359–61.
12. Mc Auliffe N, Harmon D. Ultrasound-guided hematoma block in fractured neck of femur. Reg Anesth Pain Med. 2009;34(1):80–1.
13. Abbasi S, Mollaie H, Hafezimoghadam P, et al. Diagnostic accuracy of ultrasonographic examination in the management of shoulder dislocation in the emergency department. Ann Emerg Med. 2013;62:170–5.
14. Callegari L, Leonardi A, Bini A, et al. Ultrasound-guided removal of foreign bodies: personal experience. Eur Radiol. 2009;19:1273–9.
15. Bradley M. Image-guided soft-tissue foreign body extraction- success and pitfalls. Clin Radiol. 2012;67(6):531–4.
16. Tsung JW, Blaivas M, Stone MB. Feasibility of point-of-care colour Doppler ultrasound confirmation of interosseous needle placement during resuscitation. Resuscitation. 2009;80:665–8.

Ultrasound-Guided Nerve Blocks

9

Arun Nagdev, Emily Lovallo, and Brian Johnson

Introduction

Single-injection ultrasound-guided peripheral nerve blocks are ideal for pain relief from acute injuries and painful procedures. They function by targeting the nerves that innervate the site of wound or injury. Local anesthetic is injected adjacent to the nerve, and the nerve distally essentially becomes anesthetized or colloquially termed "blocked." Wound irrigation/care, exploration/removal of foreign bodies, laceration repair, incision and drainage, fracture reduction, and joint relocation are all ideal indications. Depending upon the efficacy of the ultrasound-guided nerve block, adjunctive therapies can be used to achieve maximal patient comfort.

The alleviation of pain is a central tenet of acute care treatment. Regional anesthesia (otherwise called peripheral nerve blocks) affords the clinician another tool in their armamentarium to swiftly and efficiently address pain and suffering. Physicians are well aware of the side effects of large doses of intravenous opioids especially in the elderly including hypotension, bradypnea, altered mental status, airway compromise, and even death. Regional anesthesia offers a targeted approach to alleviate pain in the acute care setting without the reliance on opioids.

There is a growing body of literature supporting the use of regional anesthesia in the emergency care setting [1]. The drainage of soft tissue abscesses, removal of foreign bodies, complex laceration repairs, fractures, and joint relocations are few of the indications for regional anesthesia. The use of ultrasound to perform peripheral nerve blocks has been shown to reduce the time of block onset and volume of anesthetic required as compared to the classic nerve stimulation and landmark-based methods [2, 3]. Furthermore, ultrasound enables more precise needle direction, minimizing the risk of intraneural injection or vascular puncture.

Ultrasound-guided nerve blocks should only be performed in patients who can consent to the procedure – meaning they are awake, are alert, and can cooperate with the neurological examination. Any patient with an allergy to local anesthetic should be excluded as well. A preexisting neurologic deficit or a new neurological deficit due to injury is a contraindication to a peripheral nerve block. While being rare, there is a small

A. Nagdev (✉)
Highland General Hospital, Alameda Health System, Oakland, CA, USA

E. Lovallo
Department of Emergency Medicine, University of Pittsburgh School of Medicine, Pittsburgh, PA, USA

UPMC Mercy and Magee Hospitals, Pittsburgh, PA, USA

B. Johnson
University of Washington – Valley Medical Center Emergency Department, Renton, WA, USA

S. Adhikari, M. Blaivas (eds.), *The Ultimate Guide to Point-of-Care Ultrasound-Guided Procedures*, https://doi.org/10.1007/978-3-030-28267-7_9

risk of peripheral nerve injury after the peripheral nerve block, and differentiating a previous neurapraxia versus a block-related peripheral nerve injury (PNI) is extremely difficult. All injuries have a risk of developing compartment syndrome with some injuries more prone than others. The concern is for a peripheral nerve block to mask the sentinel signs of compartment syndrome by removing the sensory innervation to the affected muscle and compartment. Caution is recommended in injuries at higher risk for developing compartment syndrome, such as crush injuries, high speed/force distal tibia fractures, vascular compromise, or neurological injury. Despite poor data supporting that peripheral nerve blocks can mask compartment syndrome, we recommend discussing the patient and the block with your consultative services (orthopedics, trauma surgery, etc.) before performing the block in these higher-risk injuries.

PNI is defined as persistent motor or sensory deficit and/or pain after a nerve block. PNI is an extremely uncommon outcome from an ultrasound-guided peripheral nerve block. The incidence of PNI has been suggested anywhere from 0.5% to 2.4% in the literature [4]. The true mechanism is poorly understood. Hypotheses include direct needle trauma, increased intrafascicular pressures from injection, and direct cytotoxic effects of anesthetic or metabolic stress of the anesthetic leading to nerve ischemia. To minimize the risk of PNI, we recommend three steps when performing any ultrasound-guided peripheral nerve block. First, under ultrasound guidance, the needle tip should always be close to the nerve, but however not within the nerve fascicle. Second, always inject the local anesthetic in a slow, low-pressure, deliberate fashion. If at any time it is difficult to inject the anesthetic, ensure that your needle tip has not migrated within the nerve fascicle. Typically if the needle is in the correct location, the injection should be low pressure. Also, if the patient experiences pain or paresthesias, we recommend stopping the block and withdrawing the needle tip. Third, an ultrasound-guided nerve block should not be performed in patients with any underlying peripheral neuropathy.

Ergonomics are essential for success. Appropriate patient positioning is crucial and will depend on the injury and the specific nerve block. Universally, the ultrasound machine should be placed on the opposite side of the site of the peripheral nerve block with the screen directly in the line of site of the operator. This enables the operator minimal head and body movement while visualizing both the needle insertion site and the ultrasound image of the needle during the entire procedure. Finally, some blocks require that patients be placed on a cardiac monitor with continuous pulse oximetry for the duration of the nerve block.

The site for the peripheral nerve block should be cleaned with either chlorhexidine or equivalent skin prep. At the end of the survey scan, we recommend placing a skin wheal of local anesthetic (typically 1% lidocaine) with a small-gauge needle (25–30 gauge) at the proposed peripheral nerve block needle insertion site. The ultrasound probe should be cleaned of all gel and covered with a transparent, adhesive dressing (Fig. 9.1). Sterile gel should be used as the interface between the skin and ultrasound probe. The needle gauge and length will depend on the intended peripheral nerve block and will be described for each peripheral nerve block section. There are block-specific needles with blunt tips that can be used; however, they are not necessary to perform the nerve blocks described in this chapter [5]. If choosing to perform the nerve block with a hand-on-syringe technique, you will require a control syringe to hold the local anesthetic (Fig. 9.2). If you choose to perform the nerve block with a hand-on-needle technique, then short IV tubing with an attached syringe will be needed to hold the local anesthetic (Fig. 9.3).

We recommend establishing a specific location in your setting, be it an emergency department (ED), office, clinic, intensive care unit, or other with dedicated to nerve block supplies. This simple step will reduce time needed to prepare for the ultrasound-guided nerve blocks as well as ensure all essential items are present during the procedure.

The two local anesthetics typically stocked in a variety of clinical settings are lidocaine and bupivacaine. Both can be used for peripheral

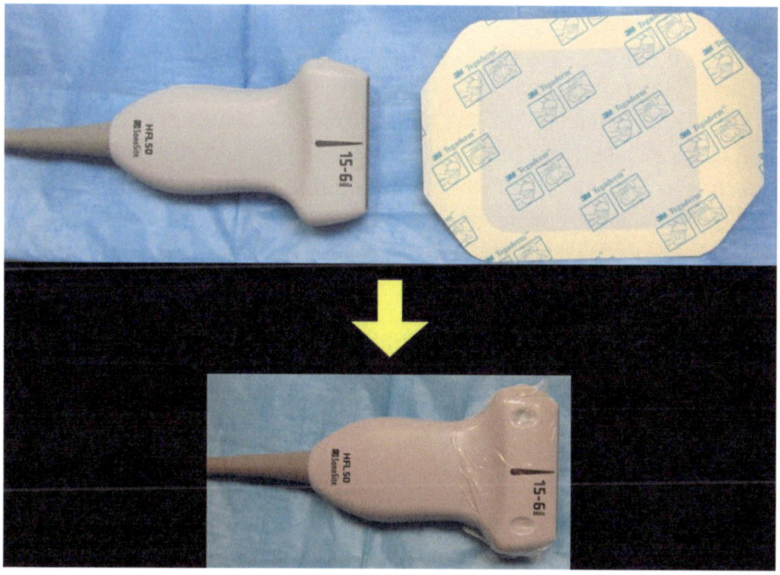

Fig. 9.1 Sterile dressing and ultrasound probe

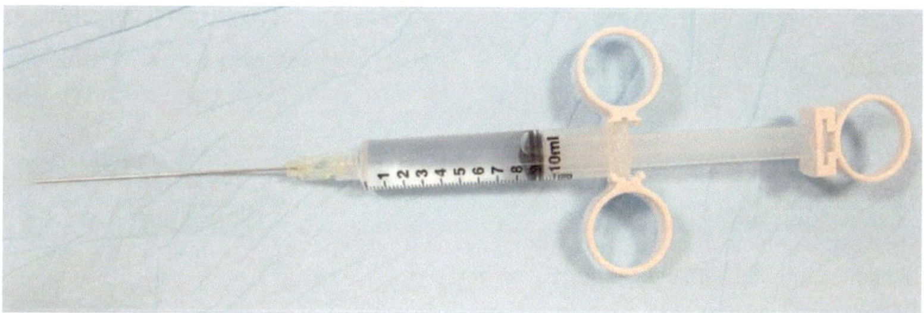

Fig. 9.2 Control syringe used for hand-on-syringe technique

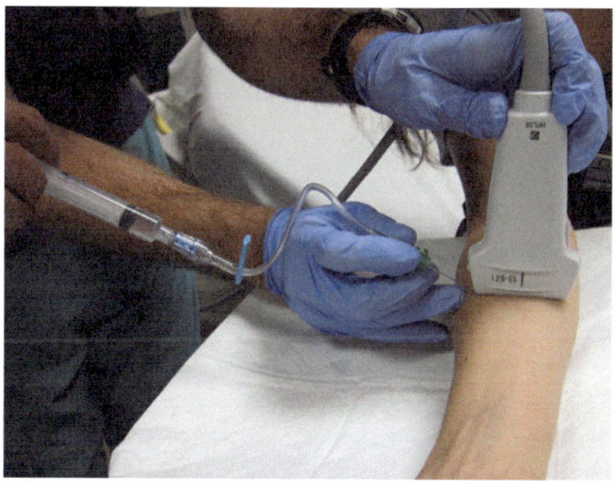

Fig. 9.3 Hand-on-needle technique

nerve blocks. For the novice provider, lidocaine is preferred over bupivacaine. Inadvertent vascular deposition of anesthetic can occur even with meticulous methods. Bupivacaine is known to be toxic to the cardiac and central nervous systems, and we recommend that providers who are not very comfortable with the subtle nuances of needle tip visualization only use lidocaine with or without epinephrine. Lidocaine has vasodilatory effects, and thus epinephrine will extend the duration of the analgesia. Even with lidocaine's shorter half-life and increased safety profile, the provider should be familiar with the signs and symptoms of local anesthetic systemic toxicity (LAST). Classically, the patient will complain of tongue numbness and light-headedness, which then progresses to muscle twitching, unconsciousness, seizures, and cardiovascular depression [6]. If bupivacaine has been inadvertently injected into the vascular system, the use of a hyperlipophilic solution (20% Intralipid; 1.5 mg/kg bolus with continued infusion of 0.25 ml/min) should be infused. We recommend 20% Intralipid be readily available when performing an ultrasound-guided peripheral nerve block. Standard safety techniques dictate the provider never injects without ultrasonographic visualization of the needle tip and always aspirates before injecting to confirm lack of vascular puncture.

Locating nerves with ultrasound requires knowledge of adjacent anatomical landmarks. Typically, nerves course through the body adjacent to fascial planes and vascular structures. Nerves are best visualized and targeted for blocks when oriented in cross section. There are subtle differences of nerve appearance based on anatomic location. Distal peripheral nerves appear on ultrasound as bundles of hyperechoic circles or "cluster of grapes" or having a "honeycombed" quality (Fig. 9.4). Employing the use of anisotropy to identify nerves is important. Anisotropy is a sonographic artifact defined as being directionally dependent. Nerves inherently have a significant amount of anisotropy. Thus, when the ultrasound probe is directly perpendicular to the nerve axis, it will appear very bright; however, when you angle or rock the transducer back and forth, the nerve will become darker and less discernible (Fig. 9.5). Proximal peripheral nerves, such as the roots of the brachial plexus, appear as individual anechoic circles that can easily be mistaken for blood vessels (Fig. 9.6). Subtle fanning of the transducer may be necessary to minimize the effects of the anisotropy and obtain the highest-quality images. We recommend that novice sonographers verify with color Doppler that the intended target is not vasculature.

There are two standard needle orientations one can employ to safely place the needle tip adjacent to the nerve.

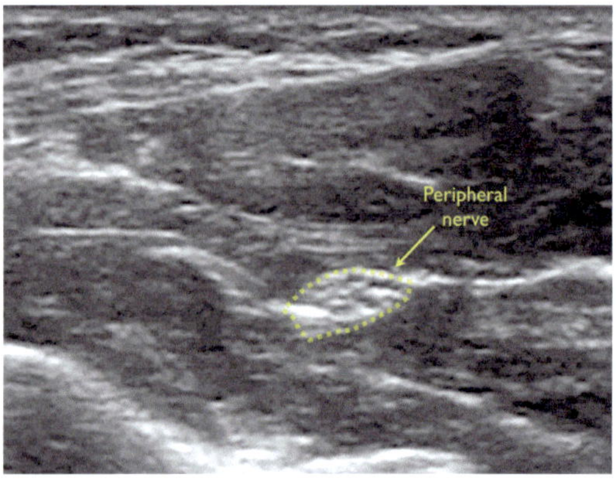

Fig. 9.4 Ultrasound image of peripheral nerve described as "honeycombed" or "cluster of grapes"

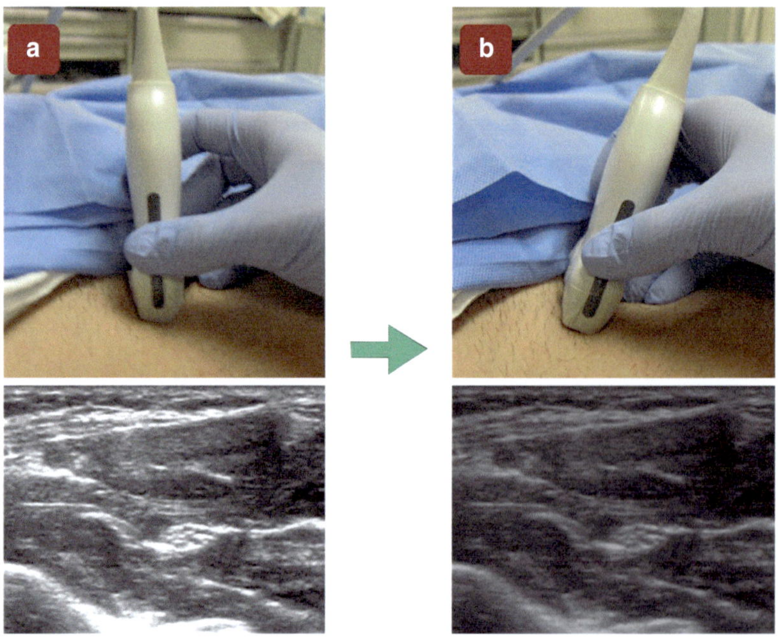

Fig. 9.5 An example of anisotropy: (**a**) probe perpendicular to nerve displaying bright, hyperechoic nerve and (**b**) probe angled away from perpendicular orientation illustrating darker, less hyperechoic nerve

In-plane needle visualization technique The needle is inserted lateral and parallel to the long axis of the transducer (Fig. 9.7). As the needle passes under the transducer, the entire length of the needle will be visualized (Fig. 9.8). The trajectory of the needle must be midline and parallel to the transducer in order to visualize the needle in its entirety. The in-plane technique for needle tip visualization is recommended for novice sonographers performing peripheral nerve blocks.

Out-of-plane needle visualization technique The needle is inserted midline and perpendicular to the long axis of the transducer at a steep angle (greater

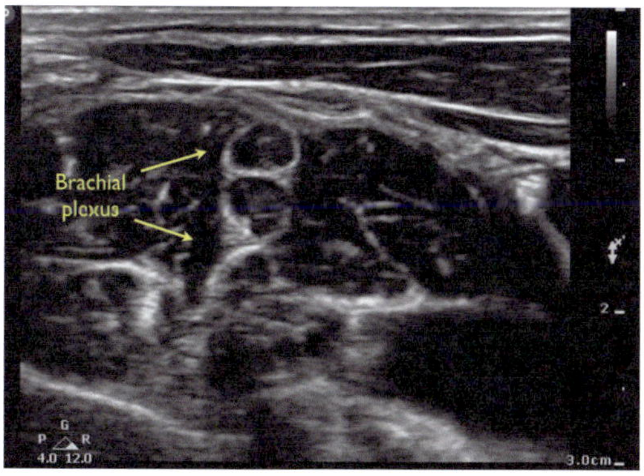

Fig. 9.6 Ultrasound image of proximal nerve bundle that can resemble vascular structures

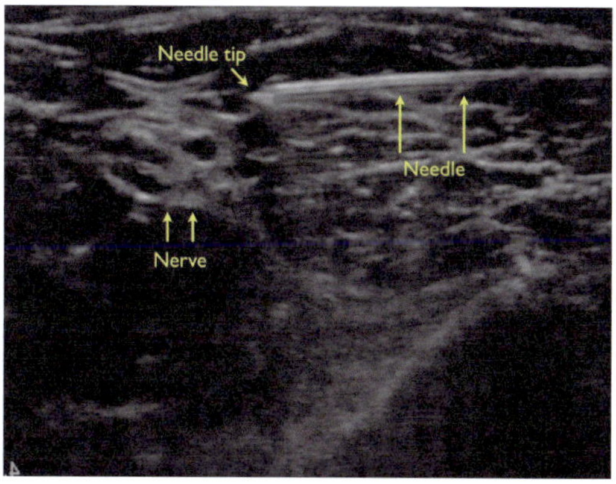

Fig. 9.8 Ultrasound image showing appropriate in-plane needle visualization technique with the entire needle visualized

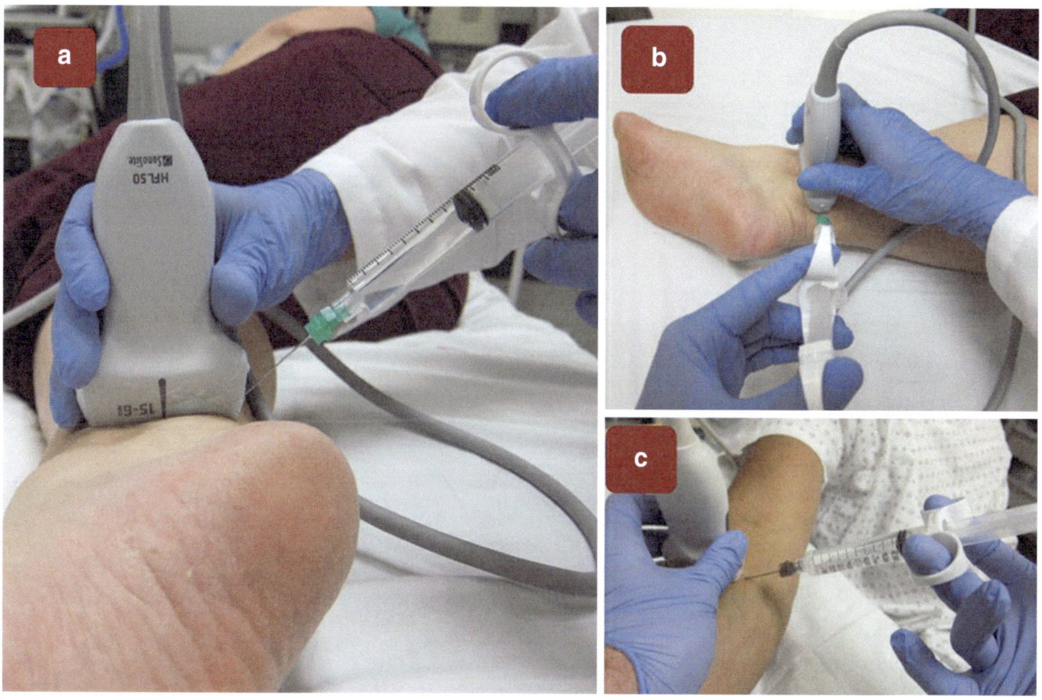

Fig. 9.7 Appropriate placement for in-plane needle visualization technique with needle positioned parallel to the long axis of the ultrasound probe. (**a**–**c**) All examples of in-plane needle visualization procedures

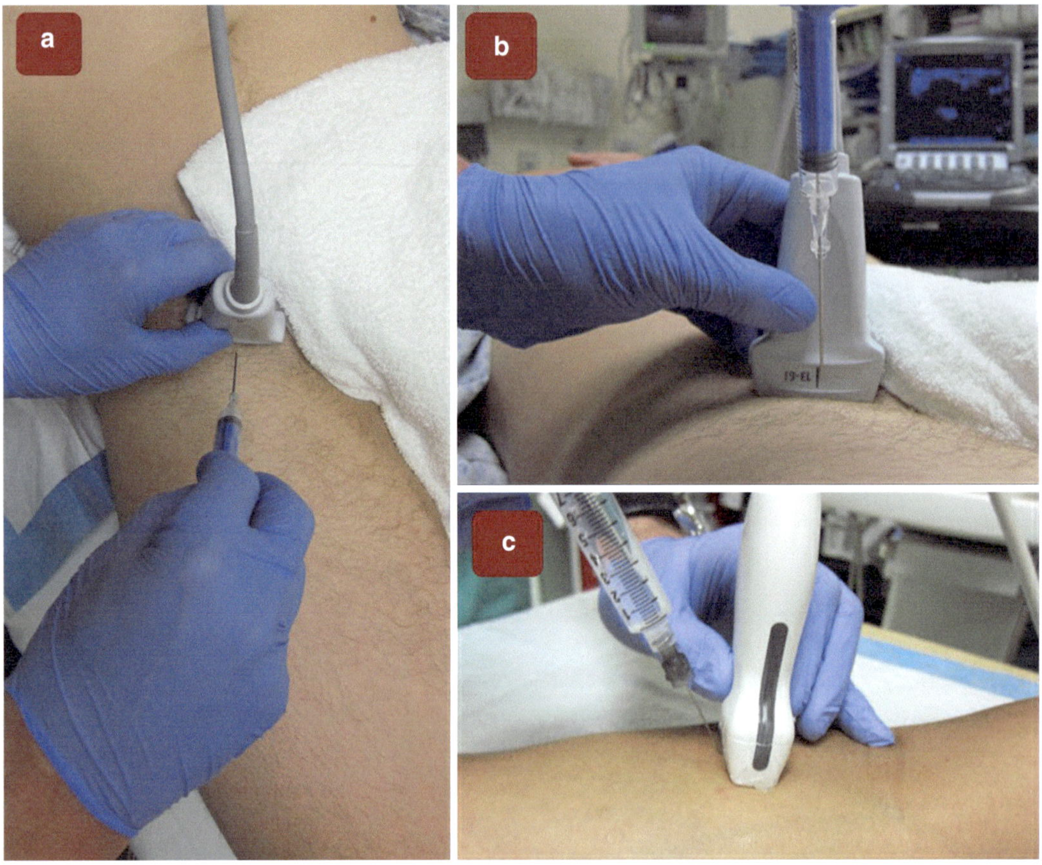

Fig. 9.9 Appropriate needle placement for out-of-plane needle visualization technique with needle positioned midline and perpendicular to the long axis of the ultrasound probe (**a**–**c**)

than 70°–80°) to the skin (Fig. 9.9). The needle tip will only be visualized as a hyperechoic dot as it passes under the transducer (Fig. 9.10). Safe and successful execution of this technique relies on confident visualization of the needle tip, which requires strong spatial motor skills with both the probe and the needle.

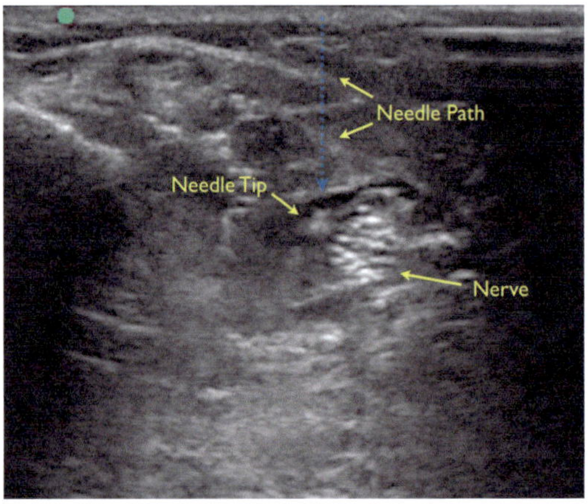

Fig. 9.10 Ultrasound image showing appropriate out-of-plane needle visualization technique with the hyperechoic needle tip visualized

There are two standard needle/syringe combinations to perform a successful peripheral nerve block.

Hand-on-syringe technique This is a single-operator technique. The provider attaches the needle typically onto a 10-ml control syringe. In this technique, the operator then is in control of the needle, aspiration, and injection of the anesthetic. The operator can appreciate the tactile feedback of this single-operator approach.

Hand-on-needle technique This is a two-person technique. The chosen needle is attached to IV tubing which is attached to the anesthetic-filled syringe. The provider holds the needle directly onto the skin surface and when in the appropriate position instructs a second operator to aspirate and then inject the local anesthetic.

It has yet to be determined which needle technique is preferred [7]. While the hand-on-needle technique affords the operator more precise needle targeting, the operator loses the tactile feedback of aspiration and injection. Furthermore, the hand-on-needle technique requires two operators to perform, and, in a busy ED setting, the hand-on-syringe technique can be performed by one operator, which might be preferred.

Post-peripheral nerve block care is extremely important. You have intentionally anesthetized part if not all of an extremity. The anesthetized extremity should be labeled with indelible marker describing the type of block performed as well as the date and time of the block completion. Nursing should be alerted that the patient has had a peripheral nerve block. Appropriate care should be applied to the extremity including appropriate padding and positioning, splinting, and ice if necessary. Consultants should also be aware that the block was performed and communicate the local anesthetic used and the expected duration of the block.

Advantages of Ultrasound Guidance

Ultrasound guidance offers many potential benefits to peripheral nerve blockade in the acute care settings. It eliminates the need for multiple needle insertions and redirections that can prolong procedure times and subject the patient to unnecessary pain and injury during peripheral nerve blockade. Specifically, ultrasound allows the operator to see target nerves, advance the needle under real-time visualization, and monitor the spread of local anesthetic. Ultrasound allows visualization of not only the nerves but other adjacent vital structures (arteries, veins, tendons, etc.) and reduces the incidence of inadvertent puncture of these structures. It avoids the unintentional injection of local anesthetic into the vasculature and minimizes the chance of local anesthetic toxicity. Overall, real-time ultrasound guidance reduces the risks of neuropathy from intraneuronal injection, systemic toxicity due to accidental intravascular injection, and other complications, such as pneumothorax, visceral injury, etc. [1]. The ability to visualize both anatomical structures and the needle under ultrasound guidance improves operator accuracy during the infiltration of anesthetic solution, which in turn leads to faster onset time, increased success rate, and reduced procedure time [1, 2]. The volume of local anesthetic required to achieve the anesthesia is considerably less than that required when using traditional landmark techniques since the operator can see the spread of local anesthetic around a nerve and can adjust the needle tip position as necessary to optimize local anesthetic distribution [1–3]. Unlike procedural sedation, ultrasound-guided nerve blocks do not require additional staff or prolonged post-procedure observation period. Ultrasound-guided nerve blocks have been shown to decrease length of stay, reduce hospital costs, and improve patient satisfaction [1–3].

Blocking the Brachial Plexus: Ultrasound-Guided Interscalene and Supraclavicular Nerve Block

The brachial plexus provides the complete motor and sensory innervation to the upper extremity. The brachial plexus includes the nerve roots of C5–T1. These nerve roots leave the cervical spine just posterior to the musculature of the neck and join with the subclavian artery and vein before entering into the upper extremity. The brachial plexus can be blocked in various locations, with this decision based on both a simple ultrasonographic anatomic surveillance and the specific injury that needs to be addressed. As the brachial plexus travels from the spinal column toward the upper extremity, the interscalene groove in the neck and just lateral to the subclavian artery in the supraclavicular fossa has been the most popular locations for regional anesthesia. The interscalene brachial plexus block will most consistently block the nerve roots of C5–C7 making this a useful choice for injuries more proximal to the mid-humerus. The supraclavicular brachial plexus block will most consistently provide analgesia for injuries from the mid-humerus to the hand. This is a simplified assumption for novice providers; in actuality the innervation of the wrist and hand is extremely complex.

Ultrasound-Guided Interscalene Nerve Block

Anatomy

The interscalene block is performed at the interscalene groove formed by the anterior and middle scalene muscles. The interscalene groove is located just below the clavicular head of the sternocleidomastoid muscle at the level of the cricoid cartilage. The medial border is the anterior scalene muscle. The lateral border is the middle scalene muscle. The C5–C7 nerve roots are quite superficial and lie between the anterior and middle scalene muscles of the neck. The C8 and T1 nerve roots are deeper and more difficult to visualize consistently. Landmarks to identify include the carotid artery and internal jugular vein medial to the anterior scalene muscle. The pleural line lies more caudal and should not be at risk of puncture if the block is done at the appropriate location, and clear ultrasonographic needle tip visualization is maintained during the procedure.

Indications

The interscalene block consistently provides anesthesia to the proximal upper extremity including the shoulder and proximal humerus. Typically, this block should be performed for pain control in patients with injuries of the proximal upper extremity (burns, proximal humeral fractures, etc.). The interscalene brachial plexus block is also ideal as either an adjunct or alternative to procedural sedation for large upper-arm laceration repairs, abscess incision and drainage, and glenohumeral reductions.

Contraindications

The interscalene block will almost always cause transient, ipsilateral diaphragm paralysis due to the fascial spread of local anesthetic over the anterior scalene muscle – anesthetizing the phrenic nerve [8]. In healthy patients without pulmonary dysfunction, the debate persists about the clinical significance of ipsilateral phrenic nerve paralysis. Ultrasound guidance has increased needle precision and lowered the amount of anesthetic volume needed to achieve a successful block, theoretically reducing the phrenic nerve paralysis [9]. We caution the use of the interscalene block in patients with poor pulmonary reserve, such as patients with severe COPD, restrictive lung disease, and severe obstructive sleep apnea. Also, the sympathetic afferent chain or recurrent laryngeal nerve can incidentally be anesthetized. This will rarely cause a temporary Horner's syndrome (ptosis, miosis, and anhydrosis) or a temporary hoarse voice. Also, the interscalene block should not be done on a patient with known contralateral laryngeal nerve palsy. Like previously mentioned for all ultrasound-guided nerve blocks, we do not recommend performing this procedure in patients with a risk for vascular injury, preexisting neurologic injury, or high risk for compartment syndrome.

Equipment/Probe Selection

A high-frequency linear probe should be used for the interscalene block. A 20–22-gauge 3.5-inch/9-cm spinal needle will be needed in most patients. Standard nerve block materials should be used and are discussed in the introduction section.

Preparation/Pre-procedural Evaluation

The patient should be placed on a cardiac monitor and positioned upright or in a semi-reclining position with the head rotated 30° away from the affected side. The ultrasound system should be placed on the opposite side of the block for easy visualization during needle manipulation. Since the interscalene block is quite superficial and will be performed in plane, place the patient in a mild decubitus position. This allows the operator a flat approach to the interscalene groove and maximize needle visualization during the entire block.

A survey scan should be performed. First, place the high-frequency linear probe in a transverse orientation on the neck of the affected side at the level of the cricoid (Fig. 9.11). Second, locate the carotid artery and internal jugular vein, and slowly slide the probe laterally until the superficial head of the sternocleidomastoid (SCM) muscle is visualized (Fig. 9.12). Third, identify the anterior and middle scalene muscles just deep to the SCM muscle. The anterior scalene muscle is the medial border of the interscalene groove, and the middle scalene muscles are the lateral border. Fourth, identify the roots of the brachial plexus that lie between the anterior and middle scalene muscles. At the interscalene groove, the C5–C7 roots of the brachial plexus are superficially wedged together and are hypoechoic round or ovoid structures vertically aligned, colloquially coined as the "traffic light" sign. The C8 and T1 nerve roots may be sonographically visualized as well; however, they lie deeper. We recommend that the clinician use color Doppler to ensure that the anechoic nerve roots are not vascular structures and that the needle path will not traverse unforeseen veins and/or arteries. Clinicians using color Doppler should be comfortable with manipulation of specific parameters (e.g., pulse repetition frequency) to ensure that the vasculature with minimal flow will be detected.

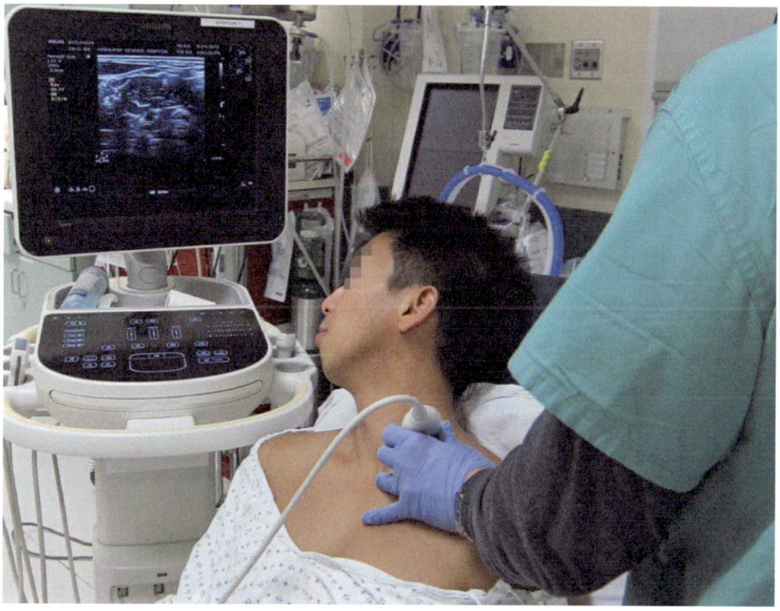

Fig. 9.11 Appropriate patient and probe positioning for interscalene nerve block

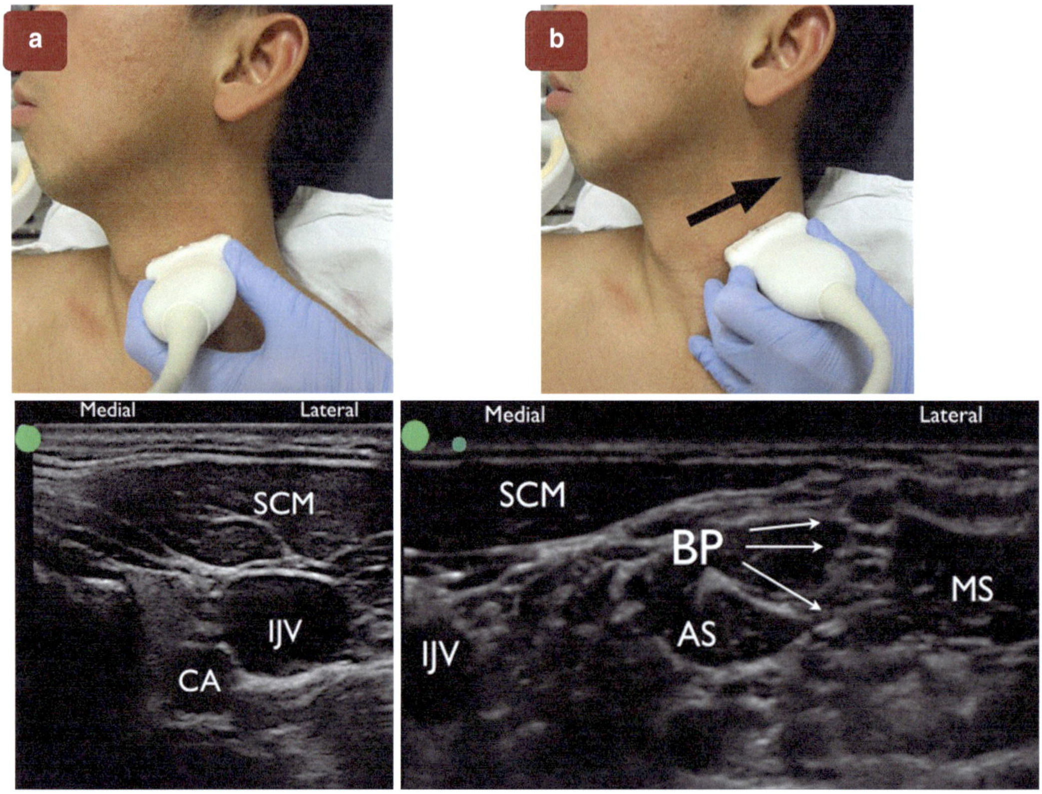

Fig. 9.12 Appropriate ultrasound probe placement for interscalene nerve block. (**a**) Identifying the carotid (CA) and internal jugular vein (IJV) and (**b**) sliding lateral to identify sternocleidomastoid (SCM), anterior scalene (AS), and middle scalene (MS) muscle with brachial plexus (BP) between scalene muscles

Oftentimes visualization of the nerve roots can be challenging at this level by simply sliding the ultrasound probe laterally in the neck at the level of the cricoid. The alternative approach involves identification of the brachial plexus in the supraclavicular fossa and then moving proximally to the interscalene groove. For this approach, first, place the transducer parallel to the clavicle in the supraclavicular fossa (Fig. 9.13). Second, aim the transducer caudally until you can visualize the subclavian artery in cross section. Third, visualize brachial plexus located laterally to the subclavian artery. Sonographically, the brachial plexus at this level will appear as a "cluster of grapes" or "honeycombed." Fourth, follow the brachial plexus in a cephalad pathway up the neck until you see the nerve roots orient in the "stop light" pattern in the interscalene groove with the medial and lateral borders of the anterior and middle scalene muscles, respectively.

Procedure

We recommend novice providers perform the interscalene brachial plexus in plane with a lateral-to-medial approach. A small skin wheal should be placed just lateral to the ultrasound probe. A 20–22-gauge 3.5-inch needle is inserted just lateral in the same direction as the transducer (in-plane technique) (Fig. 9.14). The needle tip should be clearly visualized and slowly advanced through the middle scalene muscle to the lateral border of the interscalene groove. We recommend depositing 1–2-ml aliquots slowly until the

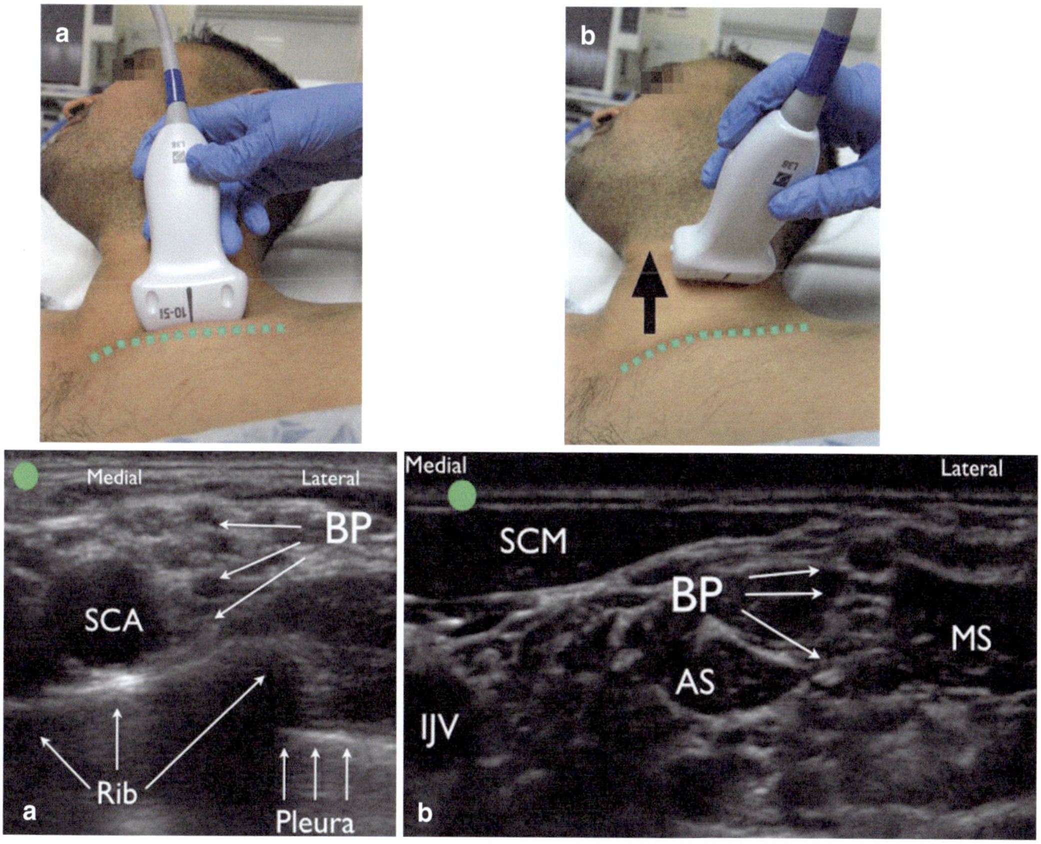

Fig. 9.13 Alternative initial placement of ultrasound probe for interscalene nerve block in the (**a**) supraclavicular fossa just above the clavicle (dotted line) identifying the subclavian artery (SCA) with the underlying rib and lung pleura and then lateral the brachial plexus (BP) and then (**b**) moving the probe cephalad to the interscalene groove to identify the brachial plexus (BP) adjacent to the anterior (AS) and middle (MS) scalene muscles with the internal jugular vein (IJV) medially and the sternocleidomastoid (SCM) above

10–20 ml is delivered. The clinician should always aspirate before placing anesthetic to ensure lack of vascular puncture as well as clearly visualize anechoic anesthetic spread on the ultrasound screen. If the needle tip is in the appropriate location, local anesthetic will track along the fascial plane between the middle scalene muscle and the nerve roots in the interscalene grove. Classically, a successful block is visualization of the "donut sign" described as hypoechoic anesthetic surrounding the brachial plexus. However, placement of the needle tip in the potential space between the brachial plexus sheath and middle scalene is often adequate for a successful block, and the "donut sign" is not necessary [10].

Complications

The ultrasound-guided brachial plexus block at the interscalene groove can be learned and performed successfully even with the close proximity of adjacent vascular structures, nerve bundles, and lung apices. Once the in-plane technique is mastered, ultrasound guidance affords precise needle tip localization and reduced anesthetic volume requirements, making the procedure relatively safe. Uncommon complications include transient phrenic nerve paralysis that causes respiratory compromise, pneumothorax, and inadvertent vascular puncture. Because of the close proximity of the

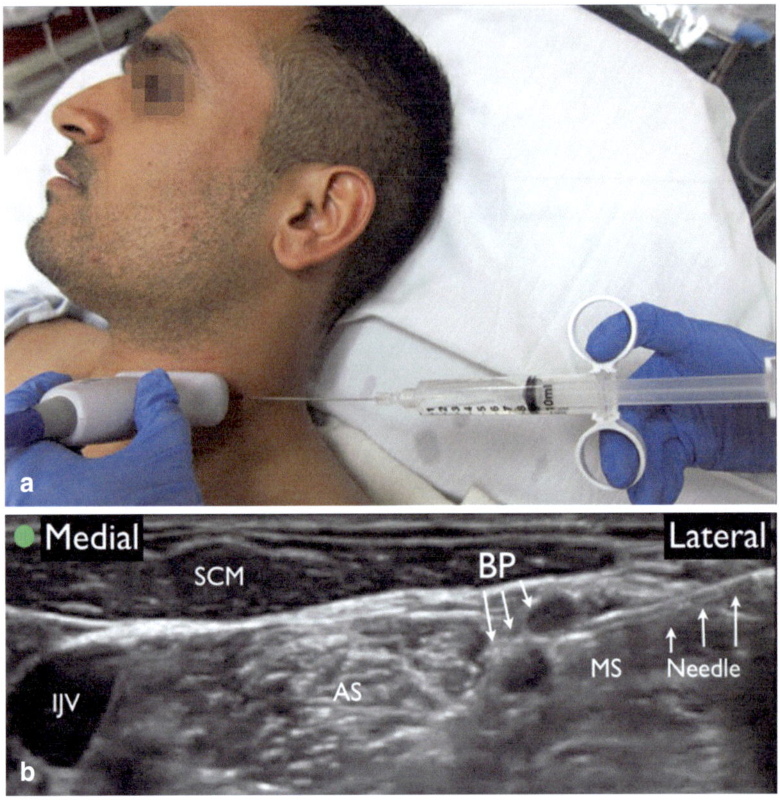

Fig. 9.14 (**a**) Correct needle and ultrasound placement for the interscalene nerve block and then (**b**) in-plane ultrasound needle placement in the potential space between the middle scalene muscle and brachial plexus

phrenic nerve (medial aspect of the anterior scalene muscle), caution should be taken when performing the interscalene brachial plexus block on patients with poor pulmonary reserve. Also, the sympathetic chain can incidentally be blocked causing a temporary Horner's syndrome. The best approach to prevent sympathetic chain injury is the injection of low volumes of anesthetic with the needle tip under the fascial plane however far from the nerve bundle. Iatrogenic pneumothorax is a theoretical risk; however, if performed at the level of the larynx and clear needle tip visualization is maintained, lung puncture will not occur. Lastly, the transverse cervical artery typically runs laterally and caudal to the brachial plexus in the interscalene groove. Rarely, this artery can course through the brachial plexus. Once you identify the interscalene groove and the brachial plexus, color Doppler should be performed to ensure this artery does not course through the brachial plexus. If the artery is present in the brachial plexus, you should not perform the block in the interscalene groove.

Pearls/Pitfalls

The ultrasound-guided interscalene nerve block will not consistently block the C8 and T1 nerve roots so that injuries to the mid/distal humerus, elbow, forearm, wrist, and hand will not achieve consistent anesthesia. For distal upper-extremity injuries, we recommend the supraclavicular brachial plexus block.

Integration into Clinical Practice

The ultrasound-guided interscalene nerve block is an excellent block for proximal upper-extremity injuries including shoulder/deltoid burns, lacerations, shoulder dislocations, and proximal humerus fractures.

Evidence

In 2008, Dr. Stone et al., in a small prospective study, showed that interscalene block decreased length of stay when compared to procedural sedation for upper-extremity emergencies [11]. Furthermore, in 2012, a study done by Dr. Blaivas et al. determined an interscalene block decreased length of stay in patients with shoulder dislocation compared to procedural sedation [12].

Key Points

- Interscalene blockade is useful for procedures around the shoulder and upper arm.
- The lateral-to-medial insertion is often chosen to prevent injury to the phrenic nerve, which is typically located anteriorly to the anterior scalene.
- Caution should be taken with patients with pulmonary dysfunction as the interscalene block causes ipsilateral phrenic nerve paralysis.

Ultrasound-Guided Supraclavicular Nerve Block

Anatomy

The supraclavicular brachial plexus block is performed in the supraclavicular fossa. At this location (adjacent to the subclavian artery), the distal trunks of the brachial plexus remain superficial and carry both motor and sensory innervations to the entire upper extremity except for the uppermost medial sensation of the arm (T2, intercostobrachial nerve). Furthermore, the suprascapular nerve and axillary nerve have both branched off the brachial plexus in the supraclavicular fossa – making this block not ideal for proximal upper-extremity injuries.

Indications

This ultrasound-guided supraclavicular brachial plexus block can be used for any injury affecting the upper extremity distal to the shoulder/proximal humerus. Common emergency medicine indications include mid- to distal humeral fractures, elbow dislocations or fractures, forearm wounds or fractures, and distal radius fractures.

Contraindications

Transient, ipsilateral phrenic nerve paralysis has been reported to occur in up to 50% of patients that received a supraclavicular nerve block without ultrasound guidance [13]. Better needle targeting and administration of lower volumes of anesthetic with ultrasound should minimize this complication. Again, we recommend proceeding with caution among patients with chronic lung pathology, such as severe COPD, restrictive lung disease, and severe obstructive sleep apnea. Because of the superficial nature of the brachial plexus in the supraclavicular fossa, there is a greater theoretical risk of iatrogenic pneumothorax. Along with determining the location of the pleura during the survey scan, clear needle tip visualization during the entire procedure will greatly reduce the rate of iatrogenic pneumothoraces. A supraclavicular nerve block should not be performed in any upper-extremity injury with a risk for vascular injury, preexisting neurologic injury, or high risk for compartment syndrome.

Equipment/Probe Selection

A high-frequency linear transducer should be used for the supraclavicular block. Based on body habitus and surface anatomy landmarks, at minimum a 21–25-gauge 1.5-inch needle can be used. For patients with large body habitus, a 20–22-gauge 3.5-inch spinal needle may be needed.

Preparation/Pre-procedural Evaluation

The patient should be placed on a cardiac monitor and positioned either in a supine position or a semi-upright position. Rotate the head 30° away from the affected side, and place either a small pillow or towel under the affected shoulder to maximize the surface area of the supraclavicular fossa. The ultrasound should be placed on the opposite side of the nerve block in clear view of the operator.

A survey scan should be performed. First, place the probe in a transverse orientation in the supraclavicular fossa parallel to the clavicle with the probe marker pointing to the patient's right (Fig. 9.15). Fan the probe caudally until the pulsating subclavian artery is identified. The brachial plexus will be located lateral to the subclavian artery and sonographically appear as a "cluster of grapes" or "honeycombed." The first rib will be deep to the subclavian artery and appear as a linear hyperechoic structure. Immediately below the first rib will be the parietal lung pleura with lung sliding. Next, place the color Doppler box over the brachial plexus to ensure no vascular structures are running with the plexus. The transverse cervical artery or dorsal scapular artery can run in the vicinity of the brachial plexus, and identification during the survey scan can prevent inadvertent vascular puncture.

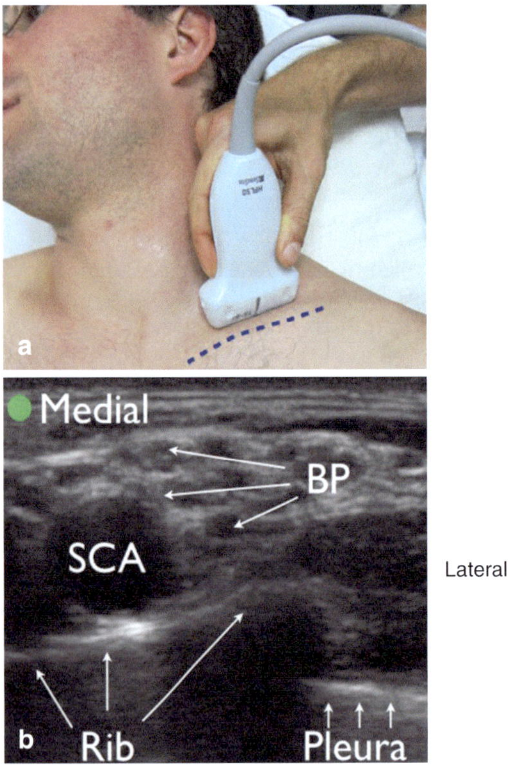

Fig. 9.15 (**a**) Correct patient and probe positioning to perform a supraclavicular nerve block with the linear probe in the supraclavicular fossa just above the clavicle (dotted line). (**b**) Ultrasound landmarks in the supraclavicular fossa including the (i) subclavian artery (SCA), (ii) brachial plexus (BP), (iii) first rib, and (iv) lung pleura

Procedure

We recommend an in-plane lateral-to-medial approach for the novice sonographer. An anesthetic skin wheel should be placed at the lateral aspect of the transducer in conjunction with the survey scan. Based on body habitus and patient position, either a 21–25-gauge 1.5-inch needle or a 20–22-gauge 3.5-inch needle is inserted lateral and in plane with the transducer at a 20–30° angle to the skin surface (Fig. 9.16). Using the in-plane

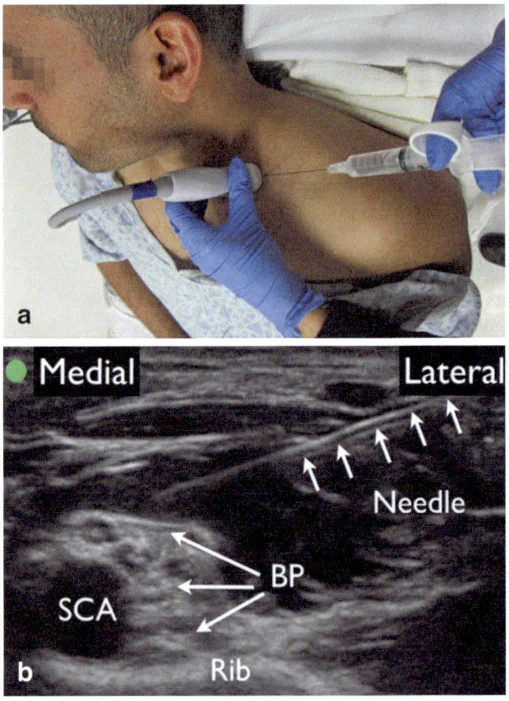

Fig. 9.16 (**a**) Appropriate ultrasound probe and needle placement for supraclavicular nerve block with (**b**) successful deposition of local anesthetic surrounding the brachial plexus (BP) with visualized in-plane needle, first rib, and subclavian artery (SCA)

technique, the needle should be advanced slowly until reaching the lateral border of the brachial plexus. Small aliquots of 1–3 ml of local anesthetic should be delivered to ensure appropriate needle position and ultrasound visualization of the anesthetic spreading around the brachial plexus. A successful block can be completed with approximately 20–30 ml of local anesthetic in total.

Complications

The brachial plexus in the supraclavicular fossa lies in close proximity to vascular structures as well as lung pleura. First, ultrasound guidance ensures appropriate needle placement minimizing the risk of vascular puncture. Furthermore, the placement of color Doppler is necessary to ensure that the transverse cervical artery or dorsal scapular artery is not running alongside the brachial plexus. Second, the lung pleura is extremely close to the brachial plexus. A very flat angle approach is necessary to minimize the risk of a pneumothorax. Ultrasound guidance will ensure appropriate needle approach. Furthermore, appropriate patient positioning is necessary to ensure the operator can enter with a flat needle angle. Third, while not as prevalent as the interscalene nerve block, transient ipsilateral Horner's syndrome can occur. Ultrasound needle targeting allows for a more precise block with smaller volumes of local anesthetic, minimizing the risk of sympathetic nerve blockade. Fourth, ipsilateral phrenic nerve paralysis occurs in 50% of patients. You should practice caution when performing this block on patients with poor pulmonary reserve.

Pearls/Pitfalls

The ultrasound-guided supraclavicular nerve block is extremely superficial with close proximity to the lung apices and subclavian artery. Appropriate patient positioning ensures a flat needle angle of approach to reach the lateral border of the brachial plexus minimizing the risk of vascular puncture or pneumothorax. Also, novice providers find it difficult to initially locate the brachial plexus. Tilting the ultrasound probe caudal can help with sonographic visualization. Furthermore, tracking the brachial plexus up and down the supraclavicular fossa to the interscalene groove can help appreciate the entire course of the brachial plexus.

Integration into Clinical Practice

The ultrasound-guided supraclavicular nerve block is an excellent block for injuries of the mid/distal humerus, elbow, forearm, and wrist. Because of the clear ultrasonographic anatomy and frequency of upper-extremity injuries, we believe that the ultrasound-guided supraclavicular brachial plexus block is an invaluable tool for the practicing emergency physician. Ultrasound guidance has greatly reduced the fear of accidental puncture of adjacent structures (lung apices and subclavian artery) and allowed integration of this very useful single injection block into clinical emergency medicine practice.

Evidence

In 2009, Perlas et al. demonstrated ultrasound-guided supraclavicular nerve blocks were safe and effective for upper-extremity injuries [14]. Ultrasound-guided supraclavicular nerve block has also been shown to be effective and safe in pediatric patients and was faster to perform compared to infraclavicular blocks [15].

Key Points

- Supraclavicular blockade is useful for emergency procedures of the upper extremity distal to the shoulder/proximal humerus.
- Given the superficial nature of this block with close proximity to the lung and vascular structures, clear needle tip visualization during the entire procedure should be performed to minimize the risk of pneumothorax and vascular puncture.

Ultrasound-Guided Superficial Cervical Plexus Nerve Block

Anatomy

The superficial cervical plexus (SCP) originates from the anterior rami of the first four cervical nerves and gives rise to four terminal branches – lesser occipital (C2), greater auricular (C2 and C3), transverse cervical (C2 and C3), and supraclavicular (C3 and C4) nerves. Collectively, the SCP provides purely sensory innervation to the skin and superficial structures of the anterolateral neck, the lateral occiput, and the sections of the ear and shoulder (Fig. 9.17). All four of these branches emerge at the midpoint of the posterior border of the sternocleidomastoid (SCM) muscle (Fig. 9.18). The deep cervical plexus is formed by the posterior rami of C1–C5 and is a purely motor plexus supplying most of the muscles of the neck as well as forming the phrenic nerve. The cervical plexus runs in the cervical nerve pathway formed by the sternocleidomastoid fascia anteriorly and paravertebral fascia posteriorly [16].

Indications

SCP innervation includes the auricle of the ear, the acromioclavicular joint, and the clavicle, all commonly injured structures, otherwise difficult to anesthetize. The SCP also provides partial innervation to deeper structures in the anterolateral neck including the carotid artery and internal jugular vein, which are more completely blocked by the deep cervical plexus. The ultrasound-guided SCP block can be used for patients with clavicle fractures, for field anesthesia prior to placing ultrasound-guided internal jugular central venous catheters and repair of ear lobe injuries, and for incision and drainage of superficial neck abscesses [17–20].

Contraindications

The SCP is made up of purely sensory branches of the cervical nerves, and care should be taken to perform the block at the appropriate cervical level (C4) with small aliquots of anesthetic under ultrasound guidance. Although there is a low risk of an inadvertent deep cervical plexus block causing phrenic nerve anesthesia and resulting in ipsilateral hemidiaphragm paralysis, the clinician should be aware of this potential complication [21, 22]. Care should be taken in patients with moderate-to-severe pulmonary dysfunction, and operators should be aware of this very small, but real, possibility.

Patient Positioning

This block is typically performed with the patient either in a supine position with the head turned or

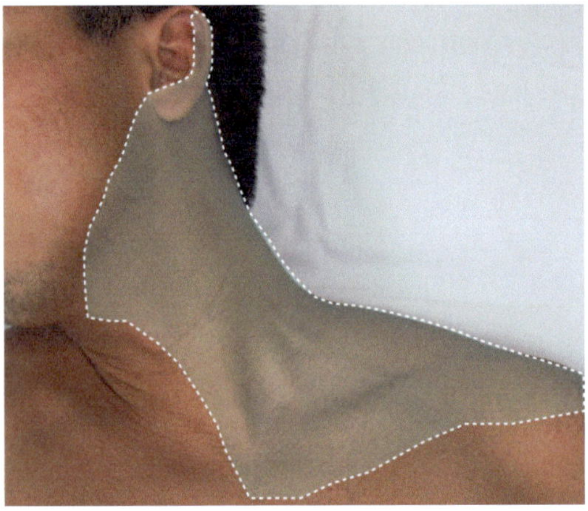

Fig. 9.17 Sensory distribution of the superficial cervical plexus

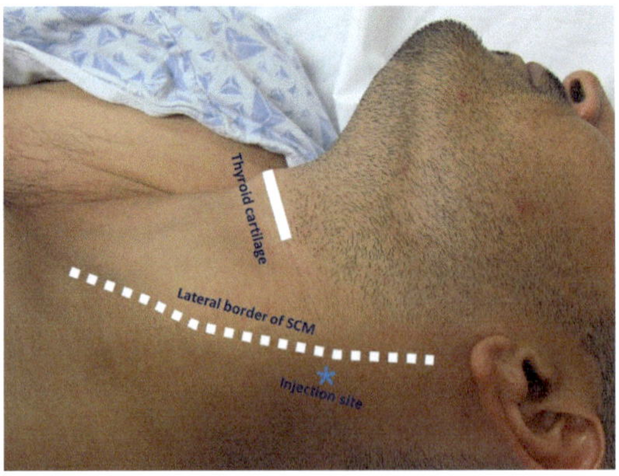

Fig. 9.18 Injection site (∗) on the neck along the lateral border of sternocleidomastoid (SCM) muscle

in a decubitus position with the side being blocked facing anteriorly (Fig. 9.19). This facilitates operator access and creates a flatter surface on which to place the probe to minimize undesired movement. Like other ultrasound-guided blocks, the ultrasound system will be contralateral to the patient, allowing the patient and the operator a clear view of the ultrasound screen.

Equipment/Probe Selection

A high-frequency linear probe should be used to image the SCP in the anterolateral neck. We recommend a 20- to 23-gauge 1.5-inch needle and a 10-ml syringe filled with local anesthetic. A 3.5-inch needle may be necessary in very obese patients.

Survey Scan

Place a linear high-frequency probe on the anterior neck at the level of the thyroid cartilage (probe marker pointing medially – toward the thyroid). At this level, locate familiar anatomy (internal jugular vein, carotid artery, thyroid, and sternocleidomastoid muscle). Slowly move the transducer cephalad to the superior pole of the thyroid (approximately the C4 level) and then laterally until the SCM muscle tapers to a beak. The SCP will be directly below the SCM muscle and just above the levator scapulae muscle at this level and will appear as a row of small hypoechoic ovoid structures (Fig. 9.20). Unlike other nerves localized on ultrasound, a clear "honeycomb" pattern will not be discernable, and the goal is to use anesthetic to gently open the space under the SCM muscle at the C4 level. Apply light pressure with the transducer to ensure superficial veins, such as the external jugular vein, are visualized if present. Color Doppler can also be applied to assess for vasculature.

Procedure

Even though the ultrasound-guided SCP block can be performed both out of plane and in plane, we recommend the later for the novice sonographer. Once the SCP is identified, a skin wheal is placed just lateral to the transducer. Enter the skin through the wheal, slowly advancing the needle just under the SCM muscle and into the fascial plane of the SCP. Because of the flat needle entry, the needle tip should be clearly visual-

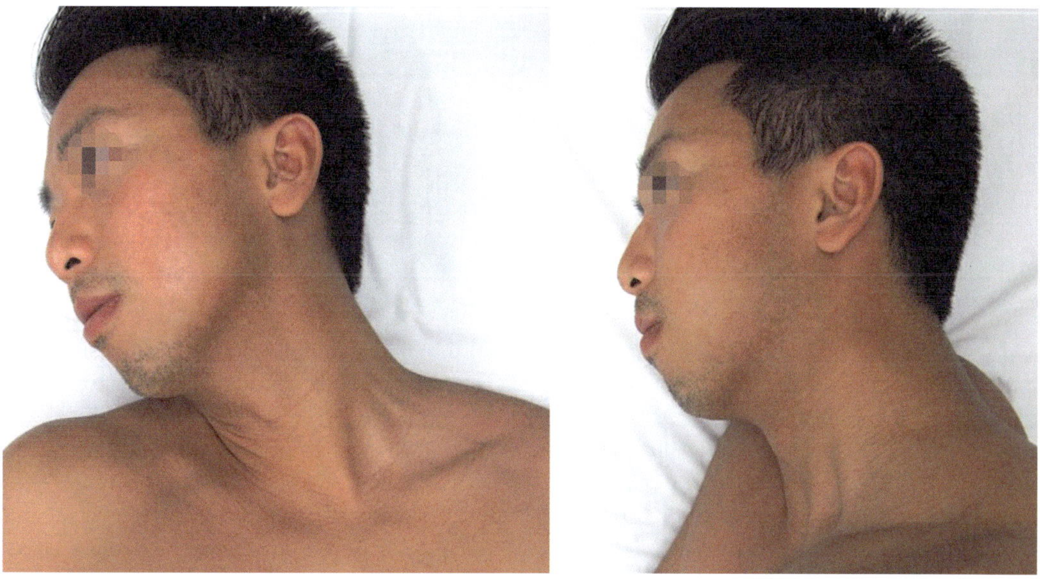

Fig. 9.19 Patient positioning supine and right lateral decubitus positions

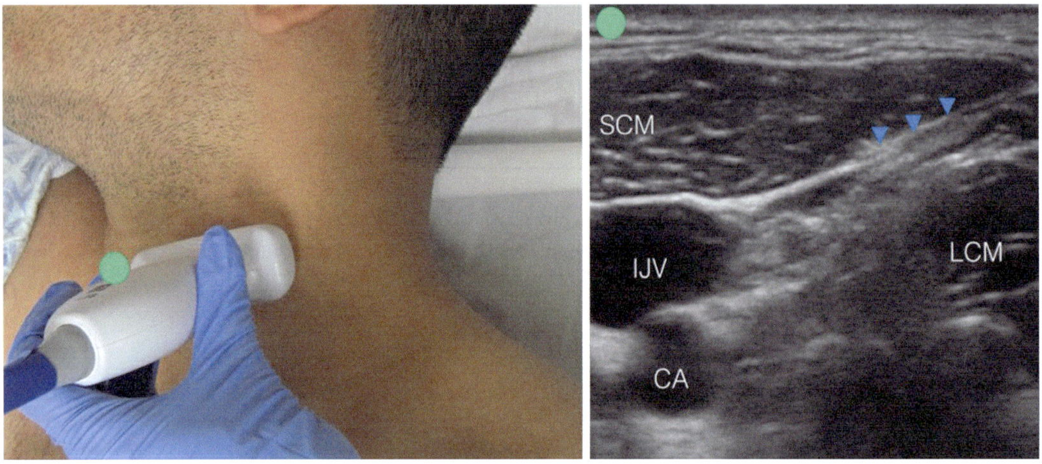

Fig. 9.20 Probe on the neck with corresponding sonoanatomy

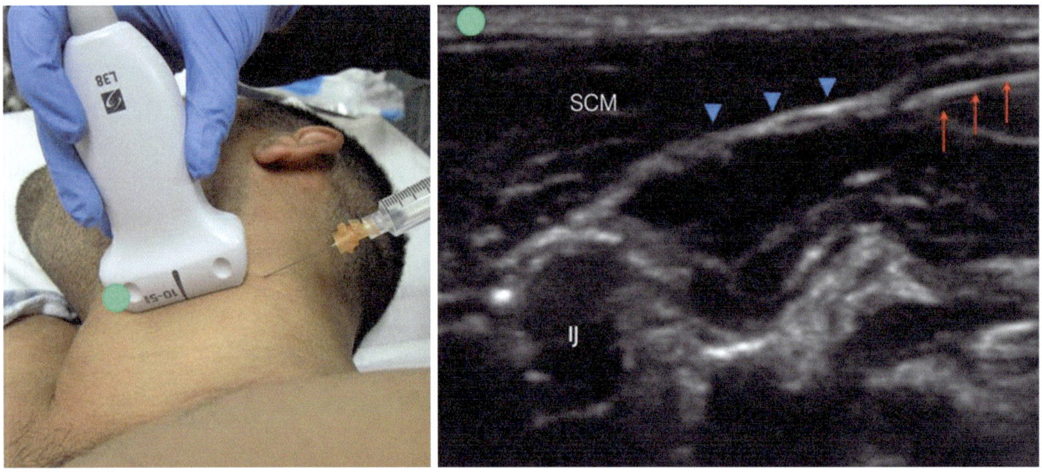

Fig. 9.21 Advancing needle toward superficial cervical plexus

ized as it approaches the SCP (through the skin, to the platysma, and to the prevertebral fascia) (Fig. 9.21). Aspirate to confirm lack of vascular puncture, and then slowly instill 1–2 ml of local anesthetic in the fascial plane between the SCM muscle and LSM. The needle tip should not transverse the midpoint of the SCM muscle to reduce chances of anesthetic traveling into the deep cervical plexus. Continue to deposit up to 8 ml of anesthetic while clear needle tip visualization is maintained.

Complications

Intravascular injection is a possibility because of the close proximity of the neck vasculature and the SCP. A flat needle angle will allow for clear needle tip visualization and reduce chances of either LAST or PNI. Deep cervical blockade can occur if the C4 level (superior pole of the thyroid) is not clearly used as the point of anesthetic injection or large amounts of anesthetic (>10 ml) are used. Transient phrenic nerve paralysis and Horner's syndrome have been reported, and we recommend sonographers confirm the approximate cervical level before anesthetic injection [23].

Pearls/Pitfalls

Using a standard step-wise approach when locating the SCP can be problematic. The sonographer should ensure that they are at the superior pole of the thyroid (C4 cervical level) before instilling anesthetic under the SCM muscle. Also, clear needle tip visualization is mandatory to ensure that anesthetic is not pushed into deeper structures. Though superficial vascular structures are uncommon in the lateral neck, we recommend using color Doppler to ensure a safe needle path prior to deposition of local anesthetic.

Integration into Clinical Practice

The ultrasound-guided SCP block is an ideal block for pain from clavicle fractures, superficial neck abscess incision and drainage, ear lobe injuries, and field block for central line placement. A simplified step-wise method for localization and clear needle visualization will allow this novel procedure to be incorporated into the clinical practice of most clinicians.

Evidence

Dr. Shteif et al., in 2008, described the use of superficial cervical plexus block to drain submandibular and submental abscesses [20]. In 2012, Dr. Herring et al. described superficial cervical plexus block effectiveness in an emergency setting for clavicle fractures [16]. Finally, in 2014, Dr. Ciftci et al. explained how the superficial cervical plexus block was safe and effective for the placement of hemodialysis catheters in children [24].

Key Points

- Superficial cervical block provides anesthesia to the auricle of the ear, the acromioclavicular joint, and the clavicle, all commonly injured structures or otherwise difficult to anesthetize.
- The operator should use a flat angle approach with the needle to ensure no deep cervical blockade.

Ultrasound-Guided Forearm Nerve Blocks

Anatomy

The median, radial, and ulnar nerves are all formed by cords of the brachial plexus. The median nerve arises from the medial and lateral cords, made up by nerve roots C5–T1. It runs down the medial side of the upper arm, crossing over the brachial artery in the antecubital fossa, and coursing anteriorly through the forearm between the flexor digitorum profundus and superficialis muscles. It supplies sensory innervation to the radial aspect of the palm, the volar aspect of the thumb and index, and long and radial aspect of the ring finger and is best visualized and blocked at the mid-volar forearm.

The radial nerve arises from the posterior cord, made up by nerve roots C5–T1. It spirals around the mid-humerus from lateral to medial, coursing anteriorly at the level of the antecubital fossa, and running radially (lateral) to the radial artery through the forearm. It supplies sensory innervation to the radial aspect of the dorsum of the hand, thumb, index finger, long finger, and radial half of the ring finger proximal to the distal interphalangeal joints and is best visualized and blocked at the distal forearm.

The ulnar nerve arises from the medial cord, made up by nerve roots C8–T1. It runs medially from the axilla down to the wrist. In the forearm, it is reliably found on the ulnar (medial) side of the ulnar artery. It supplies sensory innervation to the skin of the dorsal and palmar surfaces of the medial half of the fourth finger and all of the fifth finger and associated areas on the palm. The nerve is best visualized and blocked at the proximal forearm where it distances itself a bit from the ulnar artery [25–27].

Indications

Hand injuries are a common presentation in the emergency department. The median, radial, and ulnar nerves innervate the entirety of the hand distal to the wrist, making forearm nerve blocks ideal for exploration and repair of complex hand lacerations, fractures, burns, abscess drainage, and multiple digital injuries. Knowledge of sensory innervation of each nerve will allow the sonographer to provide targeted anesthesia based on the injury location. Specifically, the ulnar nerve block is ideal for analgesia for boxer's fractures and fourth/fifth metacarpal dislocations. Median nerve blocks are ideal in cases of palmar lacerations, since local anesthesia is often very difficult at this sensitive location. Radial nerve blocks are useful when attempting the dorsum of the hand and thenar eminence abscess drainage and for assessment of injury to the extensor mechanisms of the hand. Clinicians should be aware that forearm nerve blocks do not provide anesthesia to the wrist or forearm [28–30].

Contraindications

Injuries with a potential for compartment syndrome or presence of vascular compromise should not be blocked. Also, patients with either a preexistent or post-traumatic neurapraxia are not candidates for an ultrasound-guided forearm nerve block. Under these circumstances, forearm blocks should only be performed after discussion with consultative services (orthopedics, trauma surgery, hand surgery, etc.).

Equipment/Probe Selection

A high-frequency linear probe should be used. A small-gauge needle, such as a tuberculin, or 25-gauge needle can be used to anesthetize the skin. A 1.5-inch 21–25-gauge needle attached to a 5–10-cc syringe is ideal for the block. We generally use 3–5-ml of anesthetic agent for each forearm nerve.

Survey Scan

For the median and radial nerves, place the patient in a seated position with the arm supinated and externally rotated. For the ulnar nerve, hyper-supination facilitates visualization and approach. We recommend using a stand to support the forearm and placing the ultrasound screen across the affected extremity. Proper patient and equipment setup will allow the operator to be able to view the injection site and ultrasound screen with minimal head movement (Fig. 9.22).

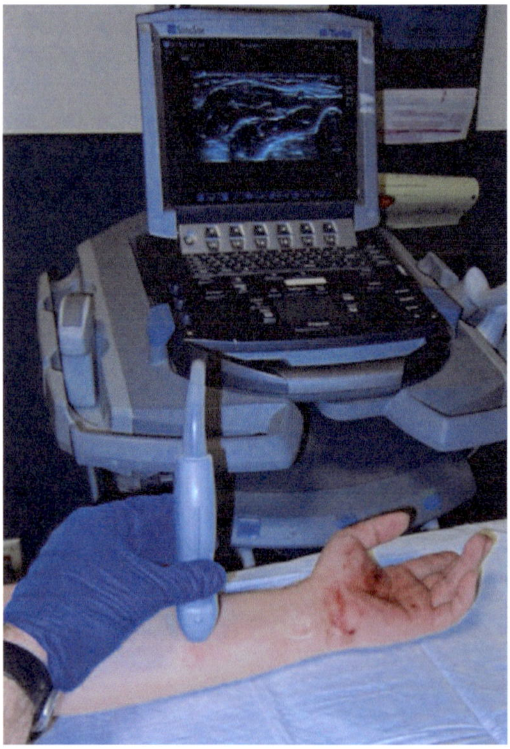

Fig. 9.22 Patient and ultrasound machine positioning

To locate the median nerve, place the ultrasound probe in a transverse orientation with the probe marker to the right of the patient. Start in the distal forearm (wrist crease) and scan proximally, looking for a honeycomb structure that lies in the fascial plane between the flexor digitorum superficialis and profundus muscles (Fig. 9.23). Also, slightly tilting the probe in a distal to proximal manner will allow for better visualization of the nerve (termed anisotropy). After the median nerve is located, inject a 1-cc lidocaine skin wheal 0.5 cm lateral to the probe for an in-plane nerve block.

For the radial nerve, place the ultrasound probe in a transverse orientation with the probe marker to the patient's right left. Start in the distal forearm (wrist crease) and look for the radial artery. The radial nerve lies on the radial aspect of the radial artery and is often difficult to identify at the wrist crease. Sliding the transducer proximally (tracing the radial artery) can help identify the small hyperechoic honeycomb-like structure that will be the radial nerve (Fig. 9.24). Unlike the ulnar nerve that commonly separates from the ulnar artery in the proximal forearm, the radial nerve commonly sits adjacent to the radial artery, making clear visualization difficult for the novice sonographer. Slightly tilting the probe in a distal to proximal manner will allow for better visualization of the nerve. After the radial nerve is located, inject a 1-ml lidocaine skin wheal 0.5 cm lateral to the probe.

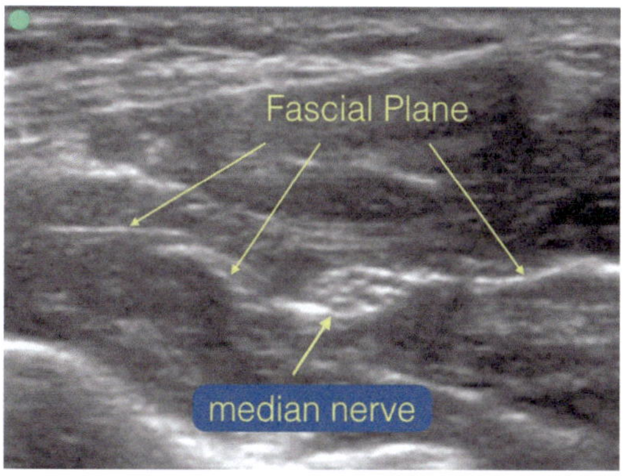

Fig. 9.23 B-mode image of median nerve in the forearm between the flexor digitorum superficialis and profundus muscles

For the ulnar nerve, place the ultrasound probe in a transverse orientation with the probe marker to the right of the patient. Start in the distal forearm (wrist crease) and locate the ulnar artery. The ulnar nerve lies on the ulnar aspect of the ulnar artery. Scanning proximally, at approximately the mid-forearm, the ulnar nerve will often separate from the ulnar artery, allowing for an ideal location for injection while minimizing risk for inadvertent intravascular injection (Fig. 9.25). Again, slightly tilting the probe in a distal to proximal manner will allow for better visualization of the nerve. After the ulnar nerve is located, inject a 1-cc lidocaine skin wheal 0.5 cm medial to the probe [31].

Procedure

For novice sonographers, we recommend an in-plane technique for the procedure, so that the needle tip can be visualized during the entire procedure. Once the provider has become more comfortable with needling technique, it may be easier to perform ultrasound-guided forearm

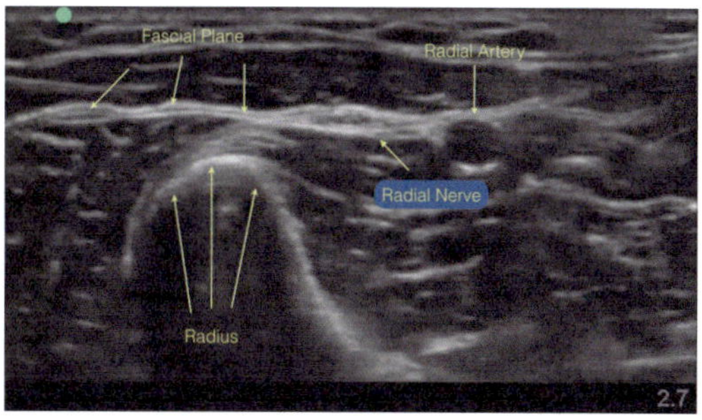

Fig. 9.24 B-mode image of radial nerve radial to radial artery

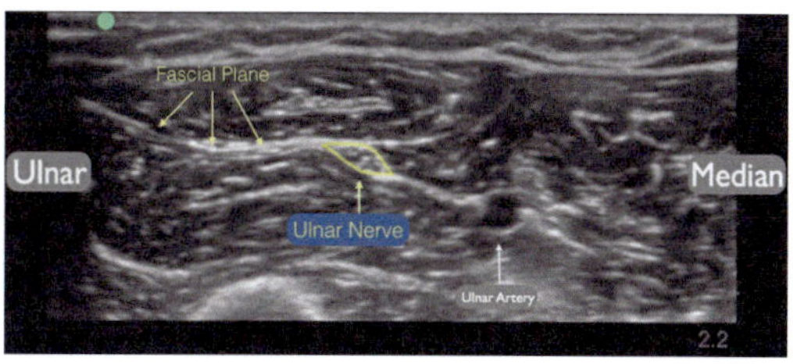

Fig. 9.25 B-mode image of ulnar nerve to ulnar artery

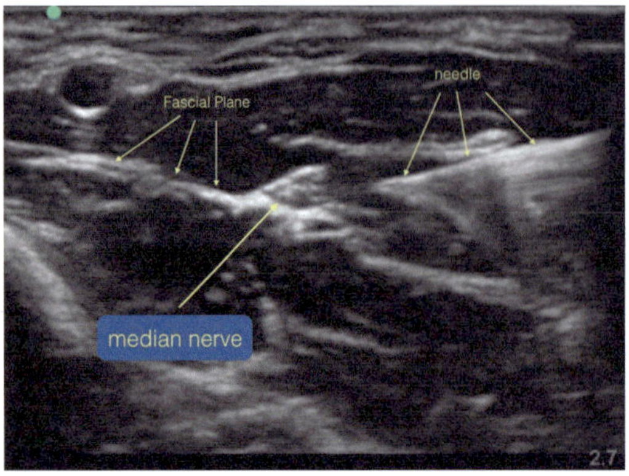

Fig. 9.26 Needle advancing toward the median nerve is seen in this B-mode image

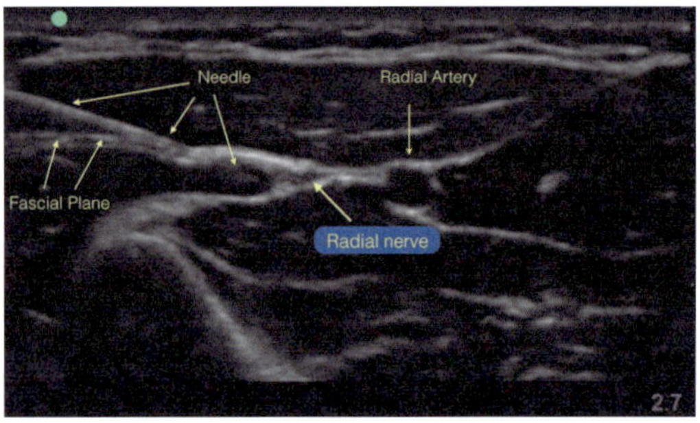

Fig. 9.27 Needle advancing toward the radial nerve is visualized

nerve blocks out of plane. This is particularly true for the ulnar nerve, which tends to be difficult to anesthetize if the patient cannot hyper-supinate the arm.

For in-plane technique, from the location of the skin wheal, enter the skin at an approximately 30-degree angle. Advance the needle in 1–2 cm increments, ensuring that the entire needle including the tip is visualized. Direct the needle tip to the fascial plane just adjacent to the targeted nerve, aspirate to ensure a lack of vascular puncture, and inject a small amount of anesthetic (0.5–1 ml). For the median nerve, the fascial plane essentially surrounds the nerve (Fig. 9.26). For the radial and ulnar nerves, the fascial plane lies on top of the nerves (Figs. 9.27 and 9.28). If anechoic fluid is not visualized on the ultrasound screen with the test injection, stop the procedure, and move the ultrasound transducer until the needle tip is clearly visualized. Once appropriate needle tip placement is achieved, the remainder of local anesthetic can be safely deposited. With experience, the operator will be able to encircle the nerve in anechoic anesthetic fluid (Figs. 9.29, 9.30 and 9.31).

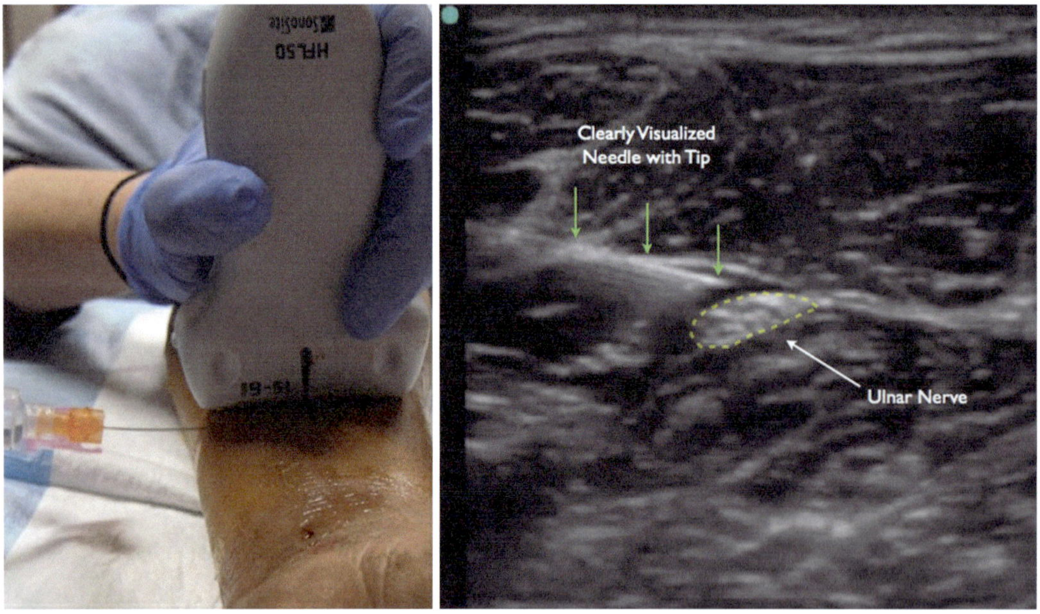

Fig. 9.28 A needle advancing toward the ulnar nerve is seen along with reverberation artifacts

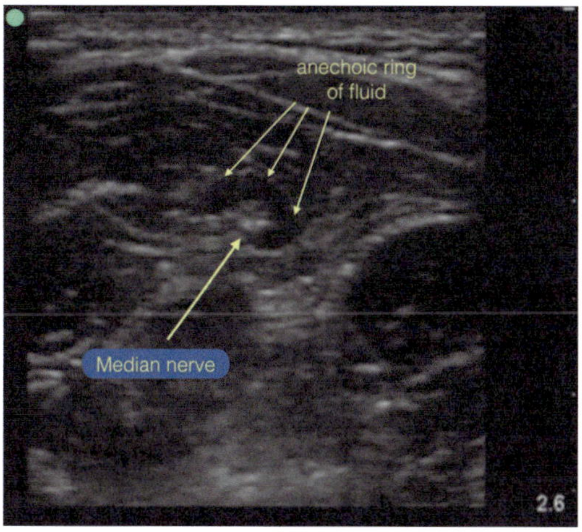

Fig. 9.29 Anechoic circle around median nerve from local anesthetic spread

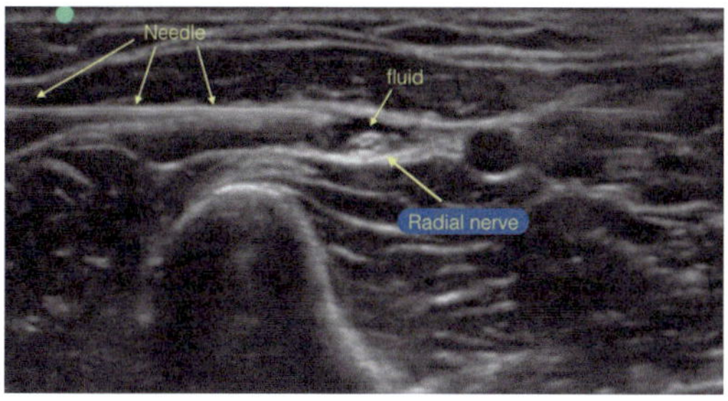

Fig. 9.30 Anechoic circle surrounding radial nerve from local anesthetic infiltration

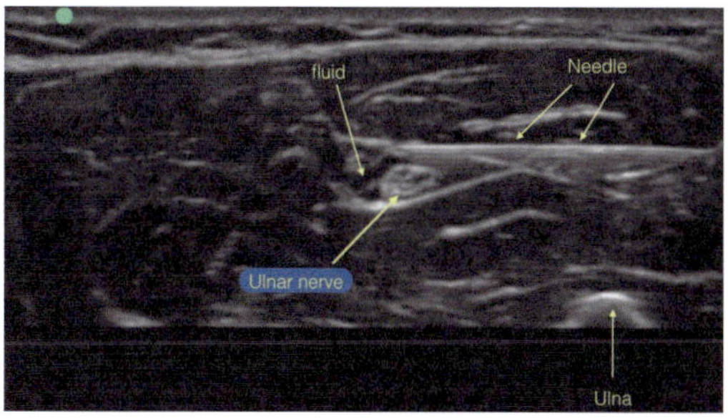

Fig. 9.31 Anechoic region adjacent to the ulnar nerve from local anesthetic spread

For out-of-plane technique, move the probe so the targeted nerve lies directly under the middle of the probe. Visualizing the nerve with a center of screen marker (M-mode line in systems that do not have this feature) may reduce the number of

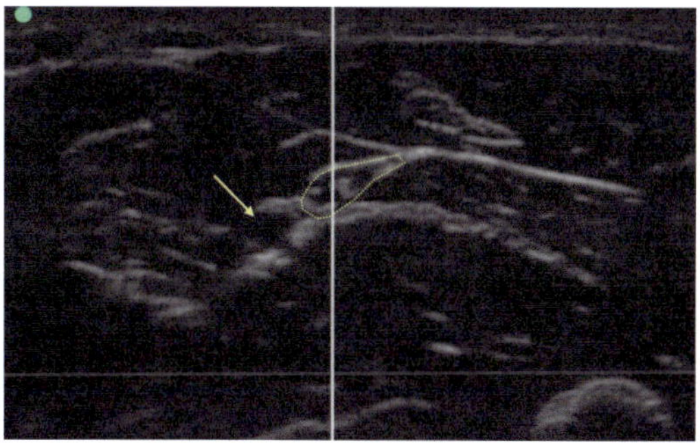

Fig. 9.32 The ulnar nerve (outlined) with M-mode (white line corresponding to middle of probe). Arrow indicates the ulnar artery

needle redirections (Fig. 9.32). Enter the skin adjacent to the midline of the transducer at a steep angle (75–80°), and note tissue displacement as the needle advances toward the nerve. By subtle fanning the probe from distal to proximal, the hyperechoic needle tip can be visualized (Fig. 9.33). Direct the needle tip to the fascial plane just adjacent to the targeted nerve, aspirate to ensure a lack of vascular puncture, and inject a small amount of anesthetic (0.5–1 ml). Once appropriate needle tip placement is achieved by visualizing an anechoic spread in the intended location, the remainder of local anesthetic can be safely deposited. The out-of-plane technique does not allow the sonographer to visualize the needle tip during the procedure, making the procedure more difficult for the novice sonographer. We recommend this technique when vascular structures are not posterior to the target nerve [31].

Complications

Potential complications are similar in this block as in others, including LAST and PNI. Sonographers should make every effort to clearly visualize the needle tip during the entire procedure during the in-plane technique.

Pearls/Pitfalls

Once the sonographer becomes comfortable with needling technique and visualizing the forearm

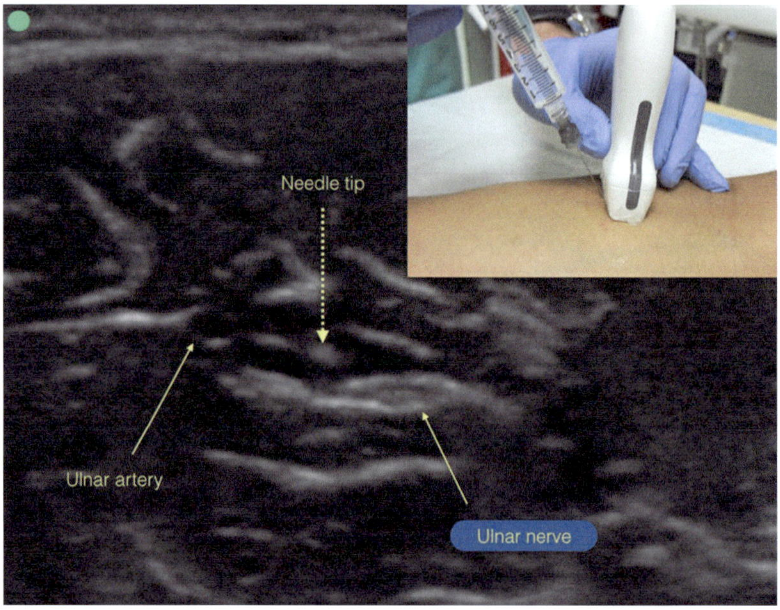

Fig. 9.33 Out-of-plane approach to the ulnar nerve – hyperechoic needle tip visualized

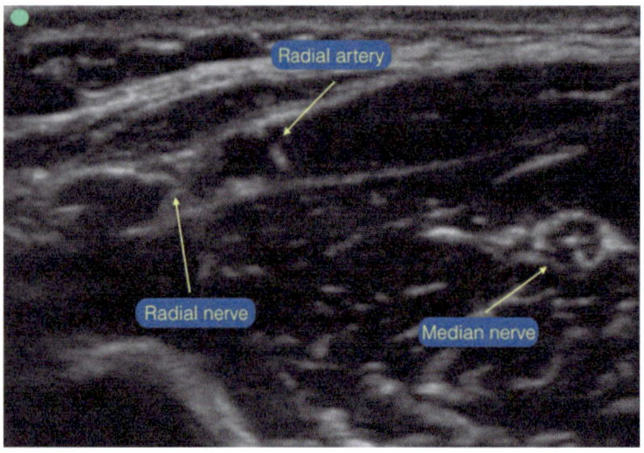

Fig. 9.34 B-mode image of both radial and median nerves in the forearm

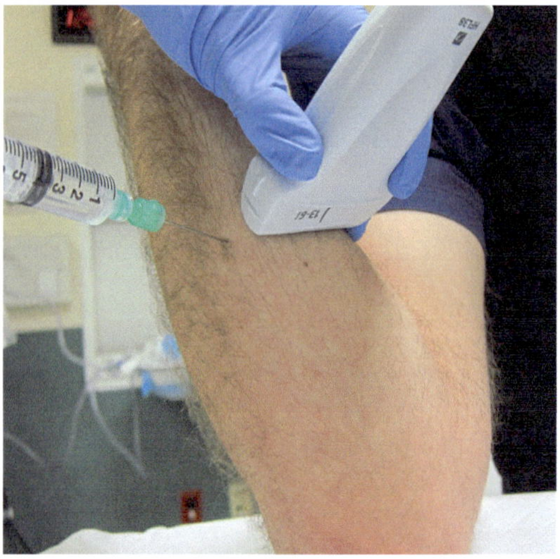

Fig. 9.35 Approach to the ulnar nerve with the elbow flexed

nerves, it is possible to block both the medial and radial nerves with one skin puncture. This is achieved by simply changing the angle of the needle and advancing from radial nerve (lateral) to median nerve (medial) (Fig. 9.34).

The ulnar nerve can be the most difficult to block due to its location on the somewhat steep angle of the medial side of the forearm. In patients who are unable to hyper-supinate their forearm, flexion of the elbow maintaining the arm in the anatomic position will allow access to the ulnar nerve with an in-plane technique (Fig. 9.35).

Evidence

In 2006, a study by Dr. Liebmann et al. showed the feasibility of ultrasound-guided forearm nerve blocks for hand procedures in the ED [31]. Furthermore, Dr. Frenkel et al. in 2015 reported on the use of forearm nerve blocks for pain control among pediatric hand injuries [32]. In 2016, Dr. Sohoni et al. demonstrated ultrasound guidance was more effective at regional blockade than landmark-based approach [33].

Key Points

- A forearm nerve block can be performed to the median, radial, and/or ulnar nerve to provide anesthesia to a portion or entirety of the distal hand and wrist.
- Forearm nerve block does not provide anesthesia to the forearm or wrist.
- If needing to block all three nerves in the forearm, the out-of-plane needle technique is technically easier to perform due to patient positioning.

Ultrasound-Guided Femoral Nerve Block

Anatomy

The femoral nerve is a branch of the lumbar plexus. It arises from the L1 to L4 ventral rami and descends toward the thigh. The femoral nerve block is performed at the inguinal crease at the level of the femoral canal. At this level, the femoral nerve is located lateral to the femoral artery directly beneath the fascia iliaca and superficial to the iliopsoas muscle.

Indications

The femoral nerve provides sensory innervation to the femur, hip joint, antero-medial thigh, knee, and medial aspect of the lower leg. The ultrasound-guided femoral nerve block (FNB) is ideal for proximal lower-extremity injuries (to the knee and above). Specifically, the femoral nerve block is an excellent adjuvant pain control agent for intertrochanteric and subtrochanteric hip fractures, femur fractures, patellar injuries, and significant wounds over the thigh or medial aspect of the lower leg from the knee to foot. The hip itself has a complex innervation pattern that involves the femoral, obturator, and sciatic nerves, and an ultrasound-guided FNB will not provide surgical anesthesia for a hip fracture. However, an ultrasound-guided FNB is an ideal tool in a multimodal pain strategy to help minimize reliance on intravenous opioids and their well-recognized complications of apnea, confusion, and hypotension, especially in elderly patients [34].

Contraindications

An ultrasound-guided FNB should not be performed on any injury to the lower extremity that is at high risk for compartment syndrome. While the risk of thigh compartment syndrome is exceedingly rare, the risk is slightly increased among patients with crush injuries and/or injuries with vascular compromise [35]. Furthermore, the femoral nerve block should not be performed for injuries or wounds with preexisting or post-injury neuropraxia. Similar to all nerve blocks, for patients unable to provide consent, hemodynamic compromise or allergy to local anesthetic should be excluded. The decision to perform a femoral nerve block should always be in conjunction with consultative services (orthopedic surgery, trauma surgery, etc.) when possible [36].

Equipment/Probe Selection

A high-frequency linear transducer (with a large footprint if possible) should be used for the femoral block. Typically a 20–22-gauge 3.5-inch spinal needle can be used. Standard nerve block materials should be used and are discussed in the introduction chapter.

Preparation/Pre-procedure Evaluation

The patient should be placed in the supine position and attached to a cardiac monitor. The ultrasound system should be placed on the contralateral side of the affected lower extremity to allow the operator easy visualization of the screen during the entire procedure.

A survey scan should be performed. First, expose the groin identifying the proximal thigh and inguinal crease (Fig. 9.36). Second, place the linear transducer in a transverse orientation in the inguinal crease with the indicator pointing to the patient's right. Third, identify appropriate landmarks (Fig. 9.37). The femoral artery (FA) is easily identified as a pulsatile vascular (anechoic) structure familiar to clinicians who have performed point-of-care deep venous thrombosis (DVT) studies. The femoral vein (FV) is just medial, non-pulsatile, and easily collapsible with mild to moderate pressure. We recommend finding the femoral nerve just above the bifurcation of the femoral artery and the profunda femoris artery. The femoral nerve will be lateral to the femoral artery and appear as a hyperechoic, "honeycombed" triangular structure. Above the femoral nerve structure will be the fascia iliaca, and below the femoral nerve bundle will be the iliopsoas muscle. In order to improve ultrasonographic visualization of the femoral nerve, fan the transducer caudally so that the angle of the ultrasound beam is perpendicular to the nerve fibers (termed anisotropy). The typical location and triangular characteristics of the femoral nerve should be used for identification and needle targeting. After needle insertion, small aliquots of either normal saline or local anesthetic will "open up" the potential space and allow for clear visualization of the femoral nerve.

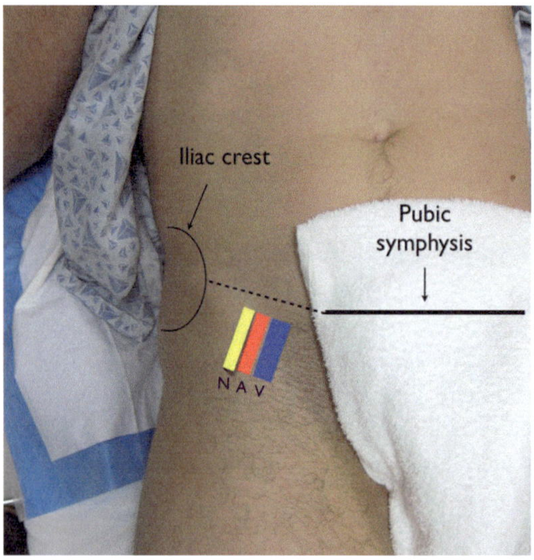

Fig. 9.36 Surface landmarks for femoral nerve block including the iliac crest laterally and the pubic symphysis medially with the femoral nerve (N), femoral artery (A), and femoral vein (V)

Procedure

We recommend the in-plane, lateral-to-medial approach for the novice clinician in order to allow for clear needle tip visualization. First, identify the appropriate location for needle insertion based on your survey scan (Fig. 9.38). The needle insertion will be approximately 1 cm lateral to the linear probe. Second, place a small skin wheal of local anesthetic at the site for needle insertion. Third, enter the skin with a 20–22-gauge 3.5-inch needle at a flat angle to ensure clear visualization of the needle tip. Fourth, using an in-plane (lateral to medial) approach, slowly advance the needle tip under the fascia iliaca and just lateral to the femoral nerve. Once under the fascia iliaca, inject small aliquots (1–2 ml) of either saline or local anesthetic. With appropriate needle placement, the aliquots should displace the fascia iliaca upward. This technique helps open the potential fascial planes and better visualize the femoral nerve bundle (especially difficult in obese or older patients). With anechoic spread of anesthetic or normal saline, needle tip repositioning is often easier and allows slow advancement of the needle tip closer to the nerve bundle. Finally, after optimal needle placement is achieved, inject in small aliquot of 3–5 ml of local anesthetic for a total of 20–30 ml. A successful block is evident by hypoechoic local anesthetic layering under the fascia iliaca and above the femoral nerve.

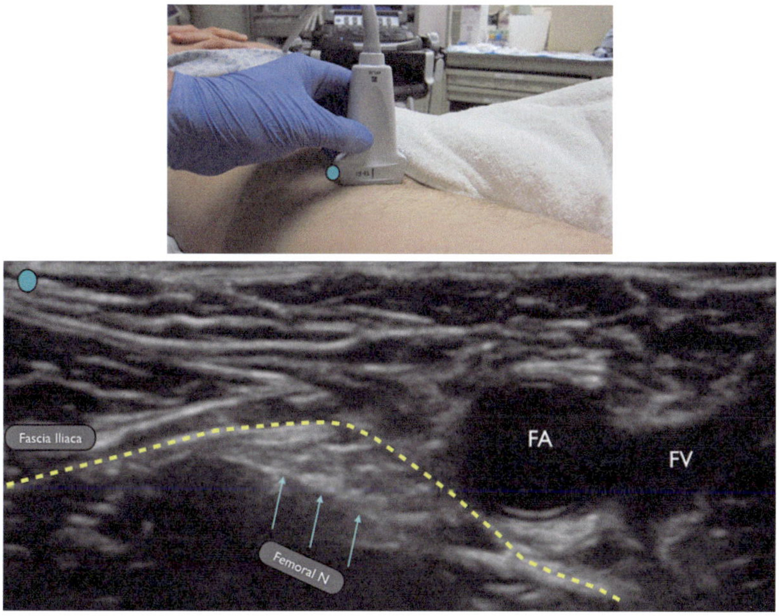

Fig. 9.37 (**a**) Appropriate placement of ultrasound probe for femoral nerve block with (**b**) ultrasound identification of the femoral nerve inferior to the fascia iliac and lateral to the femoral artery (FA) and femoral vein (FV)

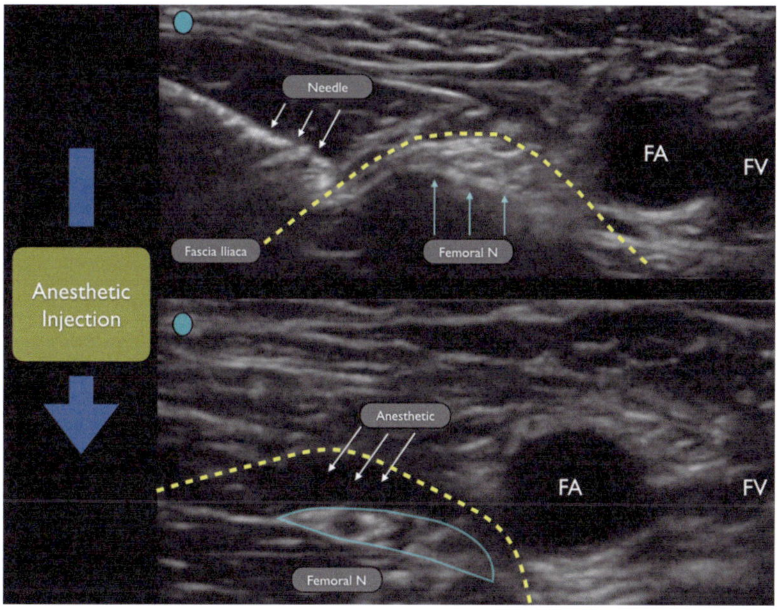

Fig. 9.38 (**a**) Correct positioning of ultrasound probe and needle for femoral nerve block and (**b**) appropriate in-plane visualization of needle below the fascia iliaca and depositing local anesthetic that is surrounding femoral nerve (FN) and far away from both the femoral artery (FA) and femoral vein (FV)

Complications

The femoral nerve is adjacent to the femoral artery and vein. Risk of vascular puncture is possible; however, maintaining sonographic needle tip visualization at all times will reduce the risk of vascular injection. There is a small risk of intraneural injection as well. Ultrasonographic needle tip visualization below the fascia iliaca, but not in the nerve fascicle, will reduce the chance of intraneural injection and associated PNI [37]. If at any point during the block, the needle tip is not visualized, halt anesthetic injection, and adjust your needle and/or probe until clear visualization is again obtained. Specifically, keeping the needle tip 1 cm lateral to the femoral nerve bundle will achieve a successful block and minimize the risk of vascular puncture or intraneural injection.

Pearls/Pitfalls

Femoral nerve blocks should be performed for hip fractures; however, they will not achieve complete/surgical analgesia given the complex innervation of the hip.

While the risk of compartment syndrome of the thigh is exceedingly small, use extreme caution in patients with crush injuries, vascular compromise, or preexisting nerve damage.

Integration into Clinical Practice

The femoral nerve block is a well-proven adjunctive to pain control for hip fractures and femur fractures and can reduce unwanted side effects from intravenous opioids.

Evidence

A study published in 2003 by Dr. Fletcher et al. demonstrated that the femoral nerve block in the ED was a safe and effective method for pain relief for a femoral neck fracture [38]. In 2007, Dr. Mutty et al. determined that the femoral nerve block was safe and effective anesthesia for diaphyseal and distal femoral fractures in the emergency department setting [39]. Dr. Beaudoin et al. in 2013 showed effective pain control and safety profile for ultrasound-guided femoral nerve block for hip fractures when compared to systemic opioids alone [34]. In 2005, Karagiannis et al. found no evidence that a femoral nerve block, in cases of femoral shaft fracture, delayed the diagnosis of compartment syndrome of the thigh [35].

Key Points

- The femoral nerve block is ideal for proximal lower-extremity injuries that are at the knee and more cephalad.
- Ultrasound-guided femoral nerve block is equally effective in providing analgesia for patients with both intracapsular and extracapsular hip fractures.
- Lateral-to-medial approach is recommended to allow for clear needle tip visualization.
- A successful block is evident by hypoechoic local anesthetic solution layering under the fascia iliaca and above the femoral nerve.

Ultrasound-Guided Distal Sciatic Block

Anatomy

The distal sciatic nerve originates from the L4 to S3 nerve roots of the lumbar-sacral plexus. The sciatic nerve initially runs deep in the posterior thigh gradually becoming more superficial as it approaches the popliteal fossa. Just proximal to the popliteal fossa, the sciatic nerve is bound by the semimembranosus and semitendinosus muscles medially and the biceps femoris muscle laterally. The large sciatic nerve bifurcates into the tibial nerve (medial) and the common peroneal nerve (lateral) approximately 7–10 cm proximal to the popliteal fossa. Although the sciatic nerve can be blocked at any location along its course, its superficial position in the region of the popliteal fossa makes this distal location ideal.

Indications

The distal sciatic nerve innervates the majority of the lower extremity below the knee, making it an ideal block for ankle and distal tibial/fibula fractures and injuries to the foot. It does not provide anesthesia to the medial aspect of the lower leg, which is innervated by the saphenous nerve (a distal branch of the femoral nerve).

Contraindications

Any injury that could potentially result in a compartment syndrome is a relative contraindication to performing a distal sciatic nerve block. High-energy injuries, such as a solitary tibial or mid-shaft tibial-fibular fracture, are known to have high rates of developing compartment syndromes. Additionally, crush injuries or any injury with associated vascular compromise should trigger a detailed discussion with consultative services (orthopedics, trauma surgery, etc.) before an ultrasound-guided distal sciatic nerve block in the popliteal fossa is performed.

Patient Positioning

If possible, the patient should be in the prone position, allowing easy access to the popliteal fossa and posterior aspect of the patient's lower extremity (Fig. 9.39a). In patients who are unable to lay prone (e.g., cervical spine immobilization), the affected extremity must be elevated and supported with mild flexion of the knee. This is best achieved by propping the foot with blankets or pillows to allow the ultrasound probe to easily fit between the popliteal fossa and the patient's bed (Fig. 9.39b). Either position will allow for the clinician to block the sciatic nerve in the popliteal fossa, with the prone position being technically much less difficult.

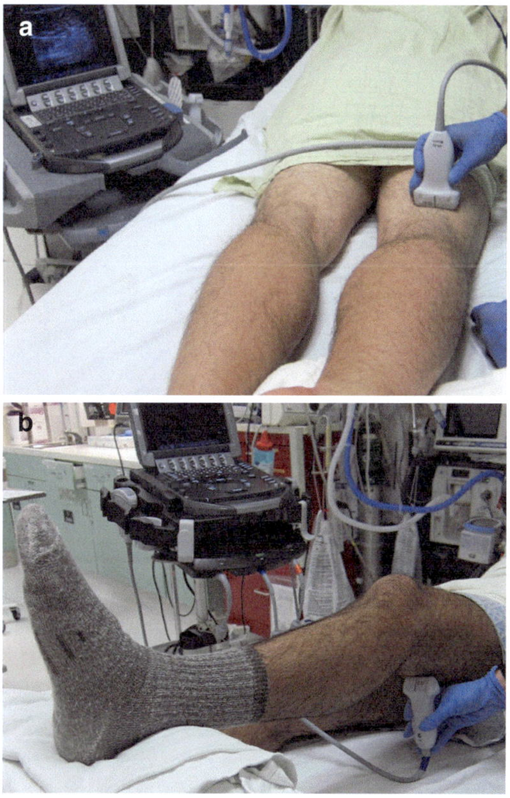

Fig. 9.39 (**a**) Patient positioning prone, which allows easy access to the popliteal fossa. (**b**) Patient positioning supine

Equipment/Probe Selection

A high-frequency linear probe should be used to image the distal sciatic nerve in the popliteal fossa. We recommend a 20- or 22-gauge 9-cm spinal needle to reach the distal sciatic nerve because of its depth and midline location in the popliteal fossa.

Survey Scan

To prepare for the block, start by placing the linear high-frequency probe with the probe marker facing the patient's right side at the popliteal crease and identify the popliteal artery and vein. The tibial nerve is commonly located just superficial to the popliteal vein and appears as a hyperechoic "honeycomb"-like structure (Fig. 9.40). If

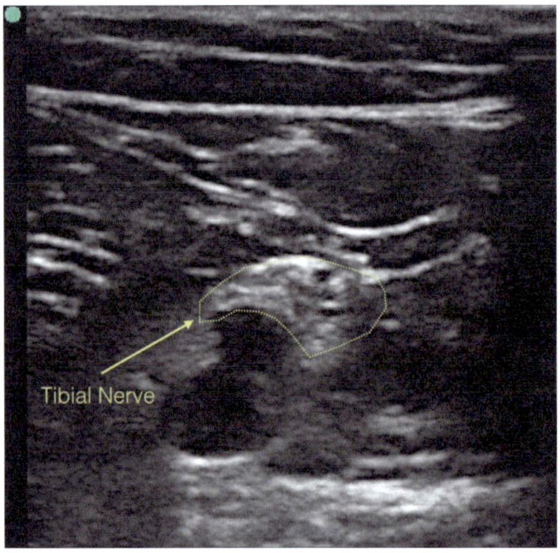

Fig. 9.40 B-mode image of the tibial nerve in the popliteal fossa

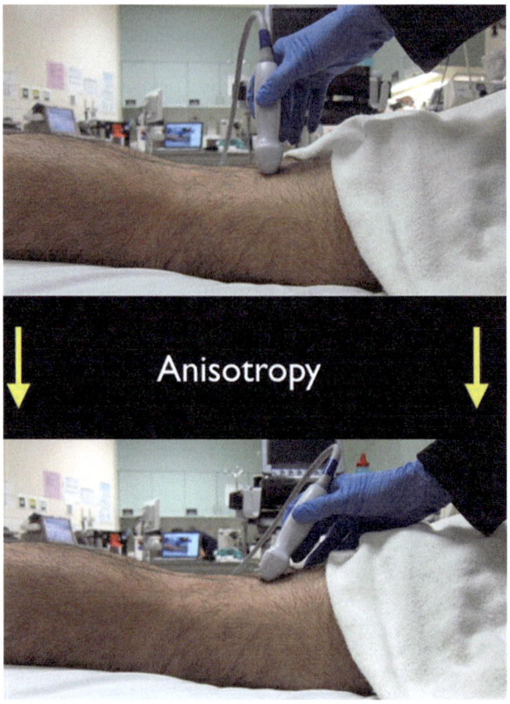

Fig. 9.41 The probe is moved caudally to obtain the most perpendicular axis to the nerve, to overcome anisotropy

you are unable to locate the neural bundle, fan the probe caudally to obtain the most perpendicular axis to the nerve, which allows for better visualization (an ultrasound phenomenon termed anisotropy) (Fig. 9.41). Once the tibial nerve is visualized, follow the nerve proximally until it joins with the common peroneal nerve (lateral) (Fig. 9.42) to form the distal sciatic nerve (Fig. 9.43). The operator should mark this location and note the depth of the nerve.

Procedure

The distal sciatic nerve is often 2–4 cm under the skin surface, making for a steep needle angle if entering the skin just adjacent to the ultrasound transducer (like most other ultrasound-guided nerve blocks). Instead, we recommend measuring the depth of the nerve during the initial survey scan and entering the lateral leg with a flat angle to ensure clear needle visualization. After placing a small skin wheal (on the lateral aspect of the thigh), fill 20 ml of local anesthetic in a syringe attached to a 20–22-gauge 9-cm spinal needle. The more lateral approach and depth of the distal sciatic nerve often necessitate the longer needle for an in-plane distal sciatic nerve block.

Even though some experienced users may prefer the out-of-plane technique, we feel that the in-plane lateral-to-medial approach is both easier and safer for the novice sonographer. Slowly advance the spinal needle maintaining a nearly parallel angle to the probe with an in-plane technique (Fig. 9.44). Since the needle will be entering the lateral thigh, the needle tip will not be visualized immediately (like in other in-plane blocks), and the operator will often have to advance the needle several centimeters until the tip will be seen entering the scanning plane (Fig. 9.45). Attempt to place the needle tip on the superficial edge of the distal sciatic nerve without penetrating the nerve bundle (Fig. 9.46). It is

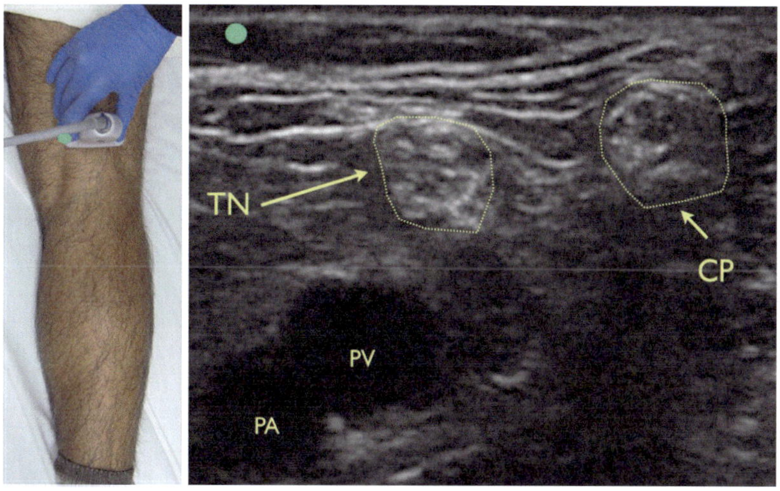

Fig. 9.42 Tibial (TN) and common peroneal (CP) nerves are seen in the near field (popliteal artery (PA) and popliteal vein (PV))

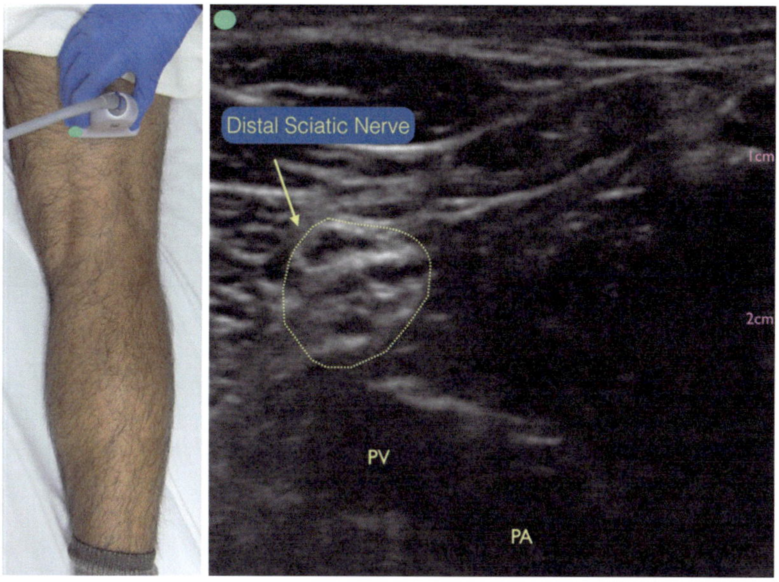

Fig. 9.43 Distal sciatic nerve in the posterior aspect of the thigh above the popliteal fossa (popliteal artery (PA) and popliteal vein (PV))

often difficult in determining whether the needle tip is either in the superficial tissue or the fascial plane of the nerve. Installing small aliquots of either anesthetic or normal saline, and visualizing its spread, can be the discriminatory test to ensure that your needle tip is in the correct location. Once in the correct location, aspirate to confirm lack of vascular puncture, and then slowly inject 2–3 ml aliquots of anesthetic until spread of anechoic fluid is noted to track around the distal sciatic nerve (Fig. 9.47). Simply fanning the probe proximally and distally without moving the needle can be a simple method to confirm tracking of fluid in the fascial plane. We do not recommend novice sonographers placing the needle tip on the inferior aspect of the nerve given its relative proximity to the popliteal vasculature.

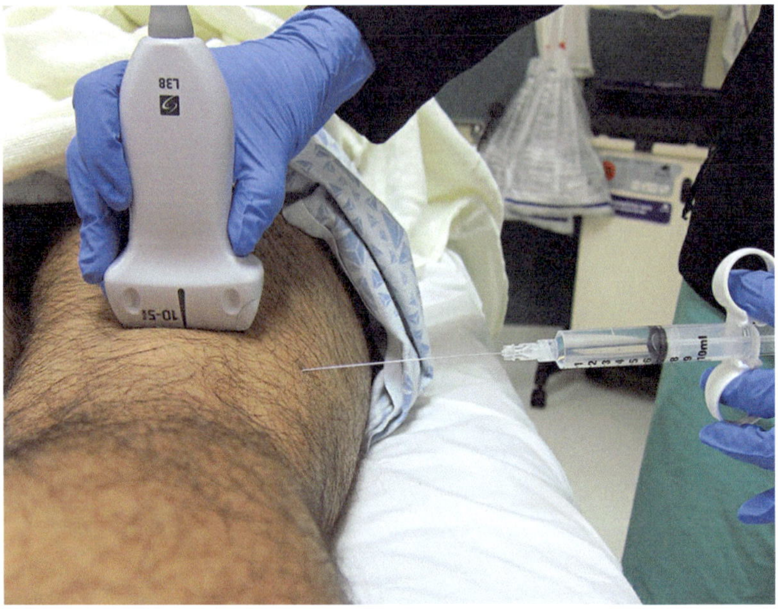

Fig. 9.44 In-plane technique probe and needle positioning (needle parallel to ground at lateral thigh)

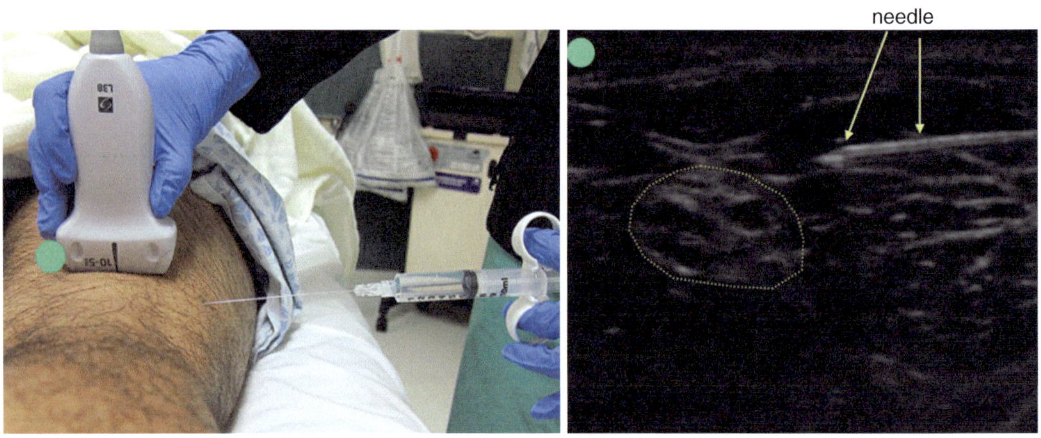

Fig. 9.45 Advancing needle toward the sciatic nerve

Complications

Intravascular injection should be a concern because of the close proximity of the popliteal vasculature and the distal sciatic nerve. A flat needle angle will allow for clear needle tip visualization and hopefully reduce chances of either local anesthetic systemic toxicity or peripheral nerve injury.

Pearls/Pitfalls

Placing the patient in prone position if possible will greatly reduce the difficulty of the block. The supine position forces the sonographer to have a vertically reversed image on the ultrasound screen as well as not having a stable place to rest the transducer during the procedure.

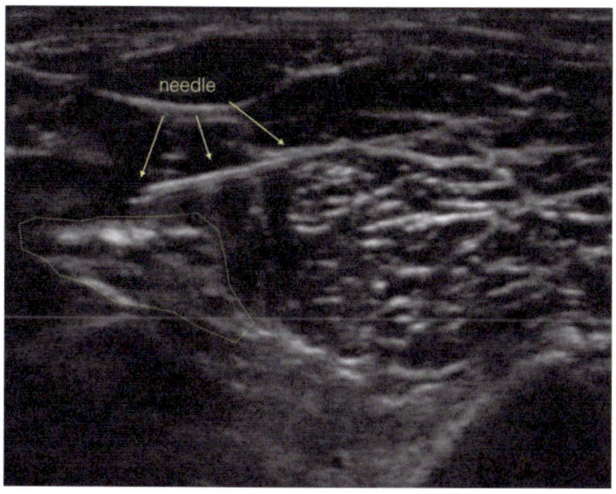

Fig. 9.46 Needle tip at superficial edge of the sciatic nerve

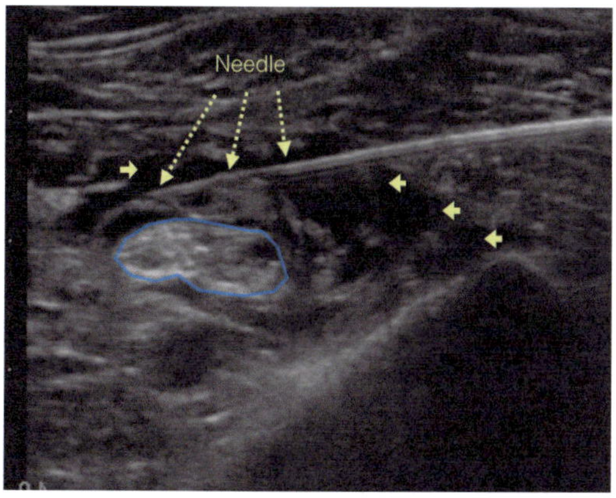

Fig. 9.47 Anechoic region around the distal sciatic nerve (encircled) from local anesthetic infiltration. Solid arrows indicate anechoic ring of local anesthetic. Dashed arrows indicate needle

Integration into Clinical Practice

The ultrasound-guided distal sciatic nerve block is the ideal block for patients with distal leg and ankle injuries (large lateral leg laceration, pain reduction from bimalleolar fractures, lower-leg burns, abscesses, etc.). Depending on the anesthetic used, the block can facilitate fracture reduction, abscess drainage or be used as an adjunct in a multimodal plan for pain control. Unfortunately, the superficial structures of the medial lower leg and ankle are not innervated by the distal sciatic nerve, and a saphenous nerve block (distal aspect of the femoral nerve) may be needed if a more complete analgesia to the lower leg is desired [40–43].

Evidence

In 2011, Dr. Herring et al. described their experience with the use of the distal sciatic nerve block for anesthesia of foot and ankle injuries in an ED [42]. In 2017, Dr. Mori et al. described a case where ultrasound-guided distal sciatic nerve block was effective and safe for ankle laceration repair in a child [44].

Key Points

- The distal sciatic nerve block is effective for distal leg and ankle injuries.
- Placing the patient in prone position will decrease the difficulty of the block.
- Distal sciatic nerve blocks are contraindicated in high-energy injuries with high risk for compartment syndrome, such as solitary tibia or mid-shaft tibial-fibular fractures.
- A flat needle angle will allow for clear needle tip visualization and reduces the chances of local anesthetic systemic toxicity and peripheral nerve injury.

Ultrasound-Guided Posterior Tibial Nerve Block

Anatomy

The posterior tibial nerve is a branch of the distal sciatic nerve. The sciatic nerve runs deep in the posterior thigh becoming more superficial at the popliteal fossa. Just proximal to the popliteal fossa, it bifurcates into the tibial nerve and common peroneal nerve. At the level of the ankle, the posterior tibial nerve travels posterior to the

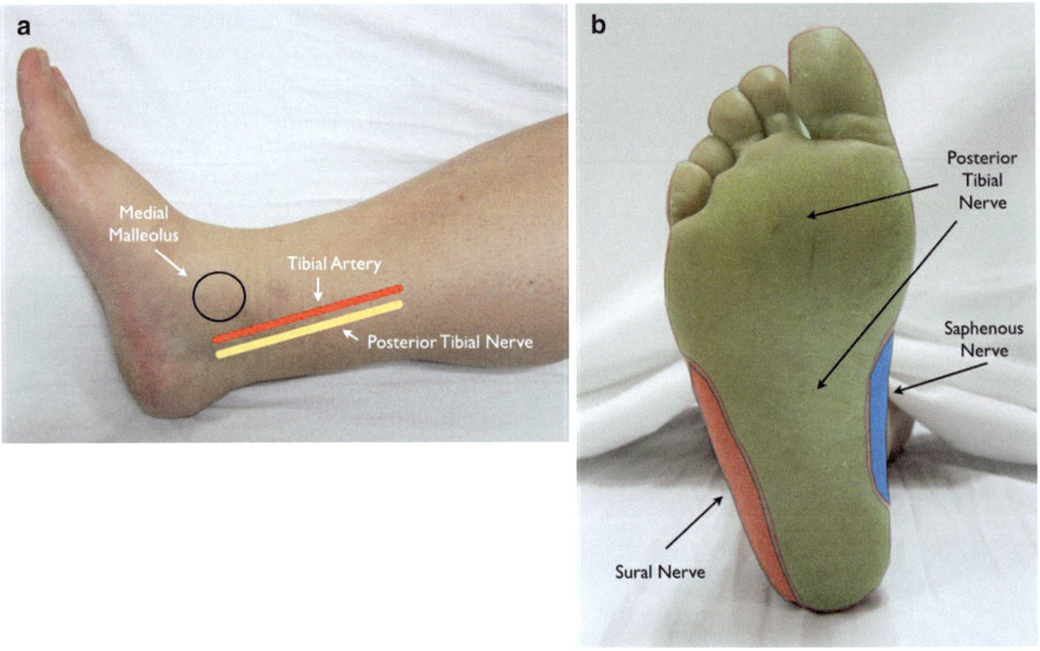

Fig. 9.48 (**a**) Surface anatomy for the posterior tibial nerve block of the tibial artery, posterior tibial nerve, and medial malleolus. (**b**) Sensory distribution of the foot (tibial, sural, and saphenous nerves)

medial malleolus and typically posterior to the tibial artery and vein (Fig. 9.48). The posterior tibial nerve provides sensory innervation to the majority of the sole of the foot. The extreme postero-lateral aspect is innervated by the sural nerve, and the extreme postero-medial aspect is innervated by the saphenous nerve.

Indications

The posterior tibial nerve block is indicated for wounds or injuries involving the sole of the foot or heel. For example, the posterior tibial nerve block is useful for definitive analgesia for laceration repair or foreign body exploration of the sole of the foot as well as pain relief from a calcaneal fracture.

Contraindications

Any injury has a potential risk for compartment syndrome. The risk is higher among crush injuries and vascular injuries. Among injuries at high risk for compartment syndrome where following a motor and sensory exam are necessary, a posterior nerve block should not be performed [45].

Equipment/Probe Selection

A high-frequency linear probe should be used. A 20–25-gauge 1.5-inch needle should be used to perform the actual nerve block.

Preparation/Pre-procedural Evaluation

The goal of patient positioning is to expose the medial ankle in a neutral position. This can be accomplished in two ways. The patient can be placed supine with the knee flexed, the hip externally rotated, and the ankle in a neutral position (Fig. 9.49). Alternatively, the patient may rest in the lateral decubitus position with the affected

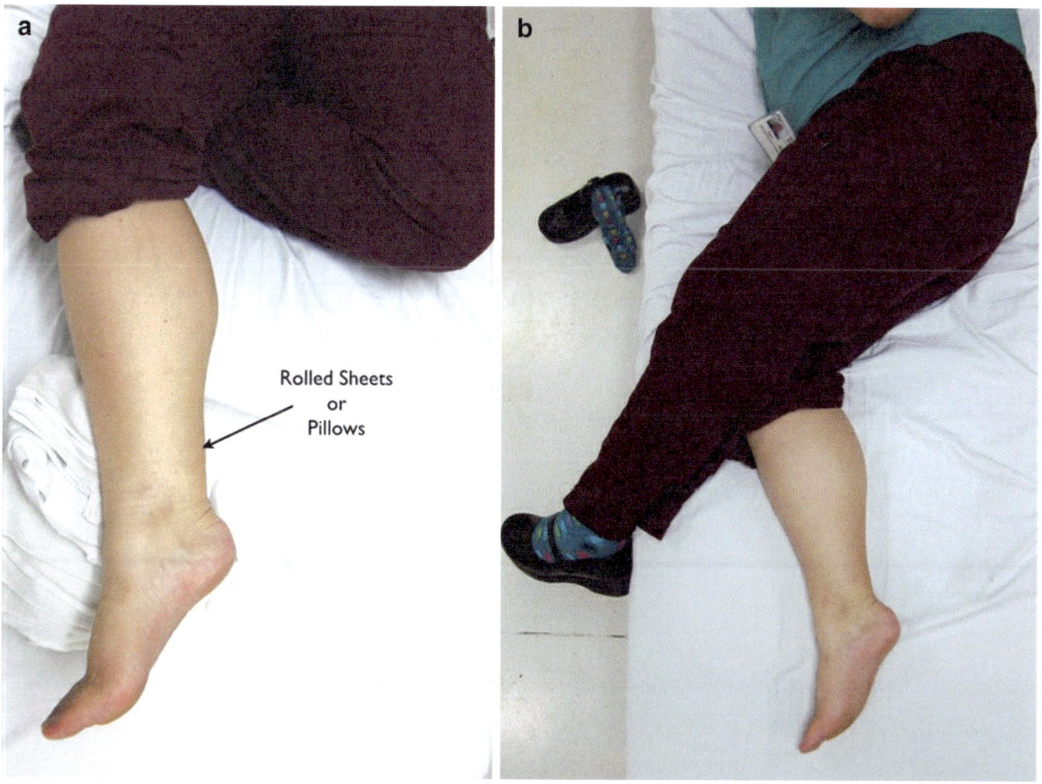

Fig. 9.49 (**a**) Appropriate patient positioning for posterior tibial nerve block with the knee flexed, the hip externally rotated, and the ankle in a neutral position. (**b**) Alternative patient positioning for posterior tibial nerve block with patient in lateral decubitus position with the affected side down, exposing the medial aspect of the ankle

side down, exposing the medial aspect of the ankle. Connect the patient to a cardiac monitor and place the ultrasound machine on the opposite side of the operator.

For the survey scan, the linear transducer should be placed in a transverse position proximal and posterior to the medial malleolus (Fig. 9.50). On the ultrasound screen, identify the medial malleolus and adjacent pulsatile tibial artery. The posterior tibial nerve will be a hyperechoic, honeycombed structure adjacent to the artery. There is significant variation in location of the tibial nerve. Color Doppler can be placed to confirm the tibial artery. Once the artery and nerve are identified, slide the probe cephalad to best visualize the tibial nerve and find where the tibial nerve is most distant from the vascular bundle.

Procedure

Using the survey scan, identify the best place for needle insertion for the block. The tibial nerve is typically very superficial and can be performed with a standard 1.5-inch needle. This block can be performed in plane or out of plane. Regardless of approach, the goal is to place the needle tip adjacent to the tibial nerve while not puncturing the vascular bundle. Furthermore, depending on technique, remember to inject a skin wheel of local anesthetic with a small gauge needle at the site of needle insertion.

For the in-plane approach, the needle will traverse either a lateral-to-medial or medial-to-lateral approach dependent on where the tibial nerve is in relation to the vascular bundle (Fig. 9.51). Typically, the tibial nerve is posterior

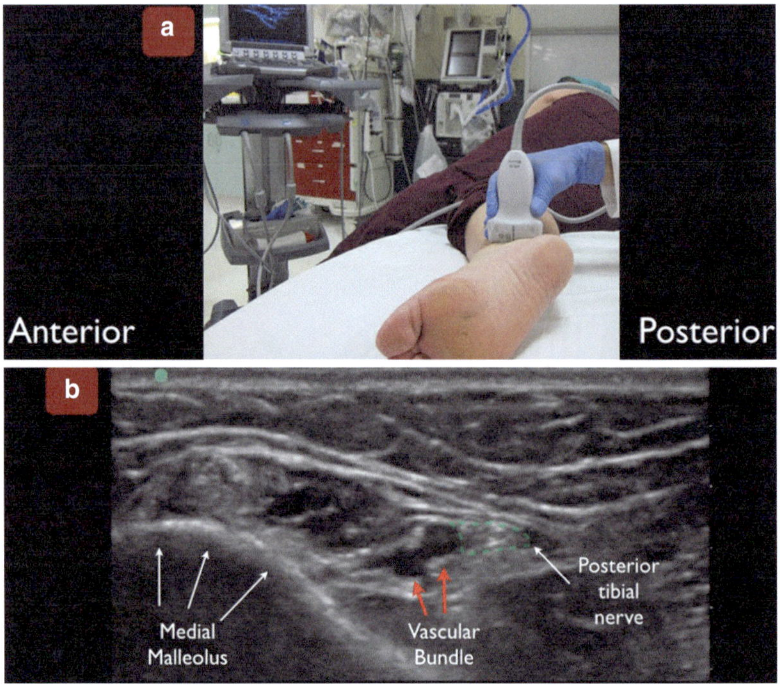

Fig. 9.50 (**a**) Proper placement of ultrasound probe for posterior tibial nerve block and (**b**) ultrasound landmarks for posterior tibial nerve block including the (i) medial malleolus, (ii) tibial artery (vascular bundle), and (iii) posterior tibial nerve

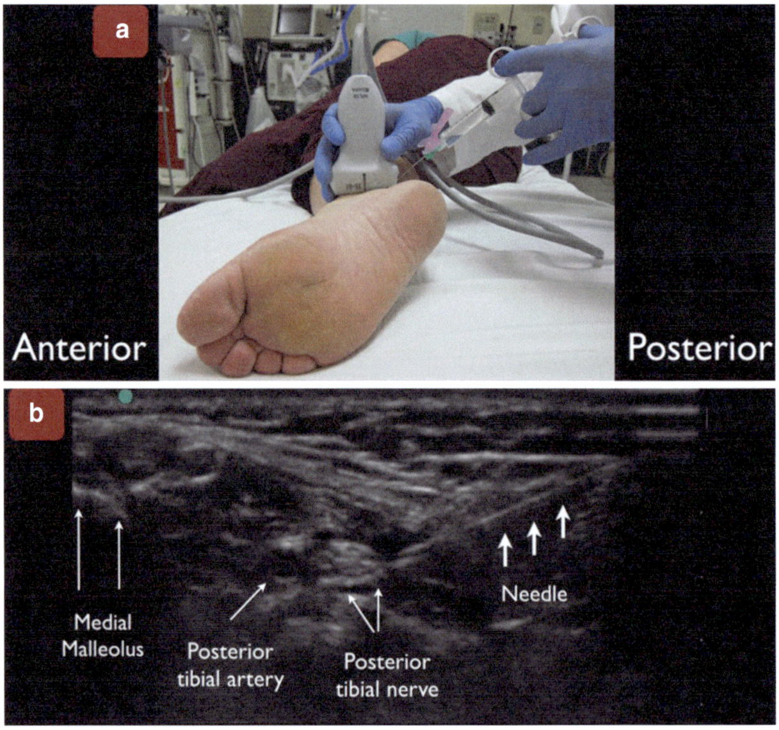

Fig. 9.51 (**a**) Appropriate ultrasound probe and needle placement for in-plane posterior tibial nerve block and (**b**) in-plane ultrasound needle visualization of posterior tibial nerve block with deposition of local anesthetic

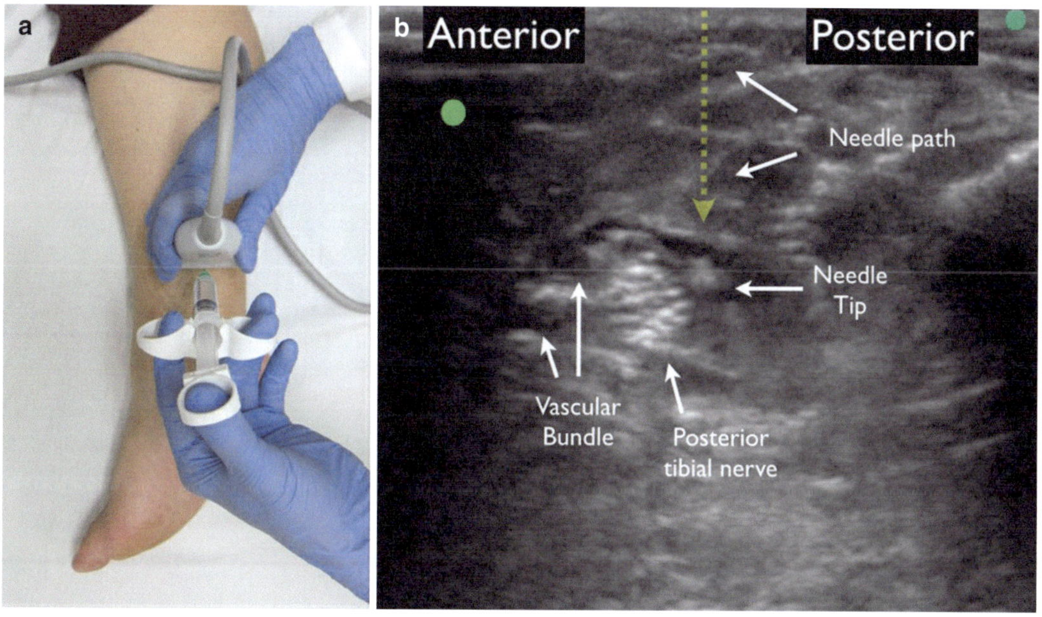

Fig. 9.52 (**a**) Appropriate ultrasound probe and needle placement for out-of-plane posterior tibial nerve block and (**b**) out-of-plane needle insertion with needle tip visualized adjacent to posterior tibial nerve with deposition of local anesthetic

to the vascular bundle, and the needle will move from lateral to medial (above the Achilles tendon). Once the needle tip is visualized adjacent to the tibial nerve, aspirate to ensure lack of vascular puncture, and inject small aliquots (1 cc) of anesthetic. Correct needle position will be indicated by visualization of local anesthetic spread surrounding the nerve as a "donut sign." A successful block can be accomplished with approximately 5–10 ml of anesthetic.

Oftentimes, the out-of-plane technique may be optimal because there is limited space between the Achilles tendon and the distal tibia. The needle should be inserted almost perpendicular to the probe, making visualization of the needle tip often difficult (Fig. 9.52). Center the probe over the tibial nerve, and insert the needle adjacent to the probe at a very steep angle (60–80°) with the tip pointed toward the probe. Pay close attention to the ultrasound screen and the tenting of the skin and tissue to ensure appropriate needle site entry in relation to the nerve and vascular bundle. Careful movements of the needle in an up and down fashion can also help appreciate the needle tip. Once again, you will only visualize the needle tip in this orientation. Once the needle tip is visualized adjacent to the tibial nerve, aspirate to ensure lack of vascular puncture, and slowly inject approximately 5–10 ml of local anesthetic. If performed correctly, the posterior tibial nerve will be shown to be surrounded by the hypoechoic local anesthetic.

Complications (Including How to Avoid)

As with any nerve block, there is an inherent risk of vascular puncture and intra neural injection. Careful use of ultrasound to always visualize the needle tip will ensure these complications are mitigated [46]. Especially if performing an out-of-plane technique, ensure your needle tip is visualized by making subtle up and down movements of the needle and watching the deformation of tissue as the needle advances.

Pearls/Pitfalls

The posterior tibial nerve is very superficial in the distal leg and can be accomplished with an in-plane or out-of-plane technique.

Integration into Clinical Practice

The ultrasound-guided posterior tibial nerve block is a great block to achieve analgesia for laceration repair or suspected foreign bodies in the sole of the foot. This block is also effective for pain relief of calcaneal fractures.

Evidence

In 2009, Dr. Redborg demonstrated that ultrasound improves the success rate of tibial nerve block at the ankle [46]. Clattenburg et al. described the utility of selective posterior tibial nerve block for treating acute calcaneal fracture pain in ED patients [47].

Key Points

- The posterior tibial nerve block is effective for injuries to the sole of the foot and calcaneal fractures.
- Oftentimes, the out-of-plane technique is the optimal approach due to limited space between the Achilles tendon and distal tibia.

References

1. Tirado A, Nagdev A, Henningsen C, Breckon P, Chiles K. Ultrasound-guided procedures in the emergency department-needle guidance and localization. Emerg Med Clin North Am. 2013;31(1):87–115.
2. Walker KJ, McGrattan K, Aas-Eng K, Smith AF. Ultrasound guidance for peripheral nerve blockade. Cochrane Database Syst Rev. 2009;(4):CD006459.
3. Chin KJ, Wong NWY, Macfarlane AJR, Chan VWS. Ultrasound-guided versus anatomic landmark-guided ankle blocks: a 6-year retrospective review. Reg Anesth Pain Med. 2011;36(6):611–8.
4. Neal JM, Bernards CM, Hadzic A, et al. ASRA practice advisory on neurologic complications in regional anesthesia and pain medicine. Reg Anesth Pain Med. 2008;33(5):404–15.
5. Prakash S, Kumar A. Needle tip and peripheral nerve blocks. J Anaesthesiol Clin Pharmacol. 2018;34(1):129–30.
6. Becker DE, Reed KL. Local anesthetics: review of pharmacological considerations. Anesth Prog. 2012;59(2):90–101, quiz 102–3.
7. Johnson B, Herring A, Stone M, Nagdev A. Performance accuracy of hand-on-needle versus hand-on-syringe technique for ultrasound-guided regional anesthesia simulation for emergency medicine residents. West J Emerg Med. 2014;15(6):641–6.
8. Urmey WF, Talts KH, Sharrock NE. One hundred percent incidence of hemidiaphragmatic paresis associated with interscalene brachial plexus anesthesia as diagnosed by ultrasonography. Anesth Analg. 1991;72(4):498–503.
9. Riazi S, Carmichael N, Awad I, Holtby RM, McCartney CJL. Effect of local anaesthetic volume (20 vs 5 ml) on the efficacy and respiratory consequences of ultrasound-guided interscalene brachial plexus block. Br J Anaesth. 2008;101(4):549–56.
10. Spence BC, Beach ML, Gallagher JD, Sites BD. Ultrasound-guided interscalene blocks: understanding where to inject the local anaesthetic. Anaesthesia. 2011;66(6):509–14.
11. Stone MB, Wang R, Price DD. Ultrasound-guided supraclavicular brachial plexus nerve block vs procedural sedation for the treatment of upper extremity emergencies. Am J Emerg Med. 2008;26(6):706–10.
12. Blaivas M, Adhikari S, Lander L. A prospective comparison of procedural sedation and ultrasound-guided interscalene nerve block for shoulder reduction in the emergency department. Acad Emerg Med. 2011;18(9):922–7.
13. Mak PH, Irwin MG, Ooi CG, Chow BF. Incidence of diaphragmatic paralysis following supraclavicular brachial plexus block and its effect on pulmonary function. Anaesthesia. 2001;56(4):352–6.
14. Perlas A, Lobo G, Lo N, Brull R, Chan VW, Karkhanis R. Ultrasound-guided supraclavicular block: outcome of 510 consecutive cases. Reg Anesth Pain Med. 2009;34:171–6.
15. De José María B, Banús E, Navarro Egea M, Serrano S, Perelló M, Mabrok M. Ultrasound-guided supraclavicular vs infraclavicular brachial plexus blocks in children. Paediatr Anaesth. 2008;18(9):838–44.
16. Herring AA, Stone MB, Frenkel O, Chipman A, Nagdev AD. The ultrasound-guided superficial cervical plexus block for anesthesia and analgesia in emergency care settings. Am J Emerg Med. 2012;30(7):1263–7.
17. Choi DS, Atchabahian A, Brown AR. Cervical plexus block provides postoperative analgesia after clavicle surgery. Anesth Analg. 2005;100(5):1542–3.

18. Sepulveda TGA, Soto NRA, Cortes AJE, Suazo GIC. Efficacy of anesthetic blockage of superficial branches of the cervical plexus. Int J Odontostomatol. 2008;2(1):77–81.
19. Shanthanna H. Ultrasound guided selective cervical nerve root block and superficial cervical plexus block for surgeries on the clavicle. Indian J Anaesth. 2014;58(3):327–9.
20. Shteif M, Lesmes D, Hartman G, Ruffino S, Laster Z. The use of the superficial cervical plexus block in the drainage of submandibular and submental abscesses—an alternative for general anesthesia. J Oral Maxillofac Surg. 2008;66(12):2642–5.
21. Pandit JJ, Dutta D, Morris JF. Spread of injectate with superficial cervical plexus block in humans: an anatomical study. Br J Anaesth. 2003;91(5):733.
22. Castresana MR, et al. Incidence and clinical significance of hemidiaphragmatic paresis in patients undergoing carotid endarterectomy during cervical plexus block anesthesia. J Neurosurg Anesthesiol. 1994;6(1):21–3.
23. Flores S, Riguzzi C, Herring A, Nagdev A. Horner's syndrome after superficial cervical plexus block. West J Emerg Med. 2015;16(3):428–31.
24. Çiftci T, Daskaya H, Yıldırım MB, Söylemez H. A minimally painful, comfortable, and safe technique for hemodialysis catheter placement in children: superficial cervical plexus block. Hemodial Int. 2014;18:700–4.
25. Boles C, Kannam S, Cardwell A. The forearm anatomy of muscle compartments and nerves. Am J Roentgenol. 2000;174:151–9.
26. Mazurek MT, Shin AY. Upper extremity peripheral nerve anatomy: current concepts and applications. Clin Orthop Relat Res. 2001;383:7–20.
27. Brown JM, Yablon CM, Morag Y, Brandon CJ, Jacobson JA. US of the peripheral nerves of the upper extremity: a landmark approach. Radiographics. 2016;36(2):452–63.
28. Ferrera PC, Chandler R. Anesthesia in the emergency setting: Part I. Hand and foot injuries. Am Fam Physician. 1994;50:569–73.
29. Salam GA. Regional anesthesia for office procedures: Part II. Extremity and inguinal area surgeries. Am Fam Physician. 2004;69:896–9.
30. McCartney CJ, Xu D, Constantinescu C, Abbas S, Chan VW. Ultrasound examination of peripheral nerves in the forearm. Reg Anesth Pain Med. 2007;32(5):434–9.
31. Liebmann O, Price D, Mills C, et al. Feasibility of forearm ultrasonography-guided nerve blocks of the radial, ulnar, and median nerves for hand procedures in the emergency department. Ann Emerg Med. 2006;48:558–62.
32. Frenkel O, Liebmann O, Fischer JW. Ultrasound-guided forearm nerve blocks in kids: a novel method for pain control in the treatment of hand-injured pediatric patients in the emergency department. Pediatr Emerg Care. 2015;31(4):255–9.
33. Sohoni A, Nagdev A, Takhar S, et al. Forearm ultrasound-guided nerve blocks vs landmark-based wrist blocks for hand anesthesia in healthy volunteers. Am J Emerg Med. 2016;34(4):730–4.
34. Beaudoin FL, Haran JP, Liebmann O. A comparison of ultrasound-guided three-in-one femoral nerve block versus parenteral opioids alone for analgesia in emergency department patients with hip fractures: a randomized controlled trial. Acad Emerg Med. 2013;20(6):584–91.
35. Karagiannis G, Hardern R. Best evidence topic report. No evidence found that a femoral nerve block in cases of femoral shaft fractures can delay the diagnosis of compartment syndrome of the thigh. Emerg Med J. 2005;22(11):814.
36. Johnson B, Herring A, Shah S, Krosin M, Mantuani D, Nagdev A. Door-to-block time: prioritizing acute pain management for femoral fractures in the ED. Am J Emerg Med. 2014;32(7):801–3.
37. Beaudoin FL, Nagdev A, Merchant RC, Becker BM. Ultrasound-guided femoral nerve blocks in elderly patients with hip fractures. Am J Emerg Med. 2010;28(1):76–81.
38. Fletcher AK, Rigby AS, Heyes FL. Three-in-one femoral nerve block as analgesia for fractured neck of femur in the emergency department: a randomized, controlled trial. Ann Emerg Med. 2003;41(2):227–33.
39. Mutty CE, Jensen EJ, Manka MA Jr, Anders MJ, Bone LB. Femoral nerve block for diaphyseal and distal femoral fractures in the emergency department. J Bone Joint Surg Am. 2007;89(12):2599.
40. Marhofer P, Harrop-Griffiths W, Willschke H, et al. Fifteen years of ultrasound guidance in regional anaesthesia: part 2—recent developments in block techniques. Br J Anaesth. 2010;104:673–83.
41. Murray JM, Derbyshire S, Shields MO. Lower limb blocks. Anaesthesia. 2010;65:57–66.
42. Herring AA, Stone MB, Fischer J, et al. Ultrasound-guided distal popliteal sciatic nerve block for ED anesthesia. Am J Emerg Med. 2011;29:e3–5.
43. Moore C. Ultrasound-guided procedures in emergency medicine. Ultrasound Clin. 2011;6:277–89.
44. Mori T, Hagiwara Y. Ultrasound-guided popliteal sciatic nerve block for an ankle laceration in a pediatric emergency department. Pediatr Emerg Care. 2017;33(12):803–5.
45. Mar GJ, Barrington MJ, McGuirk BR. Acute compartment syndrome of the lower limb and the effect of postoperative analgesia on diagnosis. Br J Anaesth. 2009;102(1):3–11.
46. Redborg KE, Antonakakis JG, Beach ML, Chinn CD, Sites BD. Ultrasound improves the success rate of a tibial nerve block at the ankle. Reg Anesth Pain Med. 2009;34(3):256–60.
47. Clattenburg E, Herring A, Hahn C, Johnson B, Nagdev A. ED ultrasound-guided posterior tibial nerve blocks for calcaneal fracture analagesia. Am J Emerg Med. 2016;34(6):1183.

Ultrasound-Guided Gastrointestinal and Genitourinary Procedures

10

Mathew Nelson, Nat Kittisarapong, Tanya Bajaj, Robert Ellspermann, Adam Ash, and Veena Modayil

Introduction

Use of bedside ultrasound to guide gastrointestinal and genitourinary procedures increases safety by allowing real-time visualization of patient anatomy. Ultrasound can be used in a static fashion to map out relevant procedural anatomy and also dynamically to visualize movement and location of needles, catheters, and tubes, ensuring that they are placed correctly and that they do not damage nerves, vascular structures, or gastrointestinal/genitourinary organs. There is an increasingly vast body of literature supporting this practice given its safety and convenience.

Advantages of Ultrasound Guidance

Ultrasound is ideal for depicting the anatomy involved with most gastrointestinal and genitourinary procedures. While bowel gas can interfere with visualization, in almost all cases, it can be moved through probe pressure and patient manipulation. Additionally, having the patient ingest water will often move interfering gas further down the gastrointestinal tract. For paracentesis, which has been performed using landmark-based approach for years, ultrasound not only makes the procedure easy and accurate but can decrease complications. Many patients who appear to have ascites on physical examination may actually have none or too little to tap which can be confirmed with bedside ultrasound. Ultrasound guidance also allows for precision of needle insertion that is beyond the capability of an experienced clinician, forced to perform aspiration of ascitic fluid using landmark technique. The use of real-time guidance and high-resolution ultrasound imaging can insure needle tips stay clear of any unintended targets and also allows precise needle insertion of difficult-to-reach areas or pockets. As seen in many other procedures performed blindly in the past, the standard of care has shifted toward real-time ultrasound guidance for these gastrointestinal and genitourinary procedures for patient safety and increased accuracy.

Ultrasound-Guided Gastrointestinal Procedures

This section will discuss the important diagnostic, therapeutic, and potentially life-saving techniques of ultrasound-guided abdominal procedures. These include ultrasound-guided paracentesis, diagnostic peritoneal lavage, gastrostomy tube (G-tube) placement, hernia reduction, and nasogastric (NG)

M. Nelson (✉) · N. Kittisarapong · T. Bajaj
R. Ellspermann · A. Ash · V. Modayil
Department of Emergency Medicine, North Shore University Hospital, Manhasset, NY, USA

S. Adhikari, M. Blaivas (eds.), *The Ultimate Guide to Point-of-Care Ultrasound-Guided Procedures*, https://doi.org/10.1007/978-3-030-28267-7_10

tube placement. The indications and contraindications of the procedures will be discussed along with the necessary equipment, setup, evaluation, and details of each procedure. Complications, pearls, and clinical pitfalls will also be addressed for the various abdominal procedures.

Paracentesis

Anatomy

Anatomy of the abdomen for ultrasound-guided procedures has several key elements: location of the stomach and other major organs, the epigastric vessels, mesentery, areas of dependency for fluid collection, and the layers of soft tissue leading to the peritoneal cavity. The epigastric blood vessels traverse the rectus abdominis muscles posteriorly and can be easily injured during blind procedures. The stomach is another site of potential complication because it is frequently distended in the acute care setting patient population. Ultrasound can help to localize it and prevent complications. A minimal fluid collection of at least 3 cm in depth is considered adequate for the paracentesis. The idea of locating the best paracentesis site should involve simultaneously locating the thinnest portion of abdominal wall and the largest pocket of underlying fluid. Evidence shows that when the patient is positioned in the left lateral oblique position, the ascites pool depth changes in patients from an average of 2.86–4.57 cm [1].

Indications

Indications for performing abdominal paracentesis in the clinical setting include the evaluation of the patient with new-onset ascites and collecting fluid for diagnostic testing and as a therapeutic intervention to relieve abdominal discomfort or respiratory difficulties in patients with massive ascites [2].

Contraindications

- A surgical abdomen is the absolute contraindication to paracentesis.
- *Relative contraindications are*:
  - Thrombocytopenia (platelet count <20 × 10 uL)
  - Coagulopathy (INR > 2.0)
  - Pregnancy
  - Distended urinary bladder
  - Overlying abdominal wall cellulitis
  - Distended bowel or massive ileus
  - Intra-abdominal adhesions [2]

Equipment/Probe Selection

A low frequency curvilinear transducer for abdominal fluid evaluation and a high frequency linear transducer to evaluate for blood vessels in the vicinity of the proposed paracentesis site are ideal. A sterile probe cover is important if utilizing dynamic guidance in place of a static guidance approach. Most of the equipment required can be found in a peritoneal lavage kit or in a specialized paracentesis kit. See the equipment as follows:

- Gloves, gown, mask, and cap
- Ultrasound machine
- Ultrasound probe cover
- Sterile gel (surgical lubricant)
- Antiseptic
- Fenestrated drape
- Surgical marking pen
- Syringes: 10 mL, 30/60 mL
- Injection needles: 25ga, 22ga
- Anesthetic
- Scalpel, #11/15 blade
- An 8F catheter over 18ga × 7.5″ needle
- Sterile 4 × 4 sponges
- Three-way stopcock
- Tubing set with drainage bag or vacuum container/bulbs
- Specimen vials (cell count, gram stain, culture) [2]

Preparation/Pre-procedural Evaluation

The patient should be positioned with the head of the bed slightly raised. The patient may be placed in the left lateral decubitus position, which can aid to sonographically identify the largest fluid pocket, although the supine position may be adequate in patients with larger fluid volumes. Scan the abdomen, and attempt to localize the thinnest layer of abdominal free wall with the largest underlying pocket of fluid, ideally at least a 3 cm column. The bladder should be identified so that

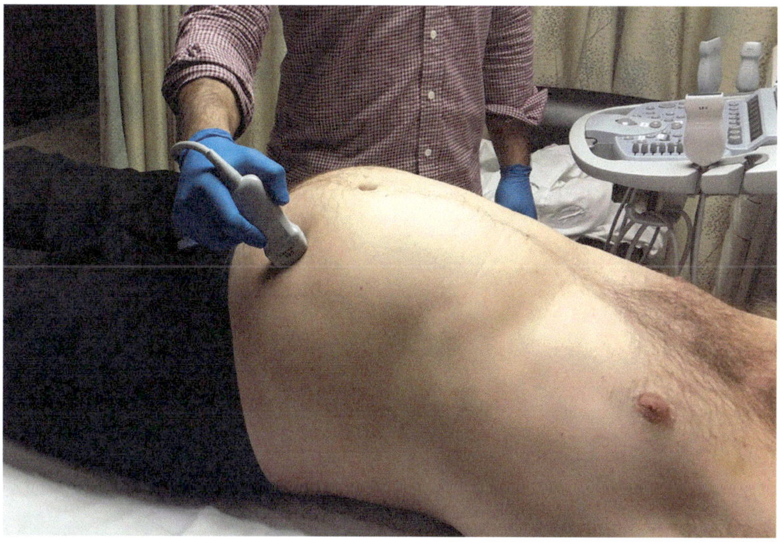

Fig. 10.1 Position of the probe for paracentesis

it may be avoided. The fluid pocket should be measured in two perpendicular planes. Use a surgical marker to identify this position. Also note abdominal wall thickness, depth of the fluid, and the clinicians anticipated angle of approach (Fig. 10.1) [1]. The area of abdominal wall proposed for needle and catheter penetration should be pre-scanned with a high-resolution linear array and color Doppler to identify any blood vessels at or near the site [3]. If vessels, especially arteries, are identified, another site should be chosen. If a site change is not possible, precise dynamic in-plane needle/scalpel/catheter guidance will be required to avoid any vasculature.

Procedure

Clean the procedure site with antiseptic (chlorhexidine, betadine, etc.), and sterilely drape the patient. Apply the sterile probe cover to the ultrasound probe. Inject a wheal of lidocaine or other anesthetic into the procedure site. Anesthetize down to the peritoneum along the desired catheter tract, always applying negative pressure when advancing the needle. Superficially incise the previously determined site with a scalpel, and slowly insert the 8F fenestrated catheter into the peritoneal cavity. The procedure is done in out-of-plane or in-plane needle visualization approach. Once past the epidermis, track the needle tip to the peritoneal wall. If using the out-of-plane approach, carefully track the catheter by fanning the probe in the direction of the catheter movement while keeping the probe in place on the patient's skin. If visualizing the catheter tip becomes difficult, attempt to place the probe and sound waves in a perpendicular orientation to the catheter tip, fanning again until you have discovered and demarcated the tip of the catheter. If using the in-plane guidance approach, the catheter and needle tip should remain visible at all times. When the tip is close to entering the peritoneal cavity (which can be visualized as tenting of tissue on ultrasound), the catheter and probe can be laterally/inferiorly/superiorly displaced with gentle pressure in order to form a discontinuous tract from the abdominal peritoneal cavity to the external environment (Z-track), and the needle can then be advanced, all the while maintaining negative pressure on the syringe piston and awaiting aspiration of fluid. After aspiration has been observed, advance the catheter. Drain the desired amount of fluid. When finished remove the catheter, apply slight pressure, and place a bandage over the procedural site (Fig. 10.2) [1, 2].

Complications

Complications from paracentesis are uncommon but may include hemorrhage (0.93%), abdominal wall and mesenteric hematomas, bladder or bowel perforation, inferior epigastric artery

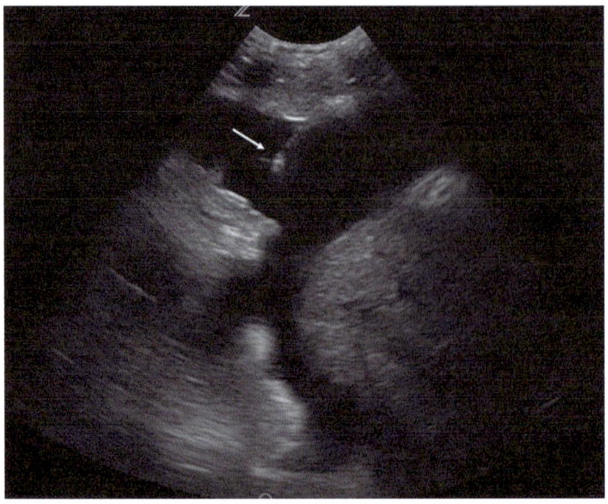

Fig. 10.2 Visualization of the needle (arrow) during a paracentesis. (Courtesy of Srikar Adhikari, MD)

aneurysm, vessel laceration (aorta, mesenteric artery, iliac artery), hypotension, infection (0.58–0.63%), and persistent ascitic fluid leak (5%). The clinician can reduce all of these with ultrasound guidance [2, 4].

Pearls/Pitfalls

- Allowing the patient to move after abdominal fluid surveying and evaluation has occurred, possibly leading to a shift in fluid and resulting in a dry tap or bowel injury
- Accidentally assuming a large fluid-containing structure like a large bladder, fluid-filled loop of bowel, bladder, or cyst is peritoneal fluid [1]

Integration into Clinical Practice

Ultrasound assists clinicians in the performance of abdominal procedures both by improving patient safety and satisfaction and by decreasing failed attempts. Paracentesis is frequently performed in high-risk populations with coagulopathies and in those who are at increased risk for infectious complications of the procedure. Ultrasound allows the clinician to identify vascular structures, both superficial and deep, at risk of being damaged during the procedure. It aids in prevention of accidental bowel and mesenteric injury by assisting in dynamic needle visualization. Ultrasound guidance brings similar benefits to diagnostic peritoneal lavage (DPL) and G-tube placement. With practice it is not difficult to become proficient with ultrasound-guided paracentesis. Inexperienced users can start with the static approach. As one becomes more accustomed to procedural ultrasound, they may begin to see the benefits of dynamic guidance and add into their clinical practice.

Evidence

In 1 prospective randomized study where 100 patients were enrolled, 56 into the ultrasound-assisted group and 44 into the traditional technique, 95% of the ultrasound group were successfully aspirated, and only 61% of the traditional group were successfully aspirated. Key pathology was noted in two of the interventional group patients (a large left lower quadrant cystic mass and a ventral hernia). Of the traditional group's 17 unsuccessful aspirations, 15 patients had a "break" in the study where they had intervention with ultrasound resulting in 13/15 successful aspirations; of the 2 remaining patients, 1 did not have enough fluid to be sampled, and the other had no fluid visualized [5]. Complications from bleeding during ultrasound-guided abdominal paracentesis are uncommon and appear to be very mild, regardless of pre-procedure INR or platelet count. Routine correction of prolonged INR or thrombocytopenia before abdominal paracentesis may not be necessary. In a 2-year study period, a total of 410 abdominal paracenteses in 163 patients were investigated. The pre-procedure INR for prothrombin time was more than 1.5 in 142 paracenteses; the pre-procedure platelet count was less than $50 \times 10^3\ \mu L^{-1}$ in 55 paracenteses. Only 2 out of 410 procedures (0.5%, 95% confidence interval = 0.1–1.8%) were associated with minor complications of cutaneous bleeding in the same patient (0.6%, 95% confidence interval = 0.1–3.4%) at different visits [6].

Key Points
- Ultrasound-guided paracentesis is safer than the traditional blind approach.
- Ultrasound-guided paracentesis increases patient satisfaction and procedural success rates.
- Visualize the tip of the procedural catheter the entire time.
- Do not let your patient shift position after the fluid contents have been surveyed.
- Do not mistakenly attempt to drain an abdominal fluid-filled structure.

Diagnostic Peritoneal Lavage (DPL)

In the setting of trauma, diagnostic peritoneal lavage has traditionally been fused in the assessment of intraperitoneal injury and bleeding. When practicing in an austere environment, physicians do not always have access to CT. Additionally, traditional trauma imaging modalities such as CT and ultrasound may yield equivocal findings.

Anatomy

Anatomy of the abdomen for ultrasound-guided procedures has several key elements: location of the stomach and other major organs, the epigastric vessels, mesentery, areas of dependency for fluid collection, and the layers of soft tissue leading to the peritoneal cavity. The epigastric blood vessels traverse the rectus abdominis muscles posteriorly and can be easily injured during blind procedures. The deep inferior epigastric artery and branches can come close to the umbilical area, and providers should maintain an awareness of the variability in apparent anatomy between patients, especially ones who have had prior abdominal surgery.

Indications

- Trauma patient in a remote location or a location that lacks computed tomography (CT)
- Hemodynamically unstable trauma patient who has a negative or equivocal FAST examination
- Should be considered in patients who have an unreliable examination or those at high risk for hollow viscus injury (HVI)
- Trauma where CT or ultrasonography detects minimal fluid or when the patient manifests fever, peritonitis, or both with concern for HVI [7–9]

Contraindications

- Any obvious need for laparotomy is an absolute contraindication.
- Unstable patient with a positive Focused Assessment with Sonography in Trauma (FAST) examination in the setting of trauma.
- Unstable patient with an open wound to the abdomen or chest at locations with trauma surgery.
- *Relative contraindications include*:
  - No training in DPL
  - Prior abdominal surgery
  - Morbid obesity
  - Second to third trimester pregnancy
  - Morbid obesity
  - Coagulopathy [2]

Equipment/Probe Selection

A low frequency curved and a high frequency linear array transducer with sterile probe cover are essential to perform DPL. Abdominal wall blood vessels will be best identified using a high-resolution linear array probe with color or power Doppler. Most of the equipment required can be found in a peritoneal lavage kit. See the equipment as follows:

- Gloves, gown, mask, and cap
- Ultrasound machine
- Ultrasound probe cover
- Sterile gel (surgical lubricant)
- Antiseptic
- Fenestrated drape
- Suture tray and suture

- Injection needles and syringe: 25ga, 22ga
- Sterile 4 × 4 sponges
- Anesthetic
- Scalpel, #15 blade
- Peritoneal dialysis set
- Intravenous (IV) pole, peritoneal dialysis tubing, and 1 liter of normal saline (NS) or Ringer's lactate (RL) solution
- Three-way stopcock
- Tubing set with drainage bag or vacuum container/bulbs
- Tape
- Specimen vials (cell count, gram stain, culture) [2]

Preparation/Pre-procedural Evaluation

The patient should lie as flat on the bed as possible. The abdomen should be mapped with the ultrasound probe at one-third the distance from the umbilicus to the pubic symphysis (PS). Make note of any hernia, blood vessel, or cystic structure that should be avoided going forward. The depth of the peritoneal cavity should be recorded during this process as well.

Procedure

A nasogastric tube and Foley catheter should be placed in order to minimize complications of the procedure prior to the start of the procedure. We will discuss closed percutaneous technique here. Patients should be placed flat on their back with the head of the stretcher at zero-degree incline. The procedure area can then be sterilely prepped with antiseptic. The IV should be flushed with the sterile fluid chosen to prepare the line free of air, and the clinician should retain the sterile cap in order to maintain a sterile column of fluid and tip of the IV tubing. DPL can be done with static ultrasound guidance after the site has been mapped prior to procedure, as recommended in the paracentesis section above. Dynamic guidance is recommended and is especially valuable when only small amount of free fluid is suspected. In the case of the latter, the sterile probe cover should be applied to the ultrasound probe, and one can evaluate the placement of the needle dynamically into the peritoneal cavity. The clinician can then begin by sterilely injecting a wheal of lidocaine or other anesthetic into the procedure site. Anesthetize down to the peritoneum along the desired needle tract. A small vertical skin incision is made one-third of the distance from the umbilicus to the pubic symphysis (approximately 2-3 cm below umbilicus). A supraumbilical incision is preferred in the presence of pelvic fracture or pregnancy. Then the needle is inserted through the linea alba and peritoneum with real-time ultrasound guidance. Ultrasound can help ensure bowel is not adherent to the anterior peritoneum. The guidewire and catheter are also inserted into the peritoneal cavity under dynamic ultrasound guidance (Fig. 10.3), thus ensuring advancement of the catheter into the peritoneal cavity and prevention of intra-abdominal organ injury. When using ultrasound guidance for this procedure, the needle tip should always be in view if using the out-of-plane approach, and the entire shaft of the needle should be in view using the in-plane approach. Upon passage of the catheter or needle into the peritoneum, aspiration of 10 ml of blood indicates a positive examination, and operative exploration is warranted. If no blood is aspirated, the liter of fluid is flushed into the

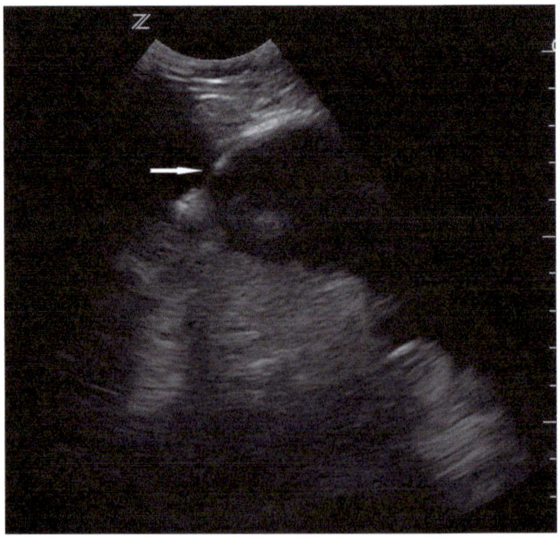

Fig. 10.3 Catheter (arrow) introduced into the peritoneal cavity under dynamic ultrasound guidance. (Courtesy of Srikar Adhikari, MD)

abdomen, and then the bag is placed below the patient in a gravity-dependent location, which will then allow the fluid to reenter the bag. The bag is then agitated, and 10–30 ml of fluid is sent for analysis, and a positive finding consists of 100,000 RBCs/mm^3; 500 WBCs/mm^3; any presence of bile, bacteria, or intestinal contents; and a serum amylase >175 IU/ml [7–9].

Complications

- Local or systemic infection
- False-positive results, resulting in unnecessary laparotomy
- Intraperitoneal injury or hematoma, which can be reduced by assistance with ultrasound monitoring the tip of the procedure needle
- Inability to recover lavage fluid (catheter into preperitoneal space, internal adhesions compartmentalizing fluid, internal contents blocking return of flow into catheter, diaphragmatic injury pooling fluid into thoracic cavity), which can be investigated by the use of ultrasound evaluating the fluid location and obstructive issues or by aiding in repositioning the catheter to recollect the fluid

Pearls/Pitfalls

- Placing fluid into the preperitoneal space
- Bladder injury secondary to neglecting to place a Foley catheter
- Fluid testing producing indeterminate results

Integration into Clinical Practice

The ultrasound-assisted DPL can limit the invasiveness of DPL and can help guide catheter placement. Given the prevalence of portable and handheld ultrasound devices, this procedure can potentially be performed in any settings where minimum requirements are met. This can be especially helpful in highly remote or austere environment and in case where patient evaluation brings severe hazards and high risk.

Evidence

Ultrasound may prove beneficial in returning the lavage fluid for testing as it can frequently be hard localize [7, 8].

Key Points

- Ultrasound can make the invasive procedure of DPL less invasive.
- Ultrasound can assist in returning fluid from the peritoneal cavity.
- Ultrasound can decrease complications arising from DPL.

Gastrostomy Tube Placement

Traditionally, gastric tube placement has been confirmed with X ray and injection of contrast into the newly replaced gastric tube. However, ultrasound can be used on a daily basis in the acute care settings to confirm placement of dislodged G-tubes decreasing time, radiation, and cost.

Anatomy

Anatomy of the abdomen for ultrasound-guided procedures has several key elements: location of the stomach and other major organs, the epigastric vessels, mesentery, and the layers of soft tissue leading to the peritoneal cavity. The epigastric blood vessels traverse the rectus abdominis muscles posteriorly and can be easily injured during blind procedures. Particular attention should be paid to the superior epigastric and superficial inferior epigastric artery branches given potential for variability between patients.

Indications

Those who are unable to safely move food from their oropharynx to the stomach are commonly those in need of a gastrostomy tube, in those that a lighted endoscope cannot pass ultrasound may prove beneficial:

- Pre-existing G-tube tract and tube was dislodged
- Oropharyngeal, esophageal, or other mass obstructing passage of an endoscope to aid in G-tube placement

Contraindications

- Uncorrected coagulopathy
- Sepsis, peritonitis, and abdominal wall infection
- Gastric outlet obstruction
- Gastroparesis
- Peritoneal dialysis

Equipment/Probe Selection

Clinicians should opt for a curvilinear transducer with sterile probe cover.

- Ultrasound
- Percutaneous endoscopic gastrostomy (PEG) tube kit
  - PEG tube
  - Guidewire
  - Nasogastric tube
  - Surgical marker
  - Partially water-filled syringe, 5 mL
  - Sterile fenestrated drape
  - Lidocaine or anesthetic of choice
  - Anesthesia
  - Needle and pigtail catheter assembly (can use one similar to the urology suprapubic pigtail catheter)
  - #11 surgical blade
  - Sterile 4 × 4 gauze
  - Sterile gel (surgical lubricant)
  - Antiseptic
  - Suture kit with iris scissors
  - Supplies for moderate sedation

Preparation/Pre-procedural Evaluation

In clinical settings, the most common indication for this procedure will be replacement of a dislodged tube with ultrasound confirmation. However, for those with upper gastrointestinal obstruction, one may need to place a percutaneous sonographic gastrostomy (PSG) tube. One can use the ultrasound to identify the stomach, which appears as an anechoic pouch with a hyperechoic rim that is the gastric mucosa. The experienced sonologist may be able to make out the gastric rugae. The thinnest layer of abdominal wall overlying the stomach can be identified. Pay special attention to the location of the colon, and map out regions where it will be safe to place the catheter without damaging the colon.

Procedure

Place the head of the bed at a 30-degree angle or greater. The patient should be administered a first-generation cephalosporin intravenously prior to beginning the procedure or some other antibiotic with gram-positive coverage for new PSG placement. After you have sterilely prepared the mapped procedure site with antiseptic, cover it with a fenestrated drape. Local anesthetic should be given to adequately anesthetize the abdominal wall. The stomach should be insufflated with water through a nasogastric tube or via direct puncture with a procedure needle. The procedure needle should be placed under direct ultrasound visualization into the gastric antrum; while holding negative pressure on the water-filled syringe piston, insert the needle until directly visualized in the stomach. If the air is aspirated into the water filled syringe prior to visualizing the needle puncture the stomach, the colon has likely been punctured. If this happens, the needle must then be redirected around the bowel and into the gastric lumen. A guidewire can then be placed through the procedure needle and a small incision is made at the skin in order to pass a trocar over the wire. While advancing the trocar, do not slowly place it into the stomach; instead, it should be advanced with a slight jab or poke in an attempt to not separate the gastric wall from the abdominal wall, and the results of this can be monitored by evaluating the trocar with ultrasound. After the trocar is advanced over the guidewire and removed, the pigtail catheter with balloon proximal to its last fenestration to enter the stomach can then be advanced over the wire. The balloon can be inflated and the stylet is removed. Successful placement can be verified with ultrasound, aspiration of gastric contents, and air insufflation. Real-time ultrasound guidance can be used to visualize a new G-tube inserted through a pre-existing stoma, through the previously fashioned tract, into the body of the stomach. This allows one to dynamically see the tube reenter the stomach and confirm accurate G-tube placement in one process (Fig. 10.4) [10–13].

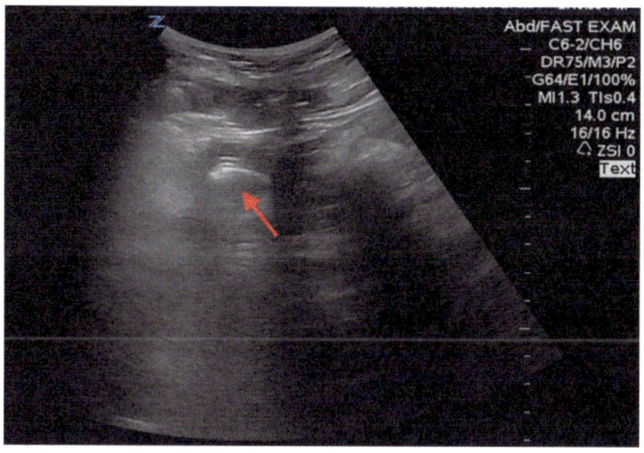

Fig. 10.4 Visualization of the gastrostomy tube (arrow) in the stomach

Complications

- Aspiration
- Peritonitis, infection, bleeding, and leakage
- Colon injury
- Oversedation leading to cardiopulmonary problems
- Placement of tube into peritoneum or abdominal wall

Pearls/Pitfalls

- The tube should be flushed and aspirated prior to completion of the procedure to ensure patency while the patient is still sedated.
- Ensure that a slight jab or poke is used when introducing the dilator and pigtail catheter.
- Ensure adequate sedation and anesthesia.

Integration into Clinical Practice

Ultrasound provides a higher degree of accuracy and safety when compared to traditional blind approaches. A practitioner can become reliant on the visualization of the tube in the antrum, aspiration of gastric contents, and the auscultation of air as reassurance of proper G-tube replacement.

Evidence

Real-time ultrasound guidance and manipulation increases provider certainty and confidence. Ultrasound allows for real-time confirmation of tube placement [10–13]. The confirmatory gastric contrast confirmatory study can be foregone and the patient safely dispositioned with a new feeding tube [7, 10–13].

Key Points

- Ultrasound assistance of the procedure is sensitive and practical for evaluating G-tube placement.
- Ultrasound helps to confirm stomach aspiration versus aspiration of bowel.

Nasogastric Tube Insertion

Nasogastric tube (NGT) insertion is one of the most commonly performed procedures in the acute care settings. The location of the NGT must be ascertained immediately after placement or with the presence of vomiting, coughing, severe retching, or a drop in oxygenation. The gold standard for proper nasogastric tube placement is the upright chest X-ray. Other methods for assessing placement include auscultation, measurement of NGT pH, colorimetric analysis of NGT carbon dioxide, and the use of sonography for direct visualization of the NGT in the stomach.

Anatomy

Placement of a NGT involves passing the flexible tube through the nares, the nasopharynx, and the oropharynx, past the larynx, and into the esophagus. The esophagus begins at the level of the cricoid cartilage; courses behind or to the left of the trachea, behind the aorta and heart in the posterior mediastinum, and through the diaphragm at the esophageal hiatus; and ends at the cardia of the stomach just below the diaphragm. Once the NGT passes into the esophagus, peristalsis will carry it into the stomach. Having the patient flex their neck will push the NGT to the posterior oropharynx allowing easier passage into esophagus. Having the patient swallow allows for the epiglottis to cover the larynx, the vocal cords to approximate together, and the larynx to pull up and forward stretching the esophageal walls to create a larger opening for the tube to go into as the first part of the esophagus relaxes. The average distance from the anterior nasal spine to the tracheoesophageal junction is about 20 cm. The average length of the muscular esophagus is about 25 cm. Ideally the tip of a nasogastric tube should lie approximately 10 cm below the gastroesophageal junction, making the ideal length for nasogastric tube insertion about 50 to 60 cm at the nasal vestibule [14].

Indications

Placement of the nasogastric (NG) tube allows for bowel decompression after intubation and in instances of acute bowel obstruction, confirmation of transdiaphragmatic hernia in trauma, lavage of pill fragments in acute overdose, or removal of blood in acute gastrointestinal bleeding.

Contraindications

Relative contraindications for this procedure include facial fractures, coagulopathy, history of esophageal strictures or caustic ingestion, esophageal varices, coma or lethargy with an unsecured airway, recent stomach or esophageal surgery, gastrectomy, and suspicion for elevated intracranial pressure.

Preparation and Pre-procedural Evaluation

An initial evaluation of the patient's bilateral nares for patency is necessary to decrease patient discomfort during the procedure. Additionally, estimation of the required length for the NGT to be placed is required to ensure intragastric placement. This is done by placing the tube up against the patient's face from the tip of the nose to the patient's ear and then from the ear to the xiphoid process. This length plus 5 cm, a total length of approximately 55–65 cm, should correspond to the proper length for intragastric insertion. Mark this length on the NGT with a permanent marker. NGT size is selected for comfort and purpose. For the commonly used Levine tube, sizes range from 2 to 18 French; 2–12 French is for neonates, infants, children, and adult patients with small nares, while 14–18 French is for the typical adult.

Equipment/Probe Selection

- Gloves
- Towels (if patient gags and vomits)
- Tincture of benzoin
- Adhesive tape
- Appropriate sized Levine nasogastric tube
- Cetacaine spray or 4% nebulized lidocaine
- Neosynephrine 0.5% or Afrin 0.5% spray
- Wall suction set up with adapter for connection to NGT tube
- Emesis basin
- Small cup of water with a straw

Procedure

Instill a topical vasoconstrictor such as neosynephrine 0.5% or Afrin 0.05% into both nares to decrease risk of epistaxis secondary to nasal trauma and wait for 5 minutes. Apply Cetacaine spray or 4% nebulized lidocaine delivered via facemask 5 minutes prior to the procedure to anesthetize the oropharynx.

Examine the patient's neck with ultrasound to view the position of the esophagus prior to NGT insertion by placing a linear, high-frequency probe (14–8 MHz) in transverse orientation, midline over the lower third of the neck, near the thyroid, with the indicator pointing to the patient's right. To the right of the screen, the trachea will appear as a hyperechoic ring with posterior shadowing lying midline under overlying thyroid tissue. To the left of the trachea, the circular esophagus will appear as a hyperechoic ring (Fig. 10.5a). Adjacent to the esophagus, the internal jugular vein and carotid artery will appear. Lubricate the NGT with sterile lubricant and/or viscous lidocaine. Have the patient flex his or her neck with the chin touching the chest, and while they are simultaneously sipping water, insert the lubricated NGT through the most patent nostril, straight back, past the posterior pharynx to the oropharynx, esophagus, and stomach as noted by the marked area on the NGT reaching the nasal vestibule. Clean the nose with the tincture of benzoin, and tape the nasogastric tube in place to the nose.

For confirmation via ultrasound, place the same linear, high-frequency probe over the same area of the patient's lower third of the neck as described above, looking for the same anatomical structures previously described, but now note that the visualized circular esophagus will appear as a hyperechoic ring with a shadowing, attenuation artifact signifying that the NG tube has been cor-

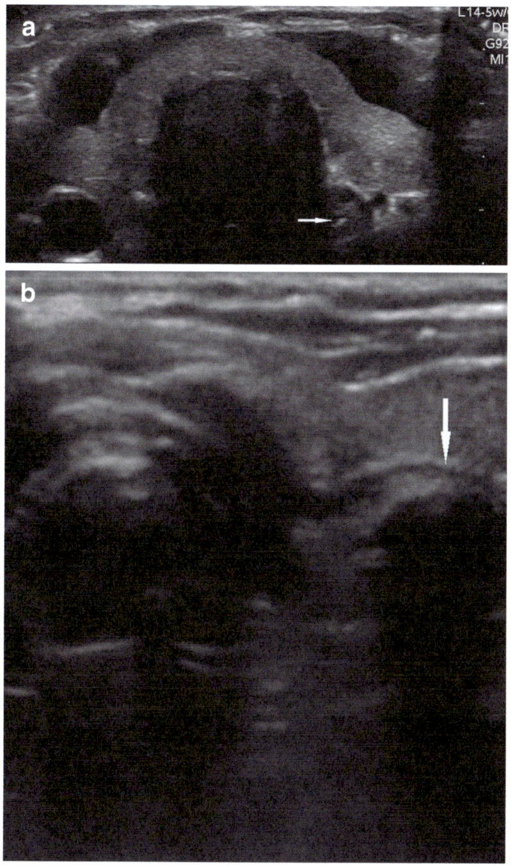

Fig. 10.5 (**a**) Visualization of the trachea, thyroid, and esophagus (arrow). (**b**) Visualization of NG tube in the esophagus with attenuation artifact (arrow)

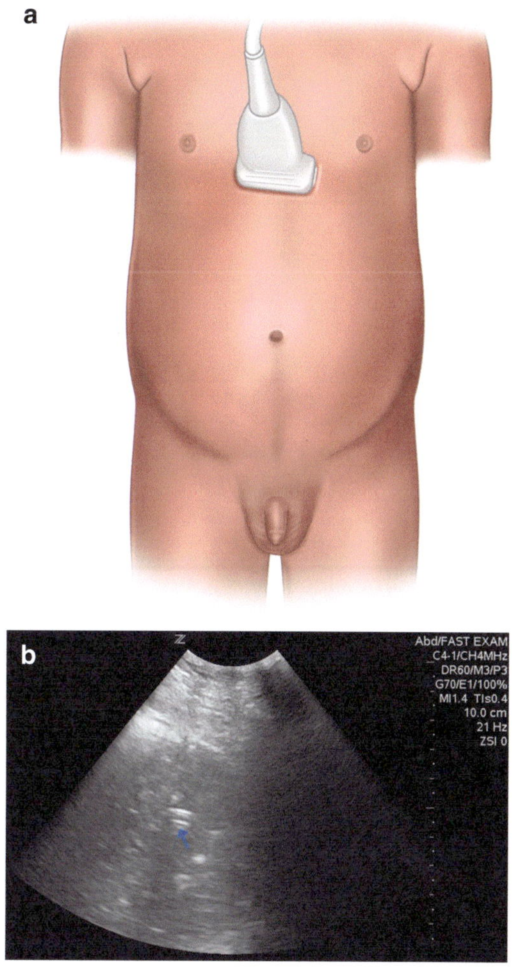

Fig. 10.6 (**a**) Position of probe on the abdomen for visualization of NG tube. (**b**) Visualization of NG tube in the abdomen as a linear hyperechoic structure (arrow)

rectly placed within the esophagus (Fig. 10.5b). To visualize and confirm that the NGT is in the stomach, place a low-frequency, curvilinear probe (6–2 MHz) in a transverse orientation with the indicator pointing to the patient's right side along the epigastrium, below the xiphoid process, and fan the probe superiorly and inferiorly (Fig. 10.6a). The NG tube will appear as a linear, horizontal, or obliquely oriented hyperechoic structure with posterior shadowing within the lumen of the stomach (Fig. 10.6b).

Complications

Complications of NGT placement may occur. Common complications include sinusitis and epistaxis due to trauma or prolonged placement. These can be avoided by properly securing and lubricating the NG tube and by using smaller tube sizes with quick removal when the tube is no longer needed. Another complication is misplacement into the pleural cavity and tracheobronchial tree and, rarely, through the cribriform plate into the brain. Although misplacement is rare, its occurrence can be catastrophic and can result in a pneumothorax, atelectasis, pneumonia, abscess formation, mediastinitis, bleeding, or even death. Other complications include esophageal, gastric, or duodenal perforation, twisting or breaking of the tube, and aspiration secondary to improper placement at the gastroesophageal junction [14, 15]. Many of these complications can be preventable by ultrasound confirmation.

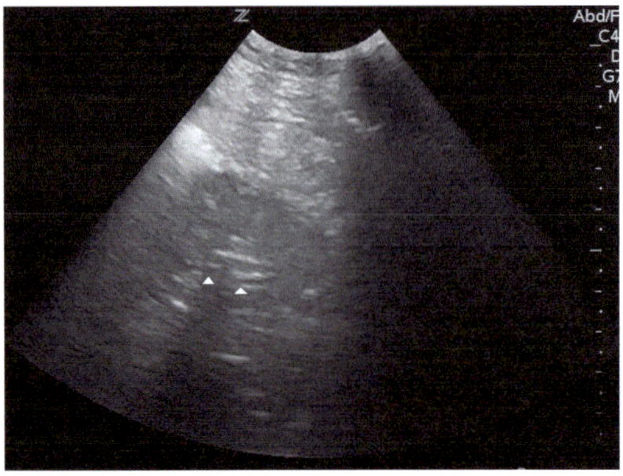

Fig. 10.7 Nasogastric tube visualized with agitated saline (swirling fog, arrowheads)

Pearls and Pitfalls

Poor visualization of the NG tube may occur in patients with large amounts of bowel gas such as those with bowel obstruction. Graded compression may be used to improve image quality; however, there may be so much gas, and visualization is still difficult.

Agitated saline may also be injected to verify placement. Position the curvilinear, low-frequency probe on the epigastrium, in a transverse orientation, indicator to the patient's right. Mix 40 ml of normal saline and 10 ml of air in a syringe, and inject it into the NG tube, watching for a hyperechoic swirling "fog" exiting the tip of the NG tube. This swirling "fog" formation confirms correct placement of the NG tube within the stomach (Fig. 10.7).

Integration into Clinical Practice

Recent studies have shown that sonographic confirmation of NGT placement in infants, neonates, and adults has a sensitivity of 95% and a specificity of up to 100% [15, 16]. Sonographic confirmation is less time-consuming (1–5 minutes) in comparison to capnography, capnometry, and pH confirmation (11–42 minutes) [15–18] and is a useful, cost-effective confirmatory adjunct to traditional methods. There are a few difficulties associated with ultrasound confirmation of nasogastric tube placement. Its use may at some point be superior to traditional methods, as it decreases the amount of radiation exposure, the time to confirmation, and, with proper training and practice, negative outcomes.

Evidence

Auscultation has been proven to be sensitive, greater than 90%, but poorly specific, 34% [13, 14]. Assessment of proper placement via auscultation has proven to be inaccurate because a proximally placed tube can be still produce the gurgling rush of air that is auscultated for confirmation. Evaluation of NGT pH has also been suggested and has a sensitivity of 86% and a specificity of 67% [13] with an ideal aspirate pH between 1 and 5.5. Unfortunately, this can also be inaccurate in patients taking acid-suppressive medications or if the tube placed is of small caliber. Use of capnography and capnometry for detection of incorrect NGT placement in the tracheobronchial tree has also been studied [17–19] demonstrating a sensitivity of 95% and a specificity of nearly 100%.

Key Points

- Ultrasound can prevent unnecessary radiation to a patient receiving a nasogastric tube.
- Visualization of the nasogastric tube can be assisted with agitated saline and graded compression of the abdomen using a curvilinear probe.
- Watch for the hyperechoic ring and attenuation artifact in the esophagus once the nasogastric tube has been placed.

Genitourinary Procedures

Ultrasound is a bedside tool that can be used for static or dynamic guidance for commonly performed genitourinary procedures. This section will cover the steps required to successfully utilize ultrasound for bladder catheterization, suprapubic aspiration, and suprapubic catheterization.

Anatomy

The genitourinary system consists of the kidneys, ureters, bladder, and urethra. The bladder is a hollow, muscular organ located posterior to the pubic bone in the anterior pelvis in adults. The bladder consists of two inlets, the ureters, and one outlet, the urethrovesicular junction. As the bladder fills with urine, it extends superiorly into the abdominal cavity. In children, the bladder is an abdominal organ between the pubis symphysis and the umbilicus. The bladder descends into the adult retroperitoneal position by approximately 9 years of age.

Dorsal Penile Block

Urological emergencies occur with relative frequency in most clinical settings. Priapism, paraphimosis, and phimosis can be extremely painful, making appropriate pain management important in these situations. The dorsal penile nerve block was initially described in anesthesia literature in 1972 by Bateman et al. and refined in 1989 by Brown and colleagues [20]. It is traditionally used to provide pain relief in infants undergoing circumcision, but in the setting of urological emergencies, it has been used in the emergency department to provide pain relief in reduction of priapism, paraphimosis, and phimosis. Traditionally this has been accomplished via landmark techniques relying on a loss of resistance (feeling a "pop" sensation) as the needle advances through Scarpa's fascia. Successful regional anesthesia requires anesthetics to be injected in close proximity to the dorsal penile nerve without damaging the nerve or any surrounding structures [21].

Anatomy

The somatosensory innervation originates in the skin of the penis, the glans, and the urethra and from within the corpus cavernosum. The ilioinguinal, genitofemoral, and posterior scrotal nerves also supply minor sensory innervation to the penis. Free nerve endings in the glans of the penis converge to form the dorsal penile nerve, which eventually become the pudendal nerve that traces back to the sacral spinal nerves. The dorsal penile nerve lies below Buck's fascia, on the dorsal surface of the corpus cavernosum (Fig. 10.8) [22]. It provides the majority of sensory innervation to

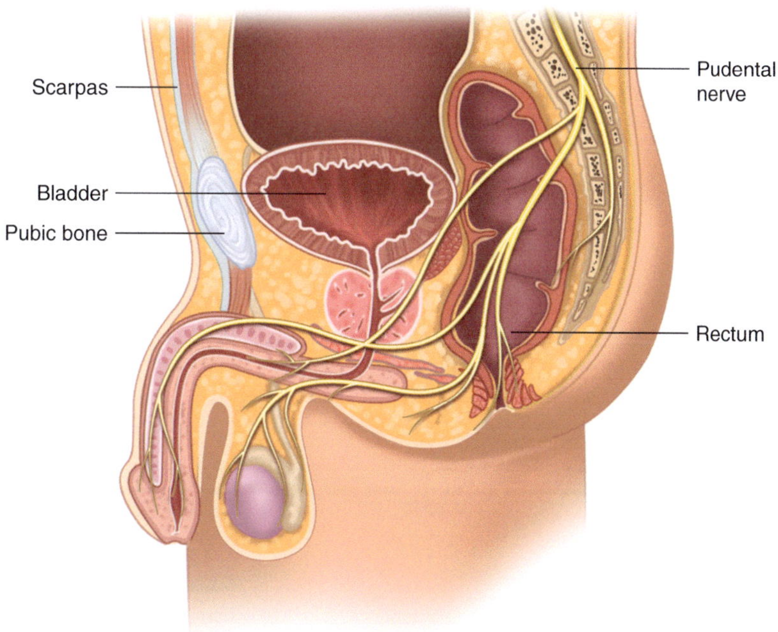

Fig. 10.8 Anatomy of the male penis and its innervation

the dorsal and ventral surfaces of the penis. This is the target nerve for adequate pain relief with the penile block.

Indications

Pain relief for infants, children, and adults presenting with phimosis, paraphimosis, priapism, and penile trauma

Contraindications

Contraindications for such a block are rare and include allergies to the anesthetic, anatomical abnormalities such as hypospadias, infection, or small cell carcinoma of the region.

Preparation and Pre-procedural Evaluation

Draw up 10 cc of 1% lidocaine using an 18G needle, and then change needle to 25 G needle in preparation for local anesthesia. Prep the patient's penis and subpubic region in sterile fashion with chlorhexidine or betadine. Place a high-frequency, linear probe (14–6 MHz) in a sterile probe cover or sterile glove with sterile lubricant applied inside the glove or cover.

Equipment/Probe Selection

- Gloves
- 10 cc syringe
- 25 G needle
- 18 G needle
- Chlorhexidine, betadine, or alcohol swabs
- Sterile lubricant
- Sterile probe cover or sterile glove for probe

Procedure

Two possible techniques utilizing a probe oriented in the transverse and longitudinal planes are possible.

In the first technique, the ultrasound probe is placed in a longitudinal fashion, midline, along the shaft of the penis with the indicator pointing toward the patient's pubic bone. Scarpa's fascia, Buck's fascia, the tunica albuginea, the pubic symphysis, and the fundiform ligament are visualized on ultrasound (Fig. 10.9a, b). A small subcutaneous wheel of 1% lidocaine is made with a 25 G, 1.5 inch hypodermic needle on the most proximal surface of the penis, midline to the probe on both sides of the penis at approximately 2 and 10 o'clock. Advance the needle into the subpubic space under real-time, dynamic ultrasound visualization, and inject 1–5 ml of lidocaine into the subpubic space on either side. In children less than 3, 1–2 ml is injected, and an additional 1 ml is added for every 3 years of age to a maximum of 5 ml [22]. The triangle forming the subpubic space is defined inferiorly by Buck's

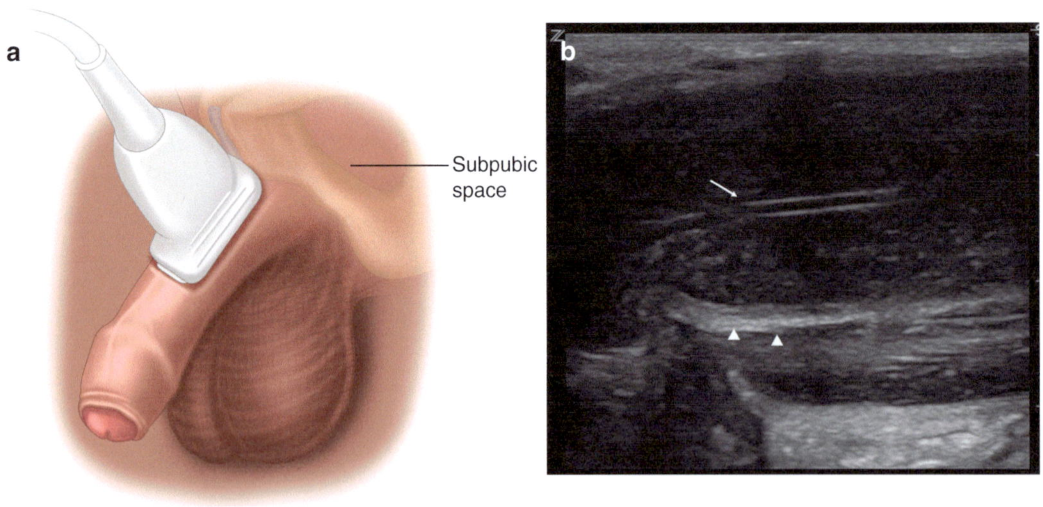

Fig. 10.9 (a) Position of probe for sagittal view of the penis. (b) Sagittal sonographic view of the penis showing corpus cavernosum, tunica albuginea, pubic bone, subpubic space (arrow-intracavernous pillar; arrowheads-penile ligament)

fascia encasing the corpus cavernosum and neurovascular bundle, superiorly by the pubic symphysis, and anteriorly by Scarpa's fascia. By rotating the probe 90° at the site of injection, visualization of the anesthetic spread is seen on ultrasound imaging as a black hypoechoic area filling adjacent to the shaft structures and on either side of the fundiform ligament. In the second technique, the high-frequency linear probe is placed in a transverse fashion indicator pointing to the patient's right (Fig. 10.10a). The penile structures of the skin, dorsal neurovascular bundle, Buck's fascia, corpus cavernosum, and tunica albuginea are visualized in cross section (Fig. 10.10b). In plane to the probe, from lateral to medial, using a 25 G, 1.5 inch hypodermic needle, inject 1–5 ml of lidocaine just underneath Buck's fascia and above the tunica albuginea (Fig. 10.11a–c). Avoid the dorsal artery and vein, which is medial to the nerve with real-time visualization of the needle showing a comet-tailed artifact on ultrasound. Local anesthetic flow, appearing hypoechoic, will displace the corpus cavernosum downward spreading circumferentially to the ventral portion of the penis.

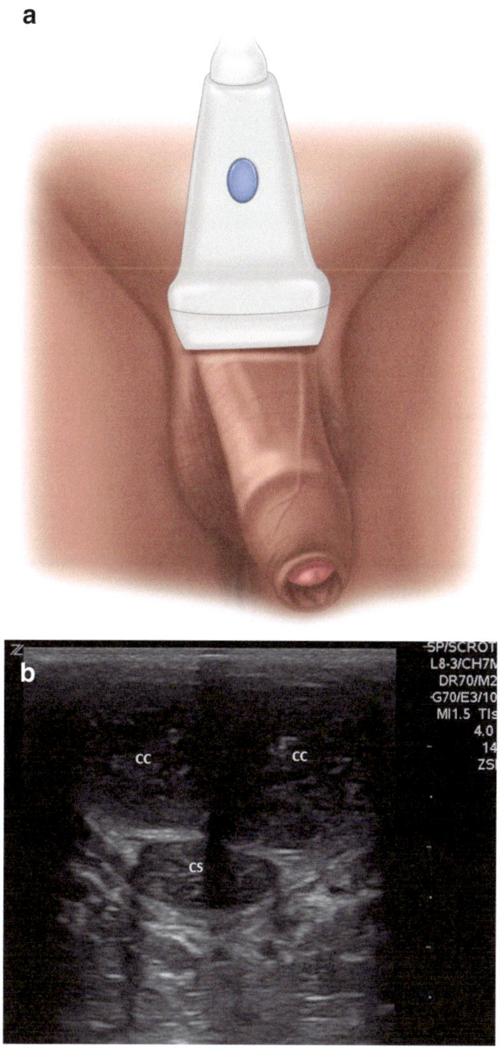

Fig. 10.10 (**a**) Position of probe for transverse view of the penis. (**b**) Transverse sonographic view of the penis depicting Buck's fascia, corpus cavernosum (cc), corpus spongiosum (cs), and tunica albuginea

Complications

Complications of the dorsal penile block include inadvertent injection into the corpus cavernosum or the neurovascular bundle, ischemia, large-volume anesthetic-induced toxicity, infection, bleeding, and hematoma formation [20, 23]. With ultrasound visualization, such complications can drastically be minimized.

Pearls and Pitfalls

Pitfalls for ultrasound-guided dorsal penile block include poor visualization of Buck's fascia and the dorsal penile nerve in the pediatric population because of the small size and the superficiality of the location. Instead, in the pediatric population, visualization of the spread of the anesthetic deep to Scarpa's fascia is the endpoint unlike most other peripheral nerve blocks that easily visualize the nerve [21]. A hockey stick probe may remedy this in some children as it provides good visualization with a smaller footprint. Anatomical variations such as hypospadias can alter visualization of the nerve and increase piercing of the wrong structures such as veins and arteries; however, color flow and power flow can be used to assist in distinguishing structures. As with all ultrasound-guided procedures, it is operator dependent and requires practice and training.

Integration into Clinical Practice

This technique shows much promise in the reduction of complications such as hematoma, poor anesthesia, ischemia, and decreased anesthetic

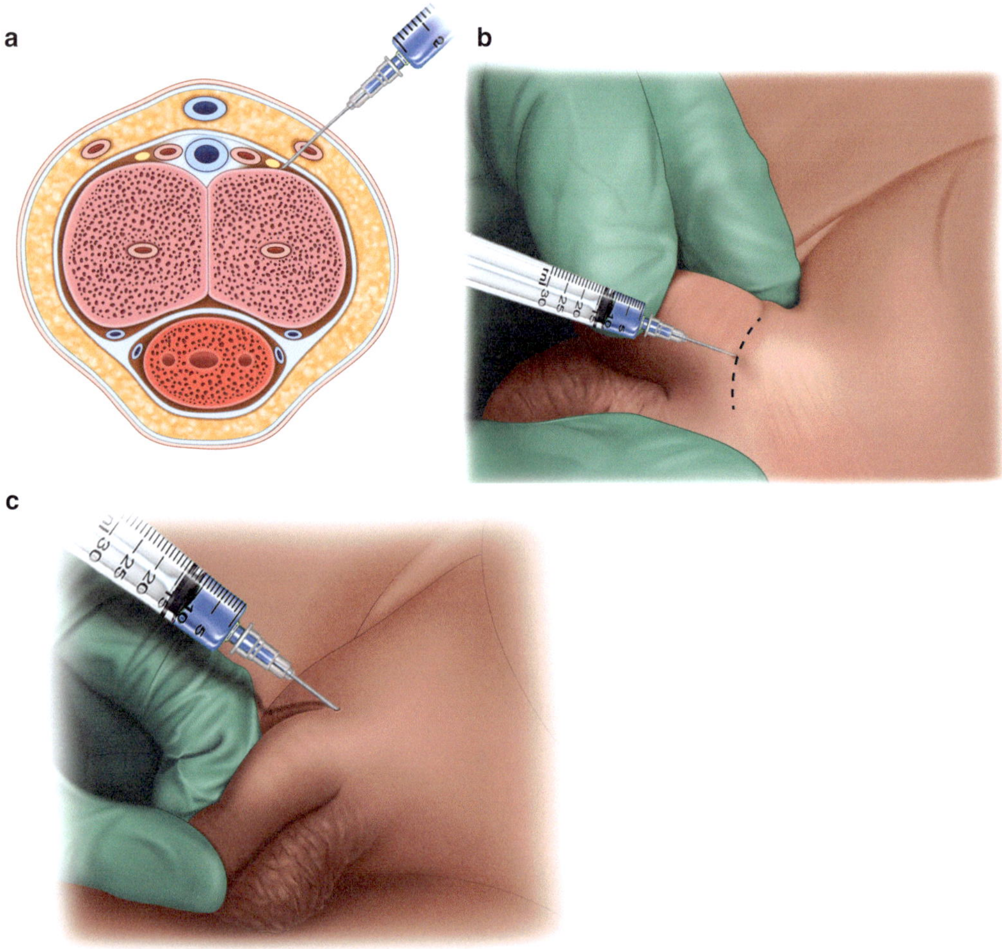

Fig. 10.11 (**a**) Illustration of the penis depicting needle location for dorsal penile block in transverse. (**b**) Position of needle for dorsal penis block. (**c**) Position of needle for dorsal penile block

volume as visualization of structures can assist the treating clinician in a procedure that is normally performed using traditional landmark techniques.

Evidence

Ultrasound guidance for regional anesthesia has shown a higher success rate than the traditional landmark technique [20, 23]. It also demonstrates a lower complication rate and a lower anesthetic volume [20, 23–25].

Key Points

- Ultrasound-guided regional block of the penis greatly reduces complications associated with blind nerve block and utilizes a smaller amount of anesthetic.
- Use a hockey stick probe if available in the pediatric population, and watch for spread of the anesthetic below Scarpa's fascia rather than trying to visualize the actual nerve as it is very small.

Ultrasound-Assisted Hernia Reduction

Of all hernias, 75% are inguinal hernias, 10% are incisional/ventral wall hernias, and 5–7% are umbilical, femoral, or other hernias. When patients present to the acute care setting with hernia pain, manual reduction is sometimes effective and can allow postponement of an operation. Regardless of type, most hernias are reduced in the same manner. An incarcerated hernia, however, is a medical emergency, and detection is crucial for bowel preservation. Incarcerated hernias that cannot be manually reduced need to emergently go to the operating suite to prevent bowel ischemia.

Anatomy

A hernia is a protrusion of abdominal contents beyond the abdominal wall (Fig. 10.12). There are *nine types of hernias*: indirect/direct inguinal, femoral, umbilical, epigastric, abdominal involving separation of the rectus abdominis, spigelian, incisional, lumbar/Petit's triangle, and internal (Fig. 10.13). A full description of each type is beyond the scope of this chapter.

Indications

Inguinal, epigastric, or incisional wall hernias causing pain

Contraindications

Toxic-appearing patient with fever; leukocytosis greater than 15,000/mm3; peritoneal signs; a dusky, black, or bluish discoloration to the viscera; and distended abdomen with signs of obstruction on X-ray

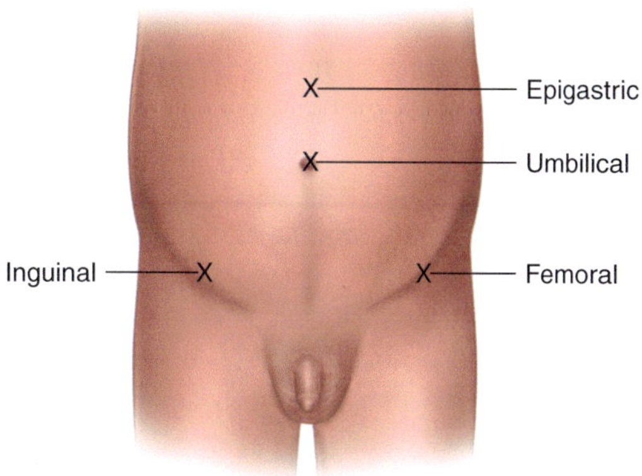

Fig. 10.13 Anatomical location of hernias

Fig. 10.12 Illustration of hernia

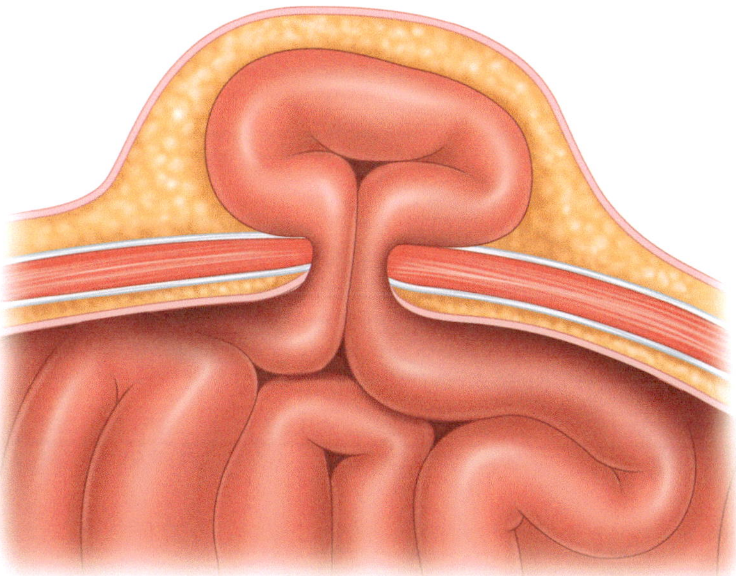

Equipment/Probe Selection

Both a curvilinear and linear transducer can be useful, and the choice depends on body habitus and patient size. A curvilinear array may be more helpful for applying directing pressure for actively reducing the hernia.

- Gloves
- IV analgesic
- Ice bags

Preparation and Pre-procedural Evaluation

Place a high-frequency linear probe (14–8 MHz) or a low–frequency curvilinear probe (6–2 MHz) on the clinically suspicious region. Depending on hernia type, identify the corresponding landmarks. For femoral, indirect, and direct inguinal hernias, this is the inguinal ligament, femoral canal, inguinal canal with content of spermatic cord or round ligament, inferior epigastric vessels, conjoint tendon, and deep and superficial inguinal rings. For epigastric, umbilical, spigelian, lumbar, or abdominal wall hernias, this is the inferior epigastric vessels, aorta, rectus abdominis, latissimus dorsi, transversus abdominis, internal and external oblique muscles, and peristalsing bowel going through the corresponding abdominal musculature. Scan patients supine, in the relaxed state, or while they are standing, during coughing, or during a Valsalva maneuver.

Criteria for ultrasound visualization of a hernia include the presence of a hernia sac (a circular cystic hypoechoic fluid-filled structure with peristalsing bowel inside) on Valsalva or cough superior to inguinal ligament (inguinal hernia), inferior to the inguinal ligament and medial to femoral vessels (femoral hernia), medial to epigastric vessels (indirect hernia), or lateral (direct hernia) to the epigastric vessels with color flow imaging (Fig. 10.14a, b) [26–30].

Procedure

To reduce the hernia, provide patient with IV analgesia, and place the patient in reverse Trendelenburg position. Locate the hernia as described above; apply a gentle graded compression, feeling for a decrease in tensity or a "give" signifying the reduction of the abdominal mass. Obtain a post-reduction ultrasound image (Fig. 10.15a–c).

Complications

Complications of reduction included an irreducible hernia that can result in an incarcerated ovary or decreased blood supply to the testicle in children resulting in testicular infarction, incomplete reduction of hernia, accidental or forced reduction of necrotic or ischemic bowel into peritoneum as visible signs of incarcerated ischemic bowel may not be obvious, and reoccurrence resulting in incarceration of the hernia.

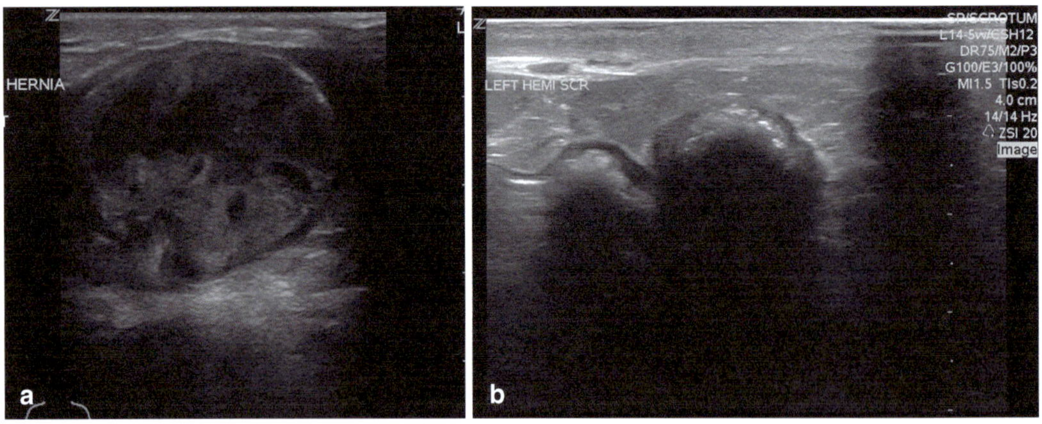

Fig. 10.14 (a) Umbilical hernia with bowel. (Courtesy of Srikar Adhikari, MD). (b) Inguinal hernia

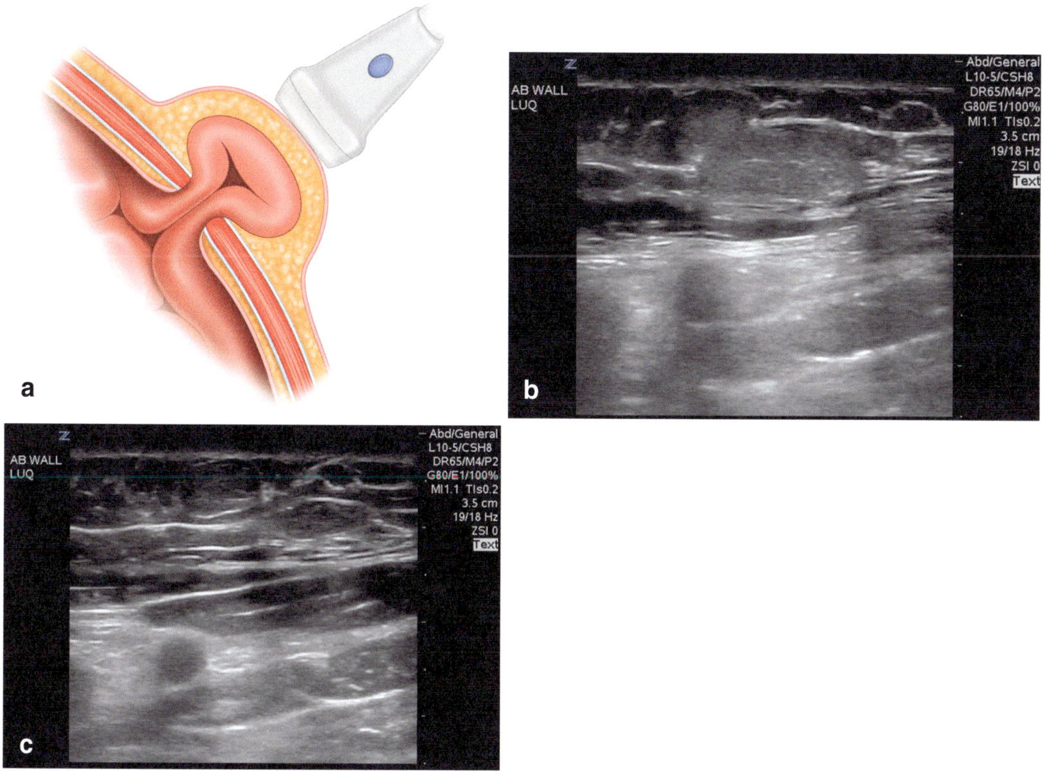

Fig. 10.15 (**a**) Probe placement for abdominal hernia. (**b**) Abdominal hernia pre-reduction. (**c**) Abdominal hernia post-reduction

Pearls and Pitfalls

Use graded compression to displace air and to assist in reduction as bowel gas and morbidly obese individuals can distort anatomy. Use color flow to identify presence or absence of blood flow. Color flow can show the position of hard to see vessels and the presence of hyperemia in a non-incarcerated hernia versus absence of blood flow in an incarcerated hernia [28, 29]. However, newly ischemic bowel may not present with the typical signs of decreased blood flow or changes in skin color.

Integration into Clinical Practice

Sonography and CT can assist in the diagnosis of a hernia, which can often be missed on typical clinical assessment. Ventral and epigastric hernias causing pain and requiring manual reduction may be difficult to identify especially on morbidly obese individuals; with ultrasound, these hernias may be more identifiable. The probe itself is a good adjunctive tool for the reduction of the hernia and for post-procedural confirmation.

Evidence

Clinically 20–30% of hernias are missed on physical exam [31]. Dynamic abdominal sonography has a positive predictive value of 91% and a negative predictive value of 97% in the detection of incisional/ventral wall hernias, a sensitivity of 86% and a specificity of 97% in the identification of direct hernias, and a sensitivity of 97% and a specificity of 86% in the identification of indirect hernias, according to 2 studies [26, 27, 31, 32].

Key Points

- Slowly scan over abdominal surface in area where patient is having tenderness to visualize hernia, looking for peristalsing fluid-filled structure.
- Use graded compression to see if hernia is easily reducible.
- Provide analgesia and muscle relaxant prior to attempt to reduce hernia, and use color flow prior to reduction to identify if bowel has blood flow.

Bladder Catheterization

Indications

Bladder Catheterization

- Management of urinary retention
- Urine output measurement in critically ill
- Management of immobilized patients
- Management of patients who are incontinent
- Management of hematuria in adults

Suprapubic Aspiration

- Safe and effective in obtaining sterile specimens in children less than 2 years of age.
- Reduced incidence of catheter-associated bacteriuria.
- Obtain urine sterilely in uncircumcised boys, tight phimosis, and girls with labial adhesions.

Suprapubic Catheterization

- When urethral catheter is contraindicated or unsuccessful
- Urethral trauma
- Neurological conditions causing bladder dysfunction
- To relieve urinary retention
- Recent urologic surgery
- Prostate enlargement
- Anatomical abnormalities
- Phimosis

Contraindications

Urethral Catheterization

- Absolute contraindication to urethral catheterization is the presence of urethral injury typically associated with pelvic trauma.
- Relative contraindication is presence of urethral strictures.

Suprapubic Aspiration/Catheterization

- Cellulitis over the bladder
- Bladder malignancy
- Anticoagulation or supratherapeutic INR
- Prior surgeries

Equipment/Probe Selection

Phased array (4–3 MHz), curvilinear (6–2 MHz), or microconvex (9–3 MHz) transducer may be useful.

Preparation/Pre-procedural Evaluation

The initial step to ultrasound-guided catheterization of the bladder is evaluating the bladder for its urinary volume. Use the curvilinear probe (6–2 or 4–3 MHz approximately) or the phased array probe (4–3 MHz approximately), and position the probe over the suprapubic area (2 cm above pubic symphysis) in transverse axis, in the midline abdomen of the supine patient (Fig. 10.16). Identify the bladder with ultrasound, and hold the probe as perpendicular as possible over it in transverse axis. In order to calculate the bladder volume, measure the maximum anterior-posterior and lateral-wall-to-lateral-wall diameters. Turn the probe 90° in the sagittal plane, and sweep through the bladder from one side of the bladder to the other. Take an additional measurement from the bladder dome to the bladder base. Save this measurement (Fig. 10.17). The bladder volume can be calculated by using the three measurements you collected above by inserting them into the following formula: $V = \text{width} \times \text{length} \times \text{depth} \times 0.75$ [33, 34]. This method is fast and reliable. However, because of the variability of bladder shape, volume measurements can have an error rate that range up to 25% [35]. The normal post-void residual volume is 100 ml or less

[34]. In addition, ultrasound has increased success rates of urethral catheterization in children. The transverse diameter, obtained in the same manner as described above, of greater than or equal to 2 cm corresponds to a bladder volume of approximately greater than or equal to 2.5 cm^3. The additional measurements in the sagittal view should be obtained and inserted into the volume formula. With a calculated bladder index volume of 2.5 cm^3, catheterization should proceed as this volume corresponds to bladder volume of 2 ml, which is the minimum amount necessary for urinalysis [36].

Procedure

Suprapubic Aspiration

Place the ultrasound machine to the right of the patient. Have the patient lie in supine position. Hold the probe in the transversely over the suprapubic area, with the marker facing the patient's right side. The bladder can usually be

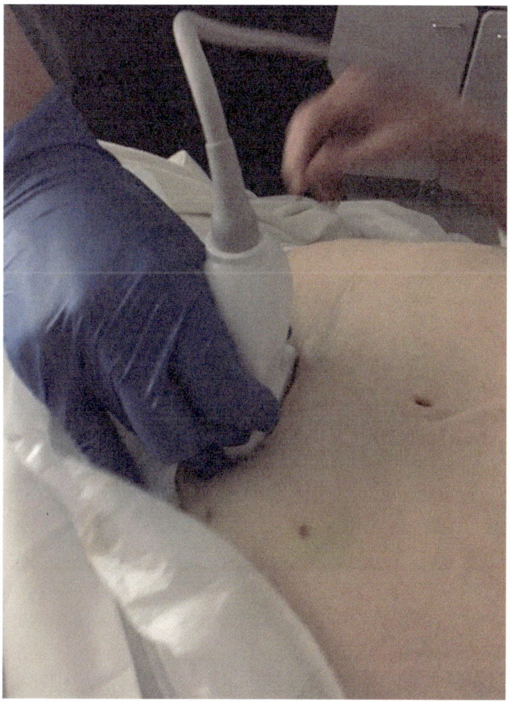

Fig. 10.16 Position of probe for bladder volume

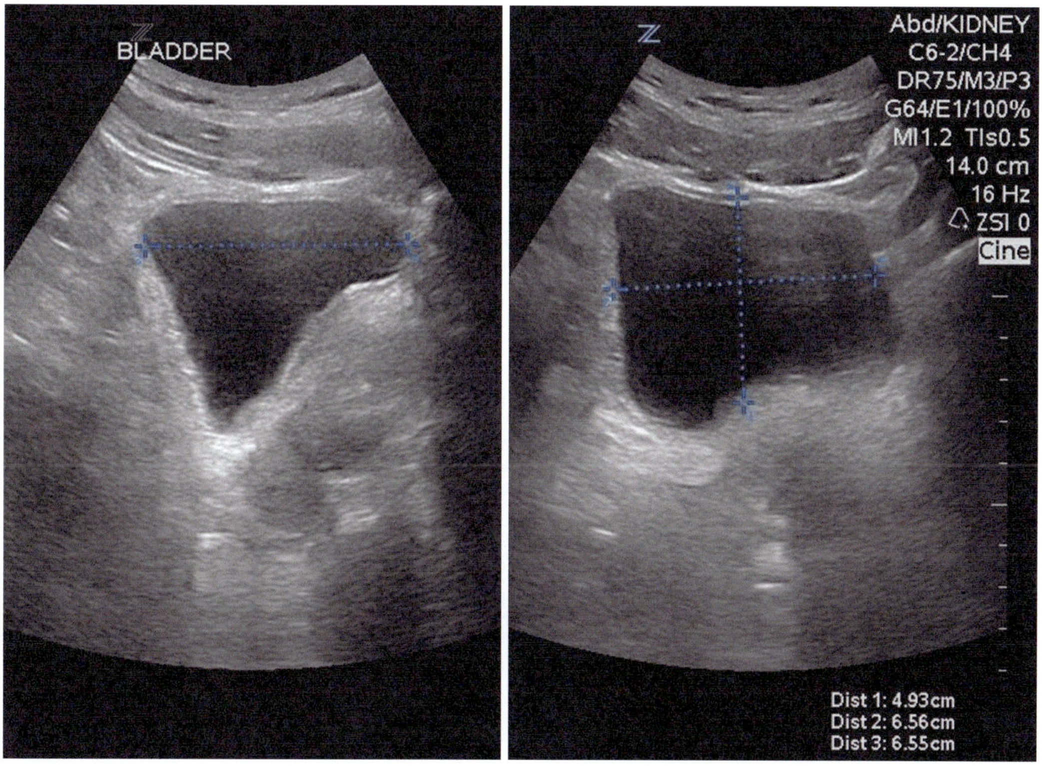

Fig. 10.17 Left: bladder measurement in sagittal axis (depth). Right: bladder measurements in transverse axis (length and width). Note the measurements are listed in the right lower corner

identified midline and deep to the anterior abdominal wall and just superior to the pubic symphysis [37]. Prep the area for this sterile procedure. Use chlorhexidine to clean the suprapubic area liberally. Inject local anesthetic both superficially and deeper into tissue in the pathway. Next apply betadine and drape the suprapubic area with a sterile drape. Apply gel to the probe, cover it with a sterile probe cover, and then apply sterile gel to the outside of the probe cover. The transverse or sagittal view may be used. Hold the probe in the chosen plane and identify the bladder. Scan through the bladder to look for the best site to puncture; the insertion site should be in the middle of the bladder where it is the largest on the screen. For a pediatric patient, select a 22-gauge needle (1.5 in) with 10 ml or 20 ml syringe attached to it. For an adult patient, select a 20-gauge needle or a spinal needle, and hold the needle midway along the length of the probe inferior to the probe. Angulate the probe slightly toward the needle while inserting it into the abdominal wall. The needle should be angled approximately 10–20° from perpendicular to the probe. Aspirate the syringe while advancing the needle which will appear as a hyperechoic focus with reverberation artifact on the ultrasound screen. Gently fan the probe back and forth from the needle insertion site to follow the needle as it enters the bladder. The bladder wall will appear to tent down as the needle pierces the anterior wall of the bladder [38]. With aspiration, urine will fill up in the syringe [39]. Once it is obtained, remove the needle, and apply gentle pressure to the puncture site. Apply a dressing to the puncture site over the area of insertion [34, 40].

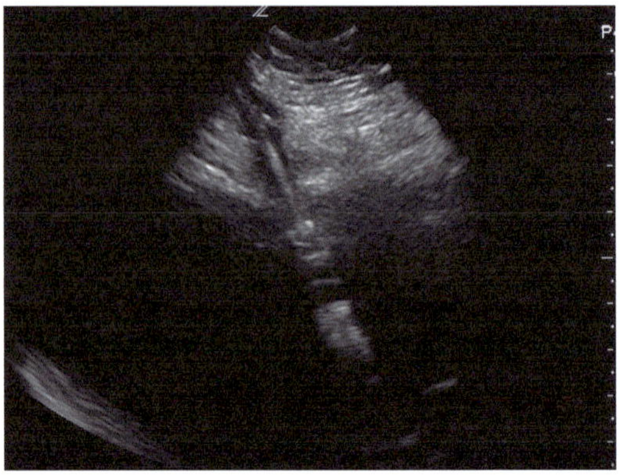

Fig. 10.18 Needle seen in bladder-suprapubic approach. (Courtesy of Srikar Adhikari, MD)

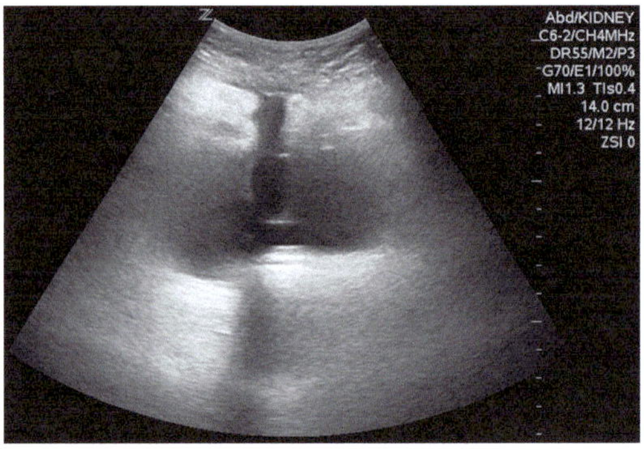

Fig. 10.19 Suprapubic catheter inside bladder with Foley balloon inflated

Suprapubic Catheter Placement

If a suprapubic catheter is going to be left in place, follow the initial steps above, but use a cystostomy kit or Seldinger technique suprapubic catheter kit. The following description assumes the use of the Seldinger technique kit, which should include a needle, guidewire, syringe, sheath with introducer, and Foley catheter. Once the needle is placed in the bladder and urine is aspirated into the syringe, detach the syringe (Fig. 10.18). Insert the J-tip guidewire through the needle into the bladder. The wire may be easily seen entering the bladder under ultrasound guidance. Remove the needle, and use the scalpel to make a small incision at the insertion site above the guidewire. Thread the peel-away sheath introducer over the guidewire into the bladder using a gentle screwing method. Remove the wire. Urine should be flowing back which again confirms you are in the bladder. Insert the Foley catheter through the introducer. Inflate the Foley catheter balloon with the 10 ml of normal saline (Fig. 10.19). Remove the peel-away sheath introducer, and pull back on the catheter until you feel some resistance. Secure the catheter tubing to the abdominal wall with sterile dressing. Attach the Foley catheter to a urinary drainage bag [34, 40].

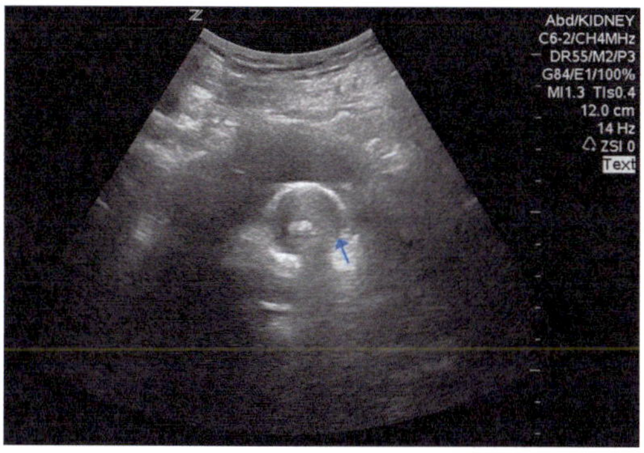

Fig. 10.20 Hyperechoic ring (arrow) inside the bladder confirms placement of Foley

Bladder Catheterization

Prepare and prep the patient prior this procedure by obtaining the bladder volume as described in an earlier section. Place the ultrasound machine to the right of the patient. Have the patient lie in supine position. Hold the probe in transverse orientation over the suprapubic area, with the marker (ridged end of the probe) facing the patient's right side. Prepare the patient in the supine position, with their legs apart and feet together (frog position). The following description assumes the use of standard Foley catheter kit. Prepare a sterile field and don sterile gloves. Check the Foley balloon for functionality. Apply generous amount of sterile lubricant to the tip of the catheter. In a female, separate the labia using the non-dominant hand. In a male, hold the penis perpendicular to patient body with the non-dominant hand. Clean the genital area with betadine swabs with non-dominant hand. Pick up catheter with dominant, sterile hand, and identify the urinary meatus. Insert the Foley until urine is noted flowing back. Inflate the balloon and gently pull back on catheter. Pick up the probe again and place it over the bladder. The Foley can be confirmed by a hyperechoic ring within in the center of the bladder (Fig. 10.20).

Complications

The risk of peritoneal perforation with or without bowel perforation can be minimized by pre-procedural identification of bowel and bladder on ultrasound. It is imperative to measure bladder volume so that you ensure there is an adequate amount of urine in the bladder to displace bowel from the anterior surface and to facilitate safe passage of the suprapubic catheter. Infectious complications can be reduced by exercising sterile technique and using sterile covers for the ultrasound probe. Tube dislodgement or misplaced catheter tube can be avoided by direct visualization of catheter placement under ultrasound guidance. Serial exams of the bladder can be performed to ensure continued placement of the catheter in the bladder and decompression [41, 42].

Pearls/Pitfalls

Keep the needle in line with the probe and in the middle of the length of the probe. For longitudinal scanning, the needle needs to be oriented exactly in the plane of the probe. Hold the probe with a palmar grip, and stabilize the palm on the abdomen of the patient to prevent sliding. Vibrating the needle in small side-to-side motions can cause deflection of adjacent tissues and may aid in highlighting the trajectory of the needle on ultrasound. Angle the probe toward the needle instead of the needle toward the probe for better visualization of the needle. Do not insert the needle or catheter in further once you have aspirated urine to minimize the risk of perforating the bowel [40].

Integration into Clinical Practice

The incorporation of point-of-care ultrasound into the performance of genitourinary procedures has decreased both complication rates and need for multiple attempts. It is an improvement from the standard landmark technique, which is currently utilized. The conventional "blind" method of placing a suprapubic catheter or suprapubic aspiration requires a full bladder to displace bowel away from the puncture site. In some patients this method fails and may lead to bowel injury, the risk of which was found to be up to 2.4% with a mortality rate of 1.8% [40].

Evidence

According to the British Association of Urological Surgeons recommendations, ultrasound should be utilized whenever possible with urinary catheterization. Ultrasound-guided suprapubic aspiration and bladder catheterization improve safety, decrease time delays secondary to nonproductive or unsuccessful attempts, and decrease both trauma and pain to the patient [39]. In one prospective study, the success rate of first attempt urethral catheterization using ultrasound was found to be 96% compared to 72% without ultrasound [43]. In addition, ultrasound can sensitively evaluate and confirm bladder distention [39].

Key Points

- Obtain a bladder volume prior to catheterization to make sure there is enough urine in the bladder to displace the abdominal contents preventing perforation.
- Watch for the hyperechoic ring representing Foley once it is placed when you visualize the bladder with the probe.

Bibliography

1. Dewitz A, Jones R, Goldstein J. Additional ultrasound-guided procedures. In: Ma OJ, Mater JR, Blaivas M, editors. Emergency ultrasound. New York: McGraw-Hill; 2008. p. 537–40.
2. Scheer D, Secko M, Mehta N. Focus on: ultrasound-guided paracentesis. In: American College of Emergency Physicians online CME. American College of Emergency Physicians; 2014. http://www.acep.org/Education/Continuing-Medical-Education-%28CME%29/Focus-On/Focus-On%2D%2DUltrasound-Guided-Paracentesis/. Accessed 13 Feb 2015.
3. Cho J, Jensen TP, Rierson K, Matthews BK, Bhagra A, Franco-Sadud R, Grikis L, Mader M, Dancel R, Lucas BP, Society of Hospital Medicine Point-of-Care Ultrasound Task Force, Soni NJ. Recommendations on the use of ultrasound guidance for adult abdominal paracentesis: a position statement of the Society of Hospital Medicine. J Hosp Med. 2019;14:E7–E15.
4. Runyon BA, AASLD Practice Guidelines Committee. Management of adult patients with ascites due to cirrhosis: an update. Hepatology. 2009;49(6):2087–107. https://doi.org/10.1002/hep.22853.
5. Nazeer SR, Dewbre H, Miller AH. Ultrasound-assisted paracentesis performed by emergency physicians vs the traditional technique: a prospective, randomized study. Am J Emerg Med. 2005;23(3):363–7.
6. Lin CH, Shih FY, Ma MH, Chiang WC, Yang CW, Ko PC. Should bleeding tendency deter abdominal paracentesis? Dig Liver Dis. 2005;37(12):946–51.
7. Isenhour J, Marx J. Abdominal. In: Marx J, Hockberger R, Walls R, editors. Rosen's emergency medicine: concepts and clinical practice. New York: Mosby Elsevier; 2009. p. 422–4.
8. Scalea TM, Boswell SA. Abdominal injuries. In: Tintinalli JE, Kelen GD, Stapczynski JS, editors. Emergency medicine: a comprehensive study guide. 6th ed. New York: McGraw-Hill; 2004. p. 1615–6.
9. Peitzman AB, Sabom M, Yearly DM, Fabian TC. The trauma manual. Hagerstwon: Lippincott Williams & Wilkins; 2002. p. 578.
10. Bleck JS, Reiss B, Gebel M, Wagner S. Percutaneous sonographic gastrostomy: method, indications, and problems. Am J Gastroenterology. 1998;93(6):941–5.
11. Brun PM, Chenaitia H, Lablanche C. 2-point ultrasonography to confirm correct position of the gastric tube in prehospital setting. Mil Med. 2014;179(9):959–63.
12. Chaves DM, Kumar A, Lera M. EUS-guided percutaneous endoscopic gastrostomy for enteral feeding tube placement. Gastrointest Endosc. 2008;68(6):1168–72.
13. Wu TS, Leech S, Rosenberg M. Ultrasound can accurately guide gastrostomy tube replacement and confirm proper tube placement at the bedside. J Emerg Med. 2009;36(3):280–4.
14. Pillai JB, Vegas A, Brister S. Thoracic complications of nasogastric tube: review of safe practice. Interact Cardiovasc Thorac Surg. 2005;4(5):429–33.
15. Chenaitia H, Brun PM, Querellou E, Leyral J, Bessereau J, Aime C, et al. Ultrasound to confirm gastric tube placement in prehospital management. Resuscitation. 2012;83(4):447–51.
16. Kim HM, So BH, Jeong WJ, Choi SM, Park KN. The effectiveness of ultrasonography in verifying the placement of a nasogastric tube in patients with low consciousness at an emergency center. Scand J Trauma Resusc Emerg Med. 2012;20:38.
17. Galbois A, Vitry P, Ait-Oufella H, Baudel JL, Guidet B, Maury E, et al. Colorimetric capnography, a new procedure to ensure correct feeding tube placement in the intensive care unit: an evaluation of a local protocol. J Crit Care. 2011;26(4):411–4.
18. Meyer P, Henry M, Maury E, Baudel JL, Guidet B, Offenstadt G. Colorimetric capnography to ensure correct nasogastric tube position. J Crit Care. 2009;24(2):231–5.
19. Chau JP, Lo SH, Thompson DR, Fernandez R, Griffiths R. Use of end-tidal carbon dioxide detection to determine correct placement of nasogastric tube: a meta-analysis. Int J Nurs Stud. 2011;48(4):513–21.
20. Sandeman DJ, Dilley AV. Ultrasound guided dorsal penile nerve block in children. Anaesth Intensive Care. 2007;35(2):266–9.
21. O'Sullivan MJ, Mislovic B, Alexander E. Dorsal penile nerve block for male pediatric circumcision--randomized comparison of ultrasound-guided vs

anatomical landmark technique. Paediatr Anaesth. 2011;21(12):1214–8.
22. Brown TC, Weidner NJ, Bouwmeester J. Dorsal nerve of penis block–anatomical and radiological studies. Anaesth Intensive Care. 1989;17(1):34–8.
23. Faraoni D, Gilbeau A, Lingier P, Barvais L, Engelman E, Hennart D. Does ultrasound guidance improve the efficacy of dorsal penile nerve block in children? Paediatr Anaesth. 2010;20(10):931–6.
24. Marhofer P, Chan VW. Ultrasound-guided regional anesthesia: current concepts and future trends. Anesth Analg. 2007;104(5):1265–9, tables of contents.
25. Rubin K, Sullivan D, Sadhasivam S. Are peripheral and neuraxial blocks with ultrasound guidance more effective and safe in children? Paediatr Anaesth. 2009;19(2):92–6.
26. Jamadar DA, Jacobson JA, Morag Y, Girish G, Dong Q, Al-Hawary M, et al. Characteristic locations of inguinal region and anterior abdominal wall hernias: sonographic appearances and identification of clinical pitfalls. AJR Am J Roentgenol. 2007;188(5):1356–64.
27. Rettenbacher T, Hollerweger A, Macheiner P, Gritzmann N, Gotwald T, Frass R, et al. Abdominal wall hernias: cross-sectional imaging signs of incarceration determined with sonography. AJR Am J Roentgenol. 2001;177(5):1061–6.
28. Bradley M, Morgan D, Pentlow B, Roe A. The groin hernia - an ultrasound diagnosis? Ann R Coll Surg Engl. 2003;85(3):178–80.
29. Gokhale S. Sonography in identification of abdominal wall lesions presenting as palpable masses. J Ultrasound Med. 2006;25(9):1199–209.
30. Korenkov M, Paul A, Troidl H. Color duplex sonography: diagnostic tool in the differentiation of inguinal hernias. J Ultrasound Med. 1999;18(8):565–8.
31. Poulose BK, Shelton J, Phillips S, Moore D, Nealon W, Penson D, et al. Epidemiology and cost of ventral hernia repair: making the case for hernia research. Hernia. 2012;16(2):179–83.
32. Torzilli G, Del Fabbro D, Felisi R, Leoni P, Gnocchi P, Lumachi V, et al. Ultrasound-guided reduction of an incarcerated Spigelian hernia. Ultrasound Med Biol. 2001;27(8):1133–5.
33. Rosh AJ. Suprapubic aspiration. In: Drugs & diseases. Medscape; 2015. http://emedicine.medscape.com/article/82964-overview#a01. Accessed 31 Mar 2015.
34. Seif D, Swadron SP. Renal. In: Ma OJ, Mater JR, Blaivas M, editors. Ma & Mateer's emergency ultrasound. New York: McGraw-Hill Companies Inc.; 2008. p. 337.
35. Dicuio M, Pomara G, Menchini Fabris F, Ales V, Dahlstrand C, Morelli G. Measurements of urinary bladder volume: comparison of five ultrasound calculation methods in volunteers. Arch Ital Urol Androl. 2005;77(1):60–2.
36. Baumann BM, McCans K, Stahmer SA, Leonard MB, Shults J, Holmes WC. Volumetric bladder ultrasound performed by trained nurses increases catheterization success in pediatric patients. Am J Emerg Med. 2008;26(1):18–23.
37. O'Brien WM. Percutaneous placement of a Suprapubic tube with peel away sheath introducer. J Urol. 1991;145(5):1015–6.
38. Noller KL, Pratt JH, Symmonds RE. Bowel perforation with Suprapubic cystostomy report of two cases. Obstet Gynecol. 1976;48(Suppl 1):67S–9S.
39. Gochman RF, Karasic RB, Heller MB. Use of portable ultrasound to assist urine collection by Suprapubic aspiration. Ann Emerg Med. 1991;20(6):631–5.
40. Jacob P, Rai BP, Todd AW. Suprapubic catheter insertion using an ultrasound-guided technique and literature review. BJU Int. 2012;110(6):779–84. https://doi.org/10.1111/j.1464-410X.2011.10882.x.
41. Aguilera PA, Choi T, Durham BA. Ultrasound-guided Suprapubic cystostomy catheter placement in the emergency department. J Emerg Med. 2004;26(3):319–21.
42. Schneider RE. Urologic procedures. In: Robert JR, Hedges JR, editors. Clinical procedures in emergency medicine. Philadelphia: W.B. Saunders Co; 2004. p. 1098–100.
43. Chen L1, Hsiao AL, Moore CL, Dziura JD, Santucci KA. Utility of bedside bladder ultrasound before urethral catheterization in young children. Pediatrics. 2005;115(1):108–11.

11 Ultrasound-Guided Percutaneous Drainage Procedures

Elaine Situ-LaCasse, Parisa Javedani, Paola Devis, and Hina Arif-Tiwari

Introduction

Patients with abscess or other abnormal fluid collection that require drainage are often evaluated in acute care settings. It has been well-documented that procedural guidance under ultrasound increases patient safety and patient satisfaction and decreases procedural time. With ultrasound guidance, there is also the benefit of seeing the fluid collection shrink in real time with aspiration. Another method of real-time procedural guidance is through interventional radiology or fluoroscopy, but that exposes the patient to large amounts of ionizing radiation. Because of the complex abdominal anatomy, it is even more critical to maintain needle visualization during the entirety of the procedure. Depending on the location of the abdominal fluid collection, ultrasound can be used for an ultrasound-guided nerve block for the analgesia in addition to being used for procedural guidance of fluid drainage.

E. Situ-LaCasse (✉)
Department of Emergency Medicine, Banner University Medical Center-Tucson, Tucson, AZ, USA
e-mail: esitu@aemrc.arizona.edu

P. Javedani
Colorado Permanente Medical Group, Denver, CO, USA

P. Devis
Medical Imaging and Gastroenterology, University of Arizona College of Medicine, Staff Interventional Radiologist, Southern Arizona Veterans Affairs Health care System, Tucson, AZ, USA

H. Arif-Tiwari
Department of Medical Imaging, University of Arizona, Tucson, AZ, USA

Incision and Drainage of Subcutaneous Abscesses

Advantages of Ultrasound Guidance

Point-of-care ultrasound (POCUS) is a useful tool to differentiate superficial cellulitis and hematoma from abscess. Ultrasound is more sensitive for detection of subcutaneous abscesses compared to computed tomography (CT) without exposing the patient to potential harmful effects of radiation. A study by Gaspari et al. demonstrated that out of 65 patients undergoing both ultrasound and CT for evaluation of suspected abscess, ultrasound demonstrated sensitivity of 96.7% and specificity of 85.7% compared to CT sensitivity of 76.7% and specificity of 91.4% for diagnosis of abscess [1]. Additionally, the training necessary to accurately diagnose presence of abscess by POCUS is readily learned in as little as 30 minutes [2].

Anatomy

POCUS can be used to evaluate the skin, subcutaneous tissue, and fascia. Both superficial epidermis and dermis can be evaluated and appear as a hyper-

S. Adhikari, M. Blaivas (eds.), *The Ultimate Guide to Point-of-Care Ultrasound-Guided Procedures*, https://doi.org/10.1007/978-3-030-28267-7_11

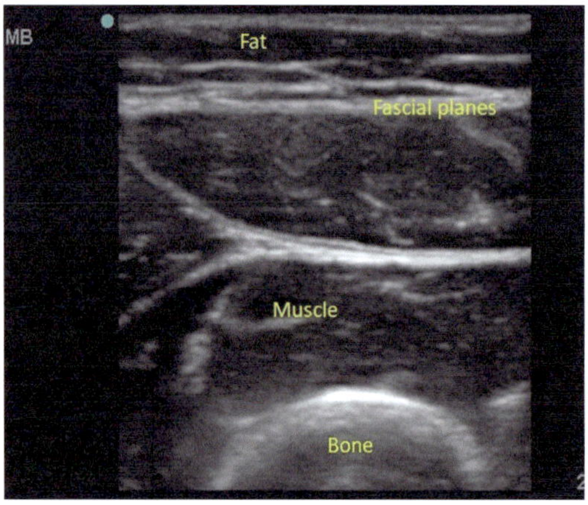

Fig. 11.1 Both superficial epidermis and dermis can be evaluated and appear as a hyperechoic layer on ultrasound. Subcutaneous tissue lies just deep to the dermis and can be visualized as hypoechoic fat lobules with hyperechoic septae. The dense fibrous membrane is the fascial layer and usually appears as a linear hyperechoic layer

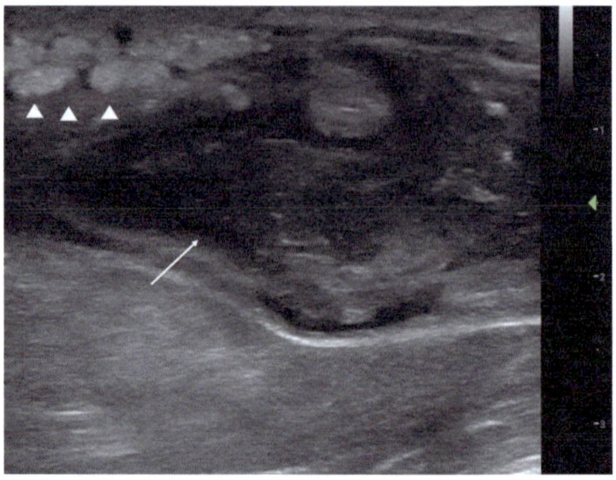

Fig. 11.2 Note the heterogeneous fluid contents with mixed echogenicities within the abscess (arrow). There is also associated cobblestoning seen in the upper left portion of the image, signifying cellulitis (arrow heads) overlying the abscess

echoic layer on ultrasound. Subcutaneous tissue lies just deep to the dermis and can be visualized as hypoechoic fat lobules with hyperechoic septae (Fig. 11.1). The dense fibrous membrane is the fascial layer and usually appears as a linear hyperechoic layer. Veins are visualized as non-pulsatile, compressible anechoic structures with hyperechoic walls. Arteries are visualized as pulsatile, non-compressible anechoic structures with hyperechoic walls. Nerves appear as a small honeycomb, hyperechoic bundle. Special attention should also be given to the underlying muscle. Subcutaneous abscesses can start in the superficial layer of the skin and penetrate through muscle fascia.

Indications

Patients with localized erythema, increased warmth, swelling, and/or discomfort of an affected body part should undergo sonographic imaging to identify pathology such as cellulitis and abscess (Fig. 11.2). In the study by Squire et al., out of 18 cases in which clinical exam did not suggest abscess, but POCUS demonstrated evidence of anechoic fluid collection, ultrasound was accurate in 17/18 (94%) of cases confirmed by incision and drainage. This suggests that patients who are found to have anechoic fluid collections by POCUS concerning for abscess should undergo incision and drainage, even if the clinical examination suggests only superficial cellulitis without abscess [2].

Contraindications

The location of concern should be evaluated with POCUS to ensure that no neurovascular structures lie in the region of interest, which would in turn warrant an alternative method for incision and drainage [2]. In addition, color Doppler can be used to ensure there is no evidence of a necrotic or cancerous lymph node, aneurysm, or pseudoaneurysm (Figs. 11.3 and 11.4). Discretion should be used in bedside incision and drainage of abscess in patients on anticoagulation or with known coagulopathic states. Abscess located in muscle, known as pyomyositis, can present similarly with erythema, pain, swelling, and tenderness on palpation of the affected region (Fig. 11.5). Pyomyositis is generally drained in the operating room.

Equipment and Probe Selection

The high-frequency (12–7 MHz) linear array probe is ideal for evaluation of superficial structures. Color Doppler can aid in identifying surrounding neurovascular structures. One percent lidocaine with or without epinephrine is a commonly used anesthetic. Chlorhexidine, a needle driver for blunt dissection, and a #11 blade scalpel should be readily available prior to starting the procedure. In more delicate areas or for smaller fluid collections, an 18- or 20-gauge needle attached to a 10 mL syringe can be used as an alternative to the #11 blade scalpel.

Of note, if the subcutaneous abscess is in a location of thick subcutaneous fat, such as the buttock, thigh, or abdominal wall, use of the low

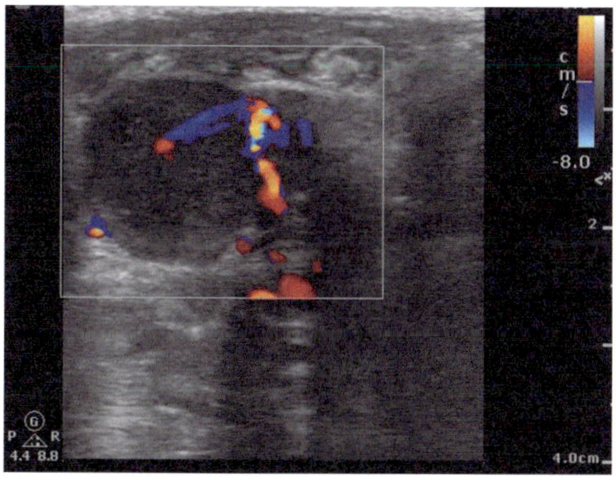

Fig. 11.3 This is an example of a metastatic cancer lymph node. The usual architecture of a normal lymph node is disrupted. There is no central hilar blood flow. The blood flow is now on the periphery. There is no change in shape with graduated compression with the ultrasound transducer to suggest fluid contents

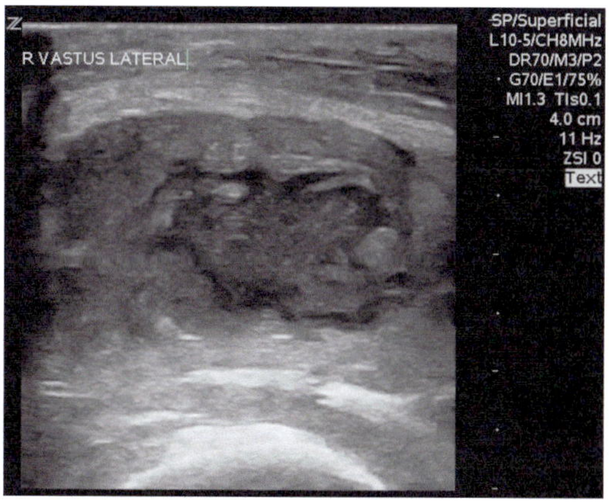

Fig. 11.5 Note the heterogeneous fluid collection that is seen within the muscle along with significant inflammation of the muscle suggesting pyomyositis

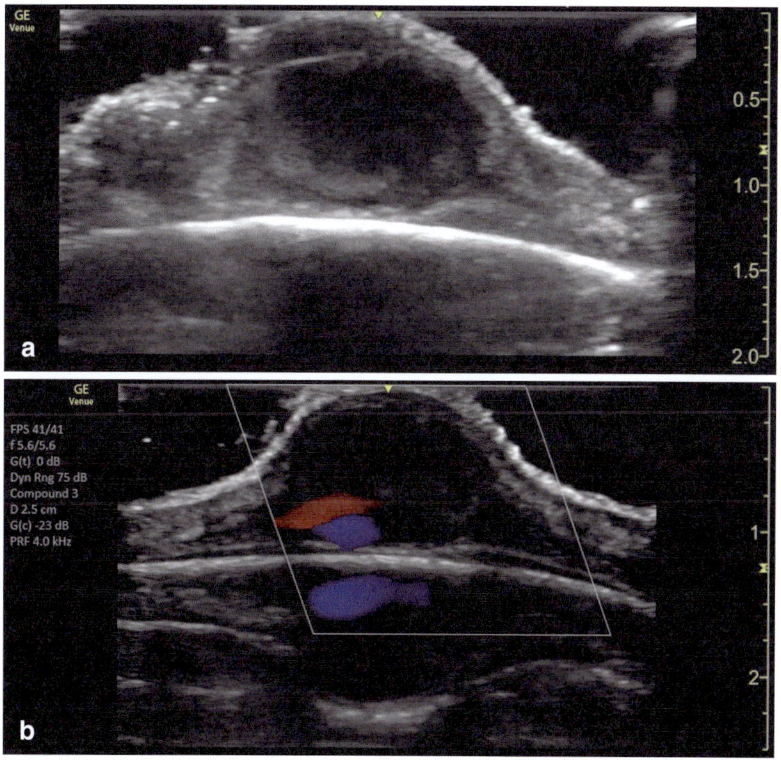

Fig. 11.4 (**a**) This superficial circular mass is pulsatile with blood contents swirling. (**b**) With color Doppler, you see the swirling flow of the blood more clearly. This example illustrates the importance of using bedside ultrasound before an incision and drainage should be performed. It also shows the importance of using color Doppler to identify blood flow

frequency curved array probe for deeper imaging may be helpful.

Preparation and Pre-procedural Evaluation

The patient should be positioned such that the affected area is easily accessible to the provider. Topical anesthetic, such as lidocaine-epinephrine-tetracaine gel, can be used over the affected area to minimize discomfort.

Procedure

Begin scanning away from the affected area to evaluate the patient's normal anatomy. Scan the entire length of the affected area in both sagittal and transverse planes using the linear array probe. An abscess will appear as an anechoic fluid collection with hyperechoic contents often with posterior acoustic enhancement. This can be distinguished from cellulitis, which has a cobblestone appearance without fluid collection (Fig. 11.2). Gentle graded compression ensures a loculated fluid collection is not missed, and color Doppler flow can be used to confirm lack of vascularity (Fig. 11.6). Furthermore, graded compression may result in swirling of abscess contents. Comparison to the contralateral side can be useful. If a fluid collection is located, the boundaries, depth from the tissue surface, and estimated size of the cavity should be noted. The sonographic appearance of a hematoma is non-specific and is challenging to differentiate from an abscess [3].

Once the abscess and surrounding anatomy have been visualized, the affected area should be cleaned with chlorhexidine and subsequently anesthetized. The probe should be covered with a Tegaderm to minimize transmission of nosocomial infections, and gel should be placed over top of the probe. Under ultrasound guidance, a small stab incision should be made using a #11 blade scalpel, and blunt dissection with a needle driver can break up loculated fluid collections. Extensive abscesses may require irrigation with normal saline to aid in breakdown of loculations. In anatomically challenging locations or for small fluid collections, needle aspiration using an 18- or 20-gauge needle attached to a 10 mL syringe can be used as an alternative to using the #11 blade scalpel (Figs. 11.7 and 11.8). Ultrasound should be used after incision and drainage is complete to verify complete evacuation of the abscess cavity.

Complications

Color Doppler can aid in the identification of neurovascular structures, lymph nodes, solid masses, etc. In addition, ultrasound should be used after the procedure to verify complete evacuation of the abscess cavity. A partially drained abscess may result in the need for further intervention.

Pearls and Pitfalls

1. The use of color Doppler during the initial evaluation and real-time ultrasound guidance

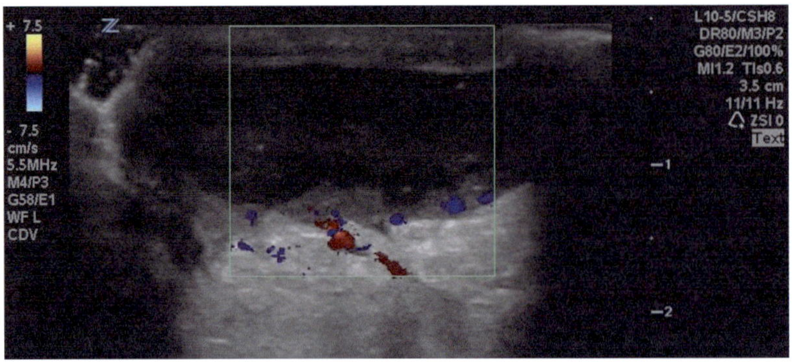

Fig. 11.6 It is normal to see scant blood flow in the periphery of an abscess, secondary to infection and inflammation. There is no central or pulsatile flow in this abscess, which makes it safe for incision and drainage

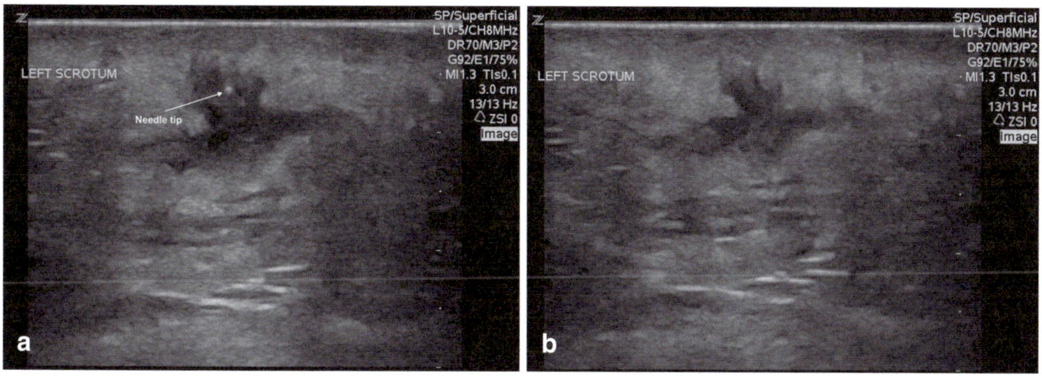

Fig. 11.7 (**a**) In sensitive areas, such as the scrotum, or if the abscess is small, needle aspiration may be preferred. In this image, you see the needle in short axis as an echogenic dot (arrow) (out-of-plane technique). (**b**) With real-time ultrasound guidance and imaging, you can see the actively shrinking abscess as purulence is aspirated

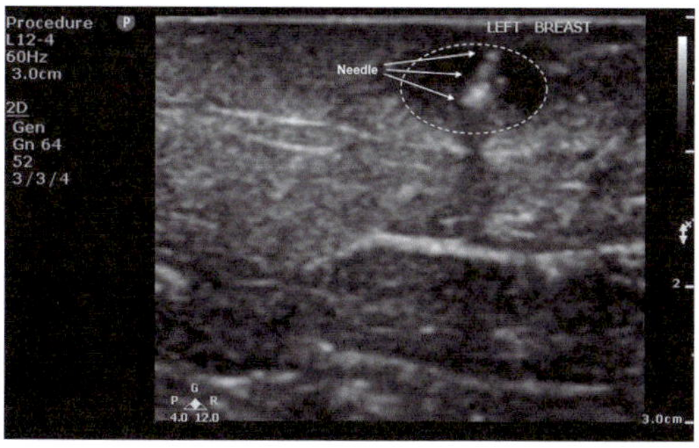

Fig. 11.8 Here is another example of needle aspiration of a left breast abscess. The dotted circle highlights the abscess in the left breast, and the arrows denote the length of the needle

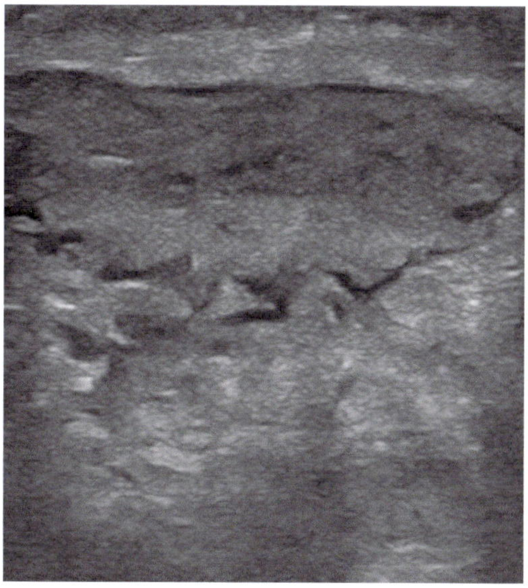

Fig. 11.9 Especially in areas of high-fat content, such as the buttocks, thighs, and, for some patients, abdominal wall, abscesses can appear isoechoic and subtle to identify under ultrasound. Note that this abscess does not have the usual obvious characteristics of a classic abscess. Compression of the area with the transducer may cause swirling of the contents to reveal pus

during the procedure can help avoid neurovascular complications.

2. Purulent material in the abscess cavity may appear isoechoic, and therefore, the use of graded compression and color Doppler can help in identification of an abscess cavity (Fig. 11.9).
3. Use of a larger 18-gauge needle is recommended for needle aspiration procedures, as purulent material may be difficult to aspirate when using a smaller gauge needle.
4. When purulent material is too viscous for needle aspiration or if the abscess cavity is too large to adequately evaluate using needle aspiration, a #11 blade scalpel can be used to create a small stab incision to allow drainage.
5. Be aware that necrotic lymph nodes appear similar to an abscess. Use gray-scale imaging and color Doppler imaging to evaluate for necrotic lymph nodes before performing an incision and drainage, and incision and drainage of necrotic lymph nodes is discouraged.

Integration into Clinical Practice

Ultrasound-guided incision and drainage of abscess and hematoma provide definitive treatment. The features to distinguish abscess from cellulitis are easily learned and can help guide management decisions about the need for incision and drainage. Furthermore, ultrasound-guided drainage provides real-time visualization of the surrounding neurovascular structures which helps reduce the incidence of complications.

Evidence

Ultrasound-guided abscess drainages are technically uncomplicated and minimally invasive. In a study by Kjær et al., subcutaneous truncal abscesses were treated successfully in 93% of their patients [4]. This approach yielded high patient satisfaction and was well-tolerated with short healing times.

Ultrasound-guided breast abscess drainages have replaced open treatment of breast abscesses, with 97% resolution rate in puerperal abscesses and 81% resolution rate for nonpuerperal abscesses [5]. Needle drainage under ultrasound decrease pain and scar formation. The evidence for using ultrasound to directly guide abscess drainage makes it suitable for outpatient settings.

Key Points

- POCUS for the diagnosis or confirmation of a subcutaneous abscess is recommended in addition to physical examination due to concern of a suspected abscess being a mass, lymph node, aneurysm, etc.
- For smaller abscesses, it is reasonable to use a large gauge needle to attempt aspiration and proceed to incision if necessary.
- In-plane technique is always preferred, if possible, to ensure the needle tip does not injury nearby structures.
- Always use color Doppler to evaluate abscesses to identify vascular or blood flow within the fluid collection.

Drainage of Subcutaneous Hematomas

Advantages of Ultrasound Guidance

POCUS is a useful tool to differentiate soft tissue swelling from hematoma, although differentiation of hematoma from abscess can be more challenging. Differentiation between a hematoma and an abscess will depend more on the clinical picture. Patients can also present with an infected hematoma, which may present with signs and symptoms of an abscess over an area of previous trauma or if the patient is prone to bleeding.

Anatomy

Pay close attention to surrounding structures, especially vasculature that may have been injured to cause the hematoma. After drainage of the hematoma that may have tamponade feeding vessels, bleeding may commence from the incision. It is also important to note the sonographic characteristics of the hematoma. Fresh blood may appear hyperechoic or isoechoic to the surrounding subcutaneous tissue, and as blood products break down over time, the blood may become anechoic with possible fibrin strands (Fig. 11.10).

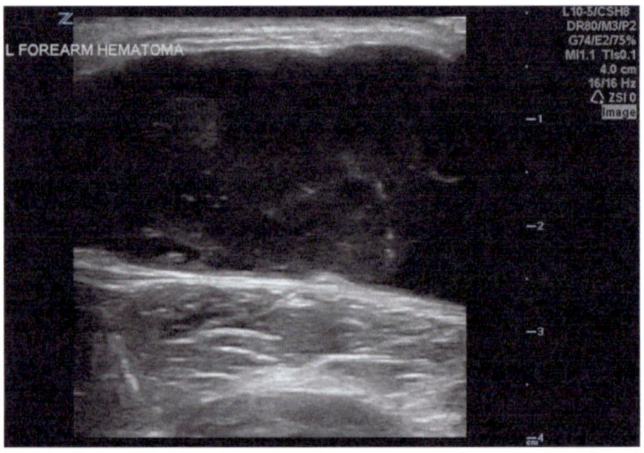

Fig. 11.10 This 4-day-old hematoma shows some heterogeneous contents, but it is mostly anechoic. It is important to incorporate clinical symptoms into diagnosing hematomas. As you can see with this image, this hematoma can certainly be confused for an abscess, but note there is no associated overlying cellulitis, which may give a clue to it being a hematoma

Indications

Patients with an area of fluctuance, induration, erythema, increased warmth, swelling, and/or discomfort should undergo ultrasound imaging to evaluate for underlying pathology. The differentiation of abscess and hematoma is largely clinical, with only very subtle differences by ultrasound. Hematoma should be clinically suspected in patient who present with history of trauma, easy bruising, thrombocytopenia, coagulopathy, anticoagulation, or recent surgery, although abscess remains on the differential diagnosis. When the pressure in the hematoma cavity exceeds that of the dermal and subdermal capillaries, there is increasing potential for overlying skin necrosis.

Contraindications

The contraindications for this procedure are very similar to those for draining abscesses. POCUS should be used to ensure that no neurovascular structures lie in the region of interest, which would warrant an alternative method for incision and drainage [2]. Use color Doppler to ensure the area in question is not a necrotic lymph node, aneurysm, or pseudoaneurysm. Discretion should be used when performing bedside incision and drainage of a hematoma in patients on anticoagulation or with known coagulopathic states, as bleeding is a concerning potential risk; patients should be counseled regarding the potential risk of bleeding prior to starting the procedure. Laboratory testing such as complete blood count to check platelet count and a coagulation panel (PTT and PT/INR) may be helpful prior to starting the procedure to further assess for bleeding risk.

Equipment and Probe Selection

As with evaluation of most superficial structures, the high-frequency (15–7 MHz) linear array probe is ideal. Color Doppler over the area in question can help identify surrounding neurovascular structures. One percent lidocaine with or without epinephrine is commonly used for anesthesia, although the use of lidocaine with epinephrine can help minimize potential bleeding if not otherwise contraindicated. Chlorhexidine, a needle driver for blunt dissection, a package of 4 × 4 inch gauze pads, and a #11 blade scalpel should be readily available. Compression dressing or an ACE bandage should also be considered for adequate pressure over the drained hematoma, since the hematoma may continue to ooze or re-bleed. The viscous nature of hematoma generally contraindicates use of needle drainage, but it is reasonable to start with a needle aspiration and convert to incision and drainage if necessary (Figs. 11.11 and 11.12).

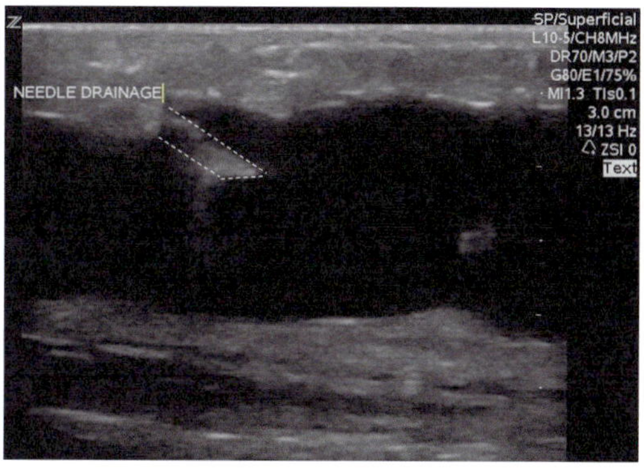

Fig. 11.11 Although the viscous nature of hematomas may preclude needle drainage, it is always reasonable to start with a needle drainage and convert to an incision if necessary. This is an example of a long-axis or in-plane technique, with visualization of the needle tip and the entire length of the needle that is in the patient. This is the preferred method for ultrasound-guided procedures. The dotted line outlines the needle and needle tip

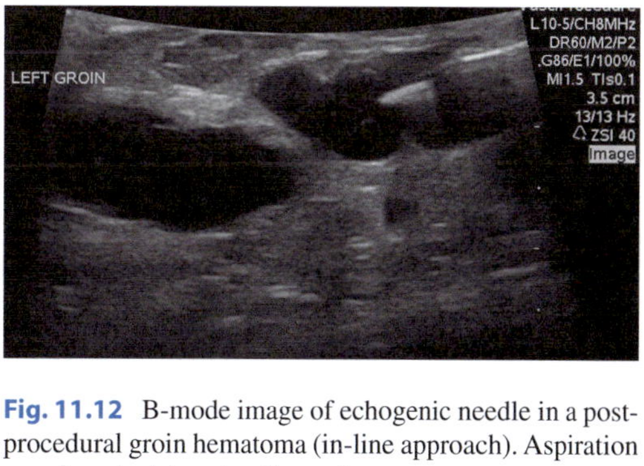

Fig. 11.12 B-mode image of echogenic needle in a post-procedural groin hematoma (in-line approach). Aspiration was done to determine if any abscess was present

Preparation and Pre-procedural Evaluation

The patient should be positioned such that the affected area is easily accessible to the provider. Topical anesthetic, such as lidocaine-epinephrine-tetracaine gel, can be used over the affected area to minimize discomfort. As mentioned previously, evaluation of the patient's platelet count and coagulation studies may be indicated. Additionally, for larger hematomas, consider a type and screen and ensure that appropriate blood products are readily available, should a bleeding emergency result. Gauze impregnated with hemostatic agents or tranexamic acid can also be at bedside to assist with bleeding control.

Procedure

Evaluate the patient's normal anatomy by initially scanning away from the affected area. Scan the entire length and width of involved area in two planes—both sagittal and transverse—using the linear array probe. Applying graded compression helps ensure a loculated fluid collection, which can be easily overlooked in the case of hematoma, is not missed. Application of color Doppler flow confirms lack of vascularity. If a fluid collection concerning for hematoma is located, note the boundaries, depth from the tissue surface, and estimated size of the cavity. The sonographic appearance of a hematoma is non-specific and is challenging to differentiate from an abscess [3].

The affected area should then be cleansed with chlorhexidine and subsequently anesthetized. The probe should be covered with a Tegaderm, and gel should be placed over top of the probe. Under ultrasound guidance, a minimal stab incision should be made using a #11 blade scalpel, and blunt dissection should be used to break up loculations, especially if there are clots or it is an infected hematoma (Fig. 11.13). Gauze pads can be used to apply pressure and evacuate any remaining clot. After incision and drainage is complete, verify complete evacuation of the hematoma cavity using ultrasonography.

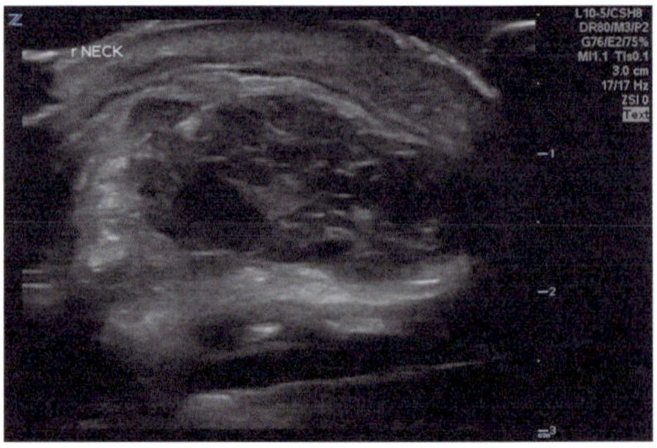

Fig. 11.13 Another possible diagnosis is an infected hematoma. A hematoma that later becomes infected. Note the heterogeneous contents of this infected hematoma. There is also thickened skin overlying this fluid collection. The patient had presented with signs and symptoms of an abscess with a history of trauma in this area. This fits with an infected hematoma

Complications

Bleeding is a potential complication associated with this procedure. Caution is advised in patients with a known bleeding diathesis or on anticoagulation. There may be persistent oozing from the incision site. It is advised to apply a compression dressing after the incision and drainage.

Pearls/Pitfalls

1. Use of color Doppler pre-procedure and real-time sonographic evaluation during the procedure can help avoid potential neurovascular complications.
2. Use of graded compression and color Doppler can help in identification of a subtle hematoma.
3. Hematomas are often comprised of viscous, clotted blood which is not amenable to needle drainage. Use of a #11 blade scalpel is recommended instead.
4. Do not underestimate the potential for blood loss in patients with known coagulopathy or in those patient predisposed to bleeding diatheses. Take appropriate precautions, and use lidocaine with epinephrine when possible to help minimize this potential complication.

5. If there is infection superimposed onto the hematoma, there may be blood, purulent drainage after the incision. Treat like an abscess and prescribe antibiotics.

Evidence

Sonographic guidance of hematomas has multiple benefits including exact positioning of the needle tip, surveying surrounding anatomy to avoid vessels, clots, soft tissue, and/or thickened synovium in the case of joint aspirations [6]. The procedure is fast and easy to perform. Because no ionizing radiation is used, this imaging modality for procedure guidance is safe for pregnant women and children [6].

This method of procedure guidance can also serve as an adjunct to other imaging-guided procedures. Reijnen et al. describe a case in which a symptomatic pseudoaneurysm was treated with endovascular repair, and ultrasound-guided needle aspiration of the hematoma was implemented [7]. The patient had no complications or recurrence of the hematoma.

Key Points

- As in the case with subcutaneous abscesses, hematomas also warrant ultrasound evaluation because of other diagnoses and the risk of infection.
- For large hematomas, especially in patients with coagulopathy, order preprocedural laboratory studies and consider and type and screen.
- It is advised to place a compression dressing over the incised area to assist with any residual oozing and drainage.

Aspiration of Symptomatic Renal Cysts

Advantages of Ultrasound Guidance

POCUS is a useful tool to differentiate simple cysts from solid or complex renal masses. The kidney is one of the most common sites of cysts in the body, with a prevalence of 20–50% in the general population with an estimated increased incidence with age [8–11].

Anatomy

POCUS should be used to evaluate the characteristics of the cyst and its surrounding anatomy prior to starting the procedure. The kidney, colon, liver (on the right), spleen (on the left), and adjacent lung should be readily identified, as these structures need to be avoided during the procedure. Renal vessels and ureter should also be identified and avoided.

Indications

Most simple renal cysts are asymptomatic incidental findings and should be left untreated. Occasionally, they may become very large. If large enough, they may cause pain, hematuria, obstructive uropathy, and even hypertension [10, 11]. It is in the latter cases when aspiration is indicated. Note that recurrence after aspiration is high and this is mostly performed to determine if the patients' symptoms are in fact caused by mass effect from the cyst. The differentiation between a simple cyst, a complex cyst, and a solid renal mass is based on imaging findings. The sonographic characteristics of a simple cyst are an anechoic lumen, well-defined back wall, acoustic enhancement deep to the cyst, and no measurable wall thickness (Figs. 11.14 and 11.15).

Contraindications

POCUS and color Doppler should be used to ensure that no vascular structures, septations, thick wall, or echogenic material lies within the cystic lesion of interest. These findings mean the cyst is complex or, in fact, a solid mass. If this is the case, it should not be drained and warrants additional advanced imaging (CT/MRI) to exclude an alternate pathology such as renal cell carcinoma. Patients on anticoagulation or with known coagulopathic states are high risk, as

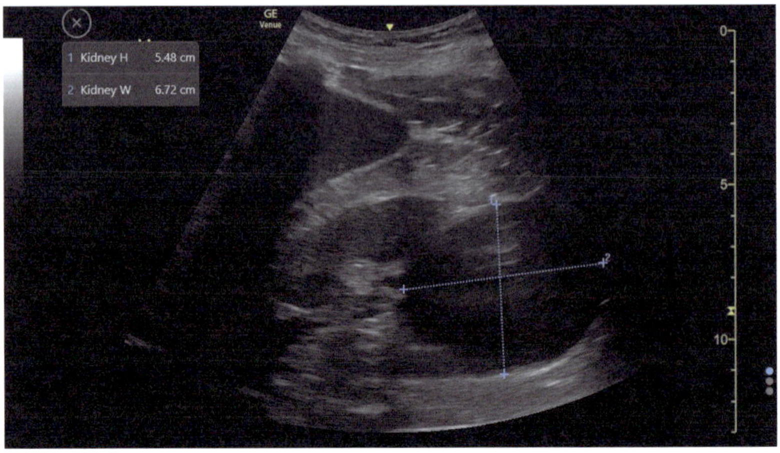

Fig. 11.14 When simple renal cysts become very large and symptomatic, drainage should be considered. The sonographic characteristics of a simple cyst are an anechoic lumen, well-defined back wall, acoustic enhancement deep to the cyst, and no measurable wall thickness, such as this example

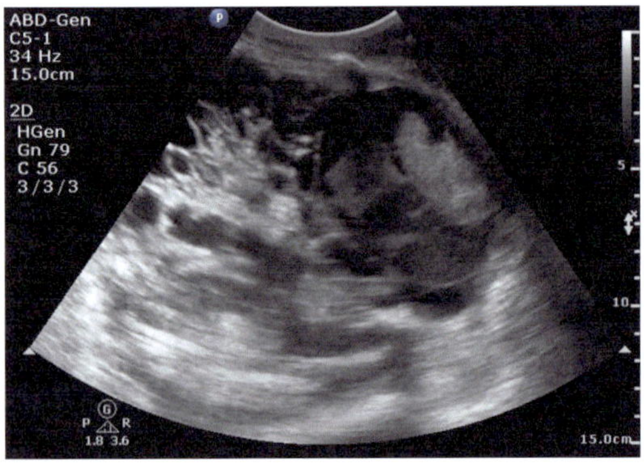

Fig. 11.15 Any time there is deviation from the description of a simple renal cyst, it is considered a complex renal cyst. In this example, the patient has polycystic kidney disease. There appears to be clusters of simple-appearing cysts, but there is also a large complex, fluid-filled renal cyst on the right side of this ultrasound image

bleeding is a concerning potential complication. All patients should be counseled regarding the potential risk of bleeding prior to starting any invasive procedure. Injury to the kidney and adjacent structures such as the ureter or colon is a possibility. These risks are minimized with the adequate use of image guidance, such as ultrasound.

Equipment and Probe Selection

As with evaluation of most deep structures, a lower-frequency, 5–2 MHz, curved array probe is ideal. Color Doppler over the lesion in question can help assess the characteristics of the cyst. Chlorhexidine, sterile towels, sterile probe cover, a needle driver for blunt dissection, a package of 4 × 4 inch and 2 × 2 inch gauze pads, an #11 blade scalpel, a 20 or 40 cc syringe, and a 19G centesis needle (7 or 14 cm length depending on the body habitus of the patient) should be readily available. One percent lidocaine with or without epinephrine is commonly used for anesthesia.

Preparation and Pre-procedural Evaluation

Evaluation of the patient's platelet count and coagulation studies is advised. The patient should be positioned prone, and the posterior flank of the affected side should be sterilely prepared with chlorhexidine and draped with sterile towels. The ultrasound probe should be covered with a sterile probe cover, and sterile gel should be used.

Procedure

Scan the entire length and width of the involved area and surrounding tissues in two planes—both sagittal and transverse—using the curved array probe. Localize the structures you want to avoid, and choose the safest, usually the shortest, route of access from the skin to the cyst.

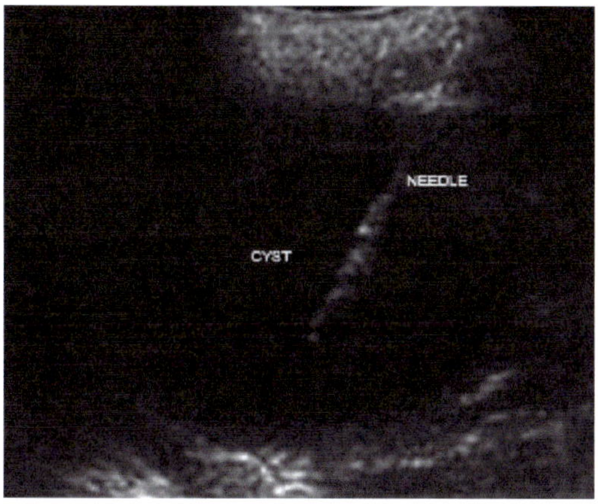

Fig. 11.16 Example of an ultrasound-guided abdominal cyst drainage. (Reproduced from book: Velasco and Hood [21]. [Figure 7.3, p. 91])

Following the administration of local anesthesia, perform a small skin nick with a #11 blade, and separate the subcutaneous soft tissues with a needle driver. Then, under direct ultrasound guidance, advance the centesis needle through the skin nick, subcutaneous tissues, into the retroperitoneum and into the cyst. Once you see the tip of the needle within the cyst, you can aspirate (Fig. 11.16). If clear fluid is aspirated, advance the outer catheter of the centesis needle, remove the sharp, and dispose it safely. Attach the 40 or 60 ml syringe to the catheter, and aspirate as much fluid as possible. Stop if the fluid becomes hemorrhagic or when you feel resistance and see a significant reduction in the size of the cyst on ultrasound. Then, remove the catheter, and place a 2 × 2 gauze and small Tegaderm over the incision. The patient should be observed for 1 hour to ensure no significant pain, discomfort, or change in vital signs, which may be signs or symptoms of a complication.

Complications

Bleeding, injury to the kidney, and injury to adjacent organs as well as infection are the potential complications of this procedure. With adequate patient selection, sterile preparation, and appropriate use of image guidance, these are greatly minimized.

Pearls/Pitfalls

1. Asymptomatic simple renal cysts should not be aspirated.
2. The ultrasound characteristics of a simple renal cyst are an anechoic lumen, well-defined back wall, acoustic enhancement deep to the cyst, and no measurable wall thickness. Care should be taken with gain settings to avoid creating false echoes or septations as well as eliminating actual ones.
3. A cystic renal lesion with a thick wall, septations (particularly if nodular), internal debris, or internal color Doppler flow is *not* a simple cyst and warrants further workup.
4. Use of real-time sonographic evaluation and color Doppler pre-procedure to assess the characteristics of a cystic renal mass can help avoid potential complications, such as potentially rupturing a renal cell carcinoma.
5. Use of color Doppler and real-time sonographic evaluation during the procedure can help avoid potential complications, such as injury to adjacent organs/structures.
6. Symptomatic cysts that arise from other organs such as the liver or adnexa should not be intervened on and may warrant additional imaging as well as specialty consultations. Cystic masses in children always warrant further workup.
7. Do not underestimate the potential for blood loss in patients with known coagulopathy or in those patients predisposed to bleeding diatheses. Take appropriate precautions to help minimize this potential complication.
8. If the patient's symptoms disappear following aspiration of the renal cyst and later recurs and the patient becomes symptomatic again, consultation to interventional radiology (for sclerotherapy) or urology (for open or laparoscopic decortication) is advised for definitive treatment.

Integration into Clinical Practice

Ultrasound-guided aspiration of renal cysts is an important tool to assess if a patient's symptoms of chronic pain, hematuria, hypertension, and/or obstructive uropathy are in fact caused by mass effect due to a large simple cyst. Note that the majority of simple renal cysts are incidental findings and asymptomatic. Asymptomatic simple renal cysts, regardless of their size, should not be treated. Real-time ultrasound-guided aspiration provides visualization of the surrounding organs and structures which helps greatly reduce the incidence of complications. Following aspiration, simple cysts often recur. If symptoms develop again with cyst recurrence, definitive treatment can be provided by interventional radiology (sclerotherapy) or urology (decortication). If this is not an option, intermittent ultrasound-guided aspiration after symptomatic recurrences may be considered to provide symptom relief. The features to distinguish a simple renal cyst from a complex cyst or solid mass are easily learned and can help guide management decisions about the need for aspiration or subspecialty workup and consultation.

Evidence

Ultrasound-guided renal cyst drainage is seen effective for ameliorating symptoms of discomfort, and the high safety profile of this image-guided procedure lends itself well for repeated drainages [9]. With further treatment techniques, such as injection of ethanol for sclerotherapy of the renal cyst epithelium, ultrasound guidance can also be used. Classic treatment is decortication through open surgery or laparoscopy, but Mohsen et al. treated 60 patients with simple renal cyst aspiration and immediate injection of ethanol for sclerotherapy via ultrasound with success [12, 13]. If there is concern for renal cyst leakage or rupture, fluoroscopy or CT can be used as adjuncts to ultrasound [14].

Key Points

- Most renal cysts are simple, and their small size does not warrant intervention.
- Renal cysts are drained for the comfort of the patient secondary to their large size.
- Thorough pre-procedural evaluation of the structures surrounding the cyst and the best, shortest approach should be pursued.
- If the renal cysts are not simple, ultrasound-guided drainage should not be pursued until the lesion is further evaluated.

Aspiration and Drainage of Intraperitoneal Fluid Collections

Advantages of Ultrasound Guidance

Despite the great advances in diagnostic imaging, there will still be a few instances when the aspiration of a fluid collection is needed to verify a diagnosis and guide therapy. If serous fluid is aspirated and cultures are negative, a seroma can be confirmed (Figs. 11.17 and 11.18). Other examples are the aspiration of pus, which confirms an abscess and may yield the specific pathogen to direct antibiotic therapy (Figs. 11.19 and 11.20); the aspiration of bile, which confirms a biloma (Fig. 11.21); and the aspiration of fluid with highly elevated lipase and amylase which confirms a pancreatic pseudocyst (Fig. 11.22).

The classic management of intraperitoneal abscesses used to be conservative (antibiotic management only) or operative drainage. With the widespread use of ultrasound for abdominal imaging starting in the 1970s and CT in the 1980s, the idea of non-surgical, image-guided management of these was introduced [15, 16]. This is now widely accepted as the treatment of choice, whenever feasible, for both spontaneous and post-surgical intraperitoneal abscesses. Percutaneous image-guided abscess drainage is associated with decreased morbidity, decreased length of drainage, and decreased

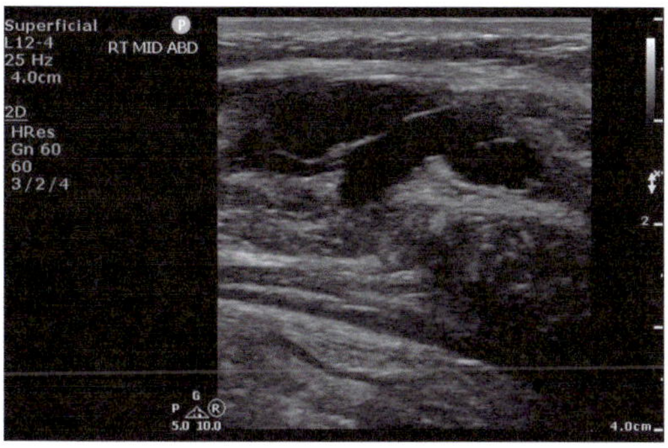

Fig. 11.17 This is an example of a seroma. The patient had spontaneously developed a fluid pocket in his abdominal wall after having abdominal surgery. There are no overlying skin changes, and upon aspiration, there was serosanguinous fluid, consistent with seroma

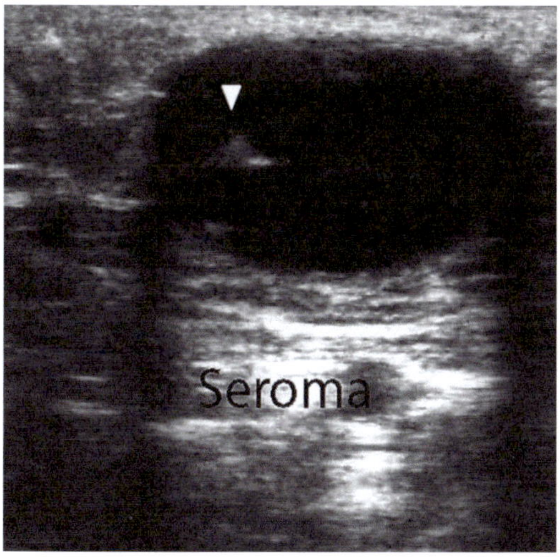

Fig. 11.18 Note the hyperechoic needle (arrowhead) in this ultrasound-guided needle drainage of an abdominal wall seroma. (Reproduced from book: Velasco and Vaince [22]. [Figure 6.10, p. 77])

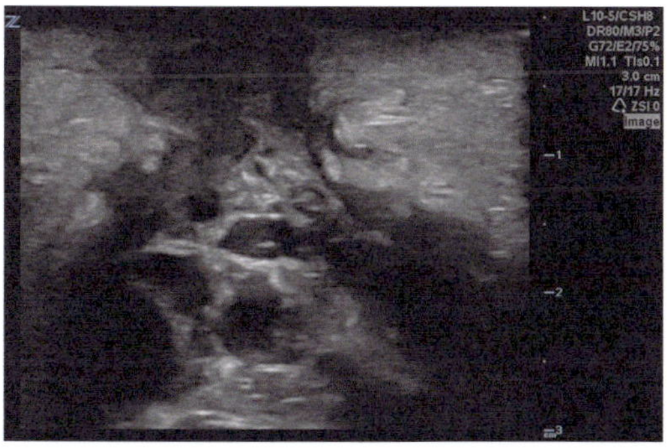

Fig. 11.19 This is an example of an abdominal wall abscess tracking deeper into the abdominal cavity to surround a recent renal transplant

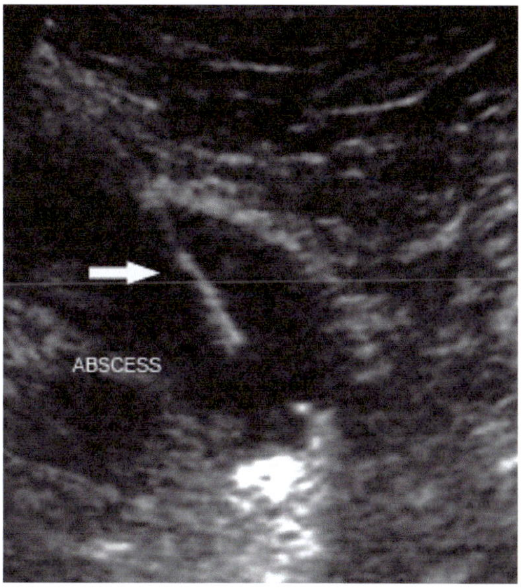

Fig. 11.20 Needle drainage of an intra-abdominal abscess with ultrasound guidance. (Reproduced from book: Velasco and Hood [21]. [Figure 7.26, p. 101])

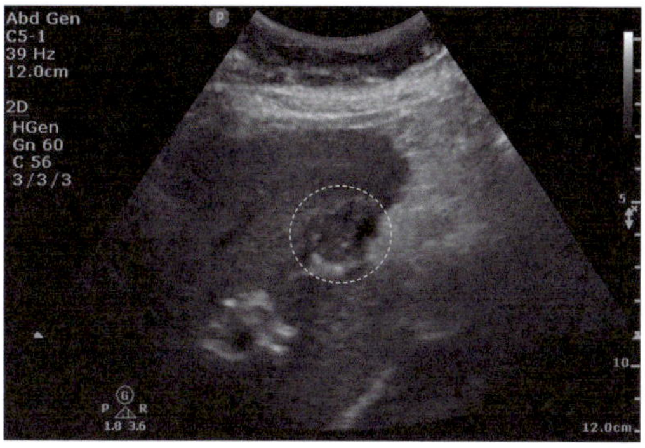

Fig. 11.21 A rare complication of laparoscopic cholecystectomy is a biloma, a collection of bile that typically is seen perihepatically. This is highlighted in this image with a dotted circle

hospital stay, when compared to open surgery [15, 16]. Also, the avoidance of surgery and anesthesia makes this a very cost-effective procedure [16].

Anatomy

POCUS should be used to evaluate the location of the loculated fluid collection and its surrounding anatomy prior to starting the procedure. The small bowel, colon, kidneys, liver, and

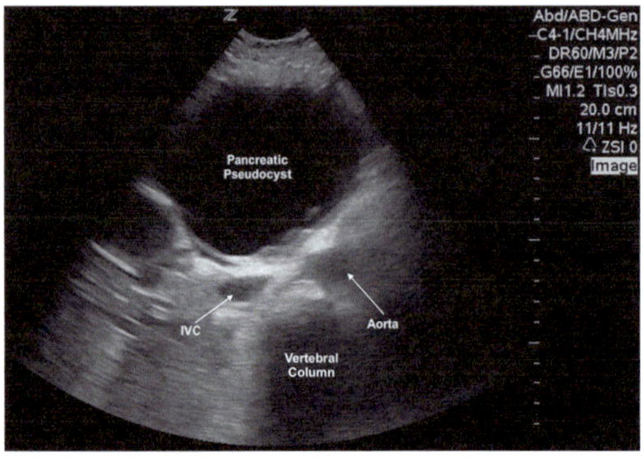

Fig. 11.22 The image is an example of a large pancreatic pseudocyst. The pancreatic tissue is not clearly seen here, but the surrounding anatomy is denoted

gall bladder, spleen, pancreas, and/or adjacent lung/diaphragm should be readily identified, as these structures need to be avoided during the procedure. Color Doppler should be used to ensure that there are no intervening vascular structures. If the target is a liver abscess, a route through some intervening liver parenchyma is preferred, to avoid capsular rupture and spillage of abscess contents into the peritoneal cavity.

Indications

Patients who present with fever, leukocytosis, +/– abdominal pain, and a localized intra-abdominal fluid collection seen on cross-sectional imaging (Ultrasound, CT, MRI) should be evaluated for the possibility of percutaneous image-guided aspiration or drain placement. The use of ultrasound has the advantage over CT in that it does not expose the patient or the operator to ionizing radiation. In some instances, overshadowing gas from bowel or within the collection itself may interfere with ultrasound imaging. In these latter cases, CT guidance may be preferred.

Contraindications

Patients on anticoagulation or with known coagulopathic states are high risk, as bleeding is a concerning potential complication; all patients should be counseled regarding the potential risk of bleeding prior to starting any invasive procedure. Injury to the bowel and adjacent solid organs or nearby vessels is a possibility. These risks are minimized with the adequate use of image guidance. On instances where there is interposing bowel or other structures, it may not be possible to perform the procedure safely. Large-volume ascites is a relative contraindication. A paracentesis may be needed prior to addressing the drainage of the loculated fluid collection.

Equipment and Probe Selection

As with evaluation of most deep structures, a lower-frequency, 5–2 MHz, curved array probe is ideal. Color Doppler over and around the fluid collection in question may help identify surrounding organs/structures. Chlorhexidine, sterile towels, sterile probe cover, a needle driver for blunt dissection, a package of 4 × 4 inch and 2 × 2 inch gauze pads, an #11 blade scalpel, a 40 or 60 cc syringe, and a 19G centesis needle (7 or 14 cm length depending on the body habitus of the patient and the depth of the fluid collection) should be readily available, as well as a specimen container to collect a sample of the aspirate. For fluid collections 5 cm or larger in diameter, a 0.035in or 0.038in guidewire, an 8 or 10 Fr all-purpose drain, and a 3.0 non-absorbable suture will be needed. One percent lidocaine with or without epinephrine is commonly used for local anesthesia. If placing a long-term drain is anticipated, intravenous pain medication such as morphine or fentanyl are advised if possible, to help provide adequate pain control.

Preparation and Pre-procedural Evaluation

Evaluation of the patient's platelet count and coagulation studies is advised. The patient should be positioned in a way that facilitates access to the affected peritoneal space. The skin overlying the fluid collection should then be sterilely prepared with chlorhexidine and draped with sterile towels. The ultrasound probe should be covered with a sterile probe sheath.

Procedure

Scan the entire length and width of the involved area and surrounding tissues in two planes—both sagittal and transverse—using the curved array probe. Localize the structures you want to avoid (bowel, adjacent organs, nearby vessels), and choose the safest, most direct, usually the shortest, route of access from the skin to the peritoneal fluid collection. Following the administration of local anesthesia, perform a small skin nick with the #11 blade, and separate the subcutaneous soft tissues with the needle driver. Then, under direct ultrasound guidance, advance the centesis needle through the skin nick, subcutaneous tissues, into the peritoneum and into the fluid collection (Fig. 11.23). Once you see the tip of the needle within the collection, you can aspirate (Fig. 11.24). If fluid is aspirated, advance the outer catheter of the centesis needle, remove the sharp, and dispose of it safely. Attach the 40 or 60 ml syringe to the catheter, and aspirate as much fluid as possible. Stop if the fluid becomes hemorrhagic or when you feel resistance and see a significant reduction in the size of the fluid collection on ultrasound. Then, remove the catheter, and place a 2 × 2 gauze and small Tegaderm over the incision. The patient should be closely monitored for a minimum of 2 h to ensure he/she suffers no significant pain, discomfort, or change in vital signs, which may be signs/symptoms of a complication.

An abscess that is 4 cm or larger in diameter will require prolonged drainage over a few days (usually up to 1 week) to completely resolve. In these cases, place the centesis needle within the collection under ultrasound guidance, as described above (Fig. 11.25). Then, once the tip of the needle is confirmed within the collection with ultrasound, advance the outer catheter of the centesis needle, remove the sharp needle, and dispose of it safely. Advance the guidewire through the catheter and coil it within the collection. Confirm adequate position of the wire with ultrasound. Then, exchange the catheter over the wire for the 8 or 10 Fr all-purpose drain. Confirm the adequate position of the drain with ultrasound, and remove the wire. Attach the drain to a suction bulb, and secure the drain with a suture. Place a sterile dressing over the dermatotomy. The patient should be observed for a minimum of 2 h to ensure he/she suffers no significant pain, discomfort, or change in vital signs, which may be signs/symptoms of a complication. Daily irrigation of the drain (to avoid clogging) with 5–10 cc of sterile saline is recommended.

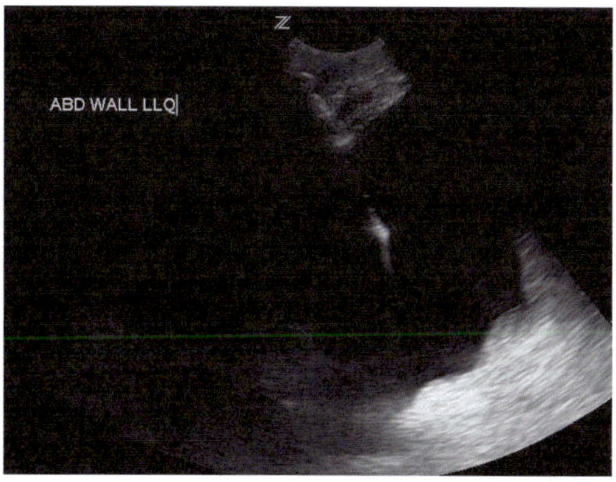

Fig. 11.23 Ultrasound-guided intraperitoneal fluid collection drainage using a low-frequency probe. Echogenic needle is seen in this B-mode image

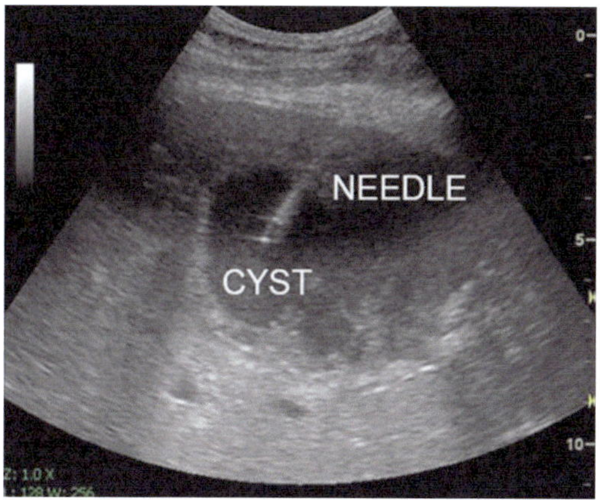

Fig. 11.24 An example of ultrasound-guided needle aspiration of an intra-abdominal cyst. (Reproduced from book: Velasco and Hood [21]. [Figure 7.23, p. 100])

Complications

Bleeding, injury to the bowel, and injury to adjacent solid organs/structures as well as infection are potential complications of this procedure. With adequate patient selection, sterile preparation, and appropriate use of image guidance, these are minimized. During drain placement, inherent risks include the spread of abscess to the adjacent spaces or

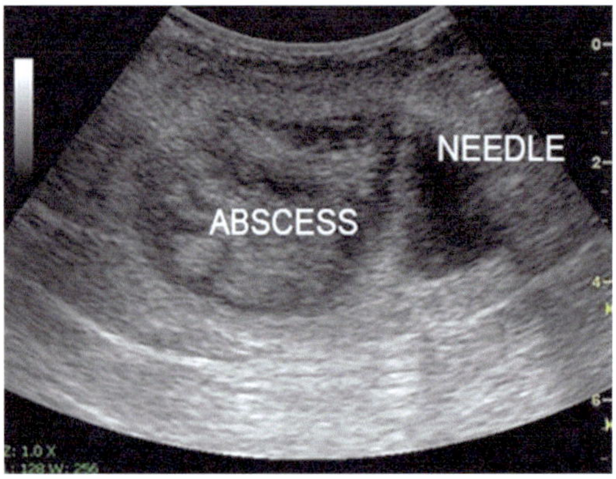

Fig. 11.25 This image shows real-time needle guidance under ultrasound to drain an intra-abdominal abscess. (Reproduced from book: Velasco and Hood [21]. [Figure 7.5, p. 92])

organs, transient bacteremia, or frank sepsis [17]. Other possible complications are abscess recurrence (when incompletely drained) and persistent output through the all-purpose drain. The latter may be a sign of a fistulous connection to the bowel, biliary tree (in the case of a biloma), or pancreatic duct (in the case of a pancreatic pseudocyst).

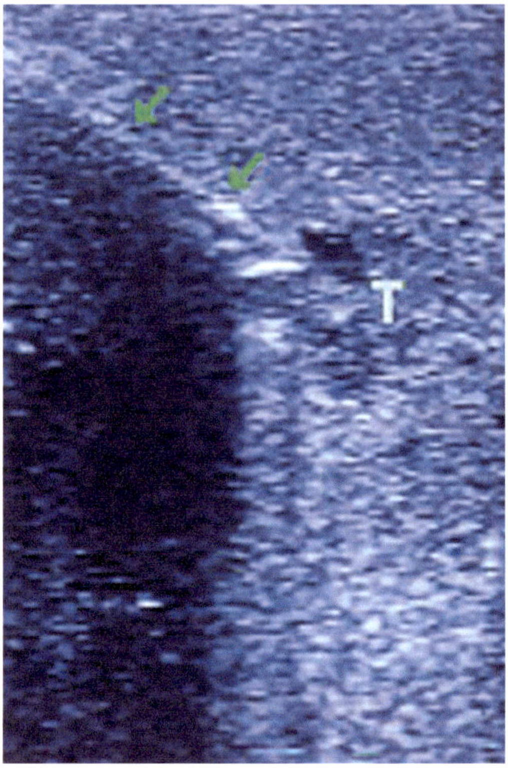

Fig. 11.26 Ultrasound-guided needle (green arrows) aspiration of a liver lesion (denoted with T). (Reproduced from book: Velasco and Hood [21]. [Figure 7.18, p. 98])

Pearls and Pitfalls

1. Use of real-time sonographic evaluation and color Doppler pre-procedure to assess the location of the loculated fluid collection can help avoid potential complications.
2. POCUS should be used to identify the small bowel, colon, kidneys, liver, and gall bladder, spleen, pancreas, and/or adjacent lung/diaphragm. These structures must be avoided during the procedure.
3. Color Doppler should be used to ensure that there are no intervening vascular structures.
4. If there is no safe route of access into the fluid collection, do not do it. Certain abscesses will require surgical management or prolonged antibiotic treatment.
5. If the target is a liver abscess, a route through some intervening liver parenchyma is preferred, to avoid capsular rupture and spillage of abscess contents into the peritoneal cavity (Fig. 11.26).
6. In the presence of free intraperitoneal fluid, a paracentesis may be required prior to the aspiration/drain placement.
7. Overshadowing gas from bowel or within the collection itself may interfere with US imaging. In these cases, CT guidance may be preferred.
8. An abscess that is 4 cm or larger in diameter will require prolonged drainage over a few days (usually up to 1 week) to completely resolve. In these cases, aspiration alone will usually not suffice and placement of a drain is required.
9. Persistent output through the all-purpose drain (>1 week) may be a sign of a fistulous connection to the bowel, biliary tree (in the

case of a biloma) (Fig. 11.27), or pancreatic duct (in the case of a pancreatic pseudocyst).
10. If a fistula is suspected, additional imaging (such as a fistulogram) and evaluation by surgery are recommended.
11. Do not underestimate the potential for blood loss in patients with known coagulopathy or in those patients predisposed to bleeding diatheses. Take appropriate precautions to help minimize this potential complication.

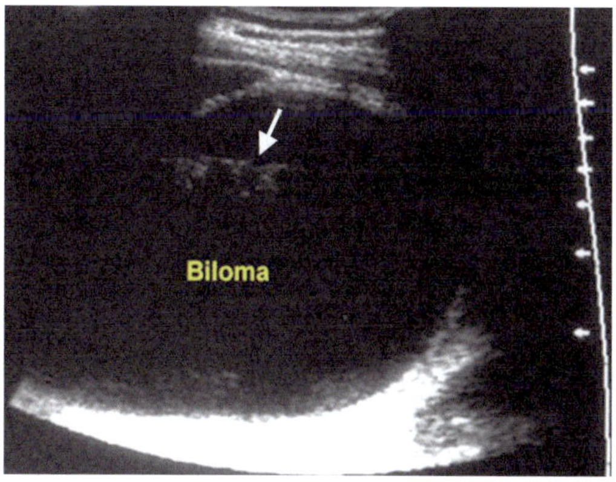

Fig. 11.27 Needle (white arrow) drainage of large biloma under ultrasound guidance. (Reproduced from book: Velasco and Hood [21]. [Figure 7.27, p. 101])

12. Be prepared to treat the patient for frank sepsis in the event this develops acutely, immediately following the procedure.

Integration into Clinical Practice

Ultrasound-guided aspiration of loculated intra-abdominal fluid collections is an important tool to verify diagnosis and guide therapy. Depending on the characteristics of the aspirated fluid, the source or cause of the fluid collection can be identified. Not only can ultrasound help guide the needle and the guidewire to the area of interest, but also watch real time aspiration and drainage, and guide placement of percutaneous drains (Fig. 11.28a,b).

Real-time ultrasound-guided aspiration/drain placement provides visualization of the surrounding organs and structures which helps greatly reduce the incidence of complications. If the window of access is not clear into the fluid collection, STOP and reconsider. CT may be a better guiding tool in this case. Complex cases will need subspecialty consultation to interventional radiology, and some inaccessible collections will require surgery. Be prepared to

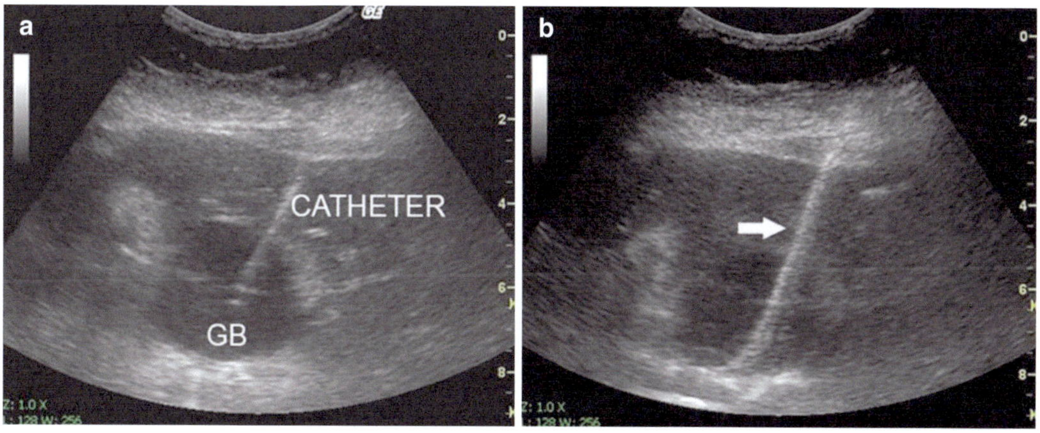

Fig. 11.28 (**a**, **b**) Examples of percutaneous cholecystostomy drains with placement confirmed via ultrasound. (Reproduced from book: Velasco and Hood [21]. [Figures 7.6, p. 92 and 7.34, p. 104])

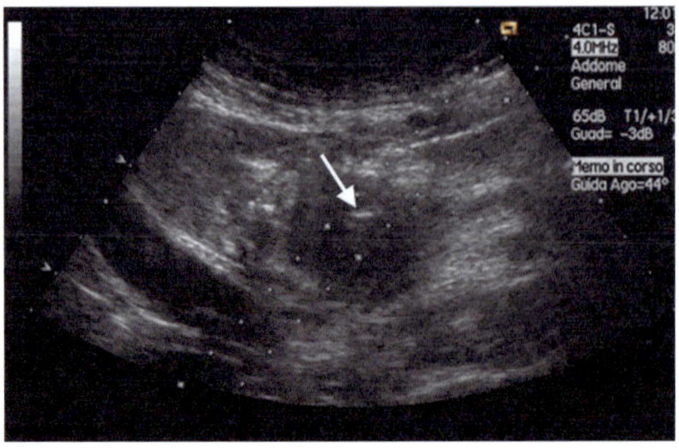

Fig. 11.29 Ultrasound-guided needle (white arrow) biopsy aspiration of a pancreatic lesion. The dotted lines denote the needle track. (Reproduced from article: D'Onofrio et al. [23]. [Figure 1, p. 3])

handle potential complications if these were to occur. Persistent output through the all-purpose drain, greater than 1 week, may be a sign of a fistulous connection. Additional imaging and surgical consultation may be warranted in these cases.

Evidence

Kassi et al. have shown that percutaneous image-guided drainage through ultrasound is feasible and effective for the treatment of abdominopelvic abscesses with a success rate of 78% [18]. Although not explained in this section, endoscopic ultrasound-guided drainage has been the standard of care for drainage of pancreatic pseudocysts [19] (Fig. 11.29). Ultrasound guidance also serves the imaging guidance modality of choice for pregnant women and children who have intra-abdominal abscesses that are amenable to percutaneous drainage [20].

Key Points

- Drainage of intra-abdominal fluid collections for analysis assists with medical management without more invasive operative management.
- In larger fluid collections, placement of a percutaneous drain for prolonged drainage may be necessary.
- Persistent output from a percutaneous drain may suggest formation of a fistula.
- In patients with a bleeding diathesis or coagulopathy, it is important to review pre-procedural laboratory studies and consider type and screen.

References

1. Gaspari R, Dayno M, Briones J, Blehar D. Comparison of computerized tomography and ultrasound for diagnosing soft tissue abscesses. Crit Ultrasound J. 2012;4(1):5.
2. Squire B, Fox J, Anderson C. ABSCESS: applied bedside sonography for convenient evaluation of superficial soft tissue infections. Acad Emerg Med. 2005;12(7):601–6.
3. Wicks J, Silver T, Bree R. Gray scale features of hematomas: an ultrasonic spectrum. AJR Am J Roentgenol. 1978;131(6):977–80.
4. Kjær S, Rud B, Bay-Nielsen M. Ultrasound-guided drainage of subcutaneous abscesses on the trunk is feasible. Dan Med J. 2013;60(4):A4601.
5. Christensen AF, Al-Suliman N, Nielsen KR, et al. Ultrasound-guided drainage of breast abscesses: results in 151 patients. Br J Radiol. 2005;78:186–8.
6. Szopinski KT, Smigielski R. Safety of sonographically guided aspiration of intramuscular, bursal, articular and subcutaneous hematomas. Eur J Radiol. 2012;81(7):1581–3.
7. Reijnen MMPJ, de Rhoter W, Zeebregts CJ. Treatment of a symptomatic popliteal pseudoaneurysm using a stent-graft and ultrasound-guided evacuation of the hematoma. Emerg Radiol. 2008;16(2):167–9.
8. Rané A. Laparoscopic management of symptomatic simple renal cysts. Int Urol Nephrol. 2004;36:5–9.
9. Skolarikos A, Laguna M, de la Rosette J. Conservative and radiological management of simple renal cysts: a comprehensive review. BJU Int. 2012;110:170–8.
10. Hemal A. Laparoscopic management of renal cystic disease. Urol Clin North Am. 2001;28:115–26.
11. Okan B, Nalbant I, Can Sener N, Yesil S, et al. Management of renal cysts. JSLS. 2015;19(1):e2014.00097.
12. Okeke A, Mitchelmore A, Keeley F, Timoney A. A comparison of aspiration and sclerotherapy with laparoscopic de-roofing in the management of symptomatic simple renal cysts. BJU Int. 2003;92:610–3.

13. Mohsen T, Gomha MA. Treatment of symptomatic simple renal cysts by percutaneous aspiration and ethanol sclerotherapy. BJU Int. 2005;96(9):1369–72.
14. Lohela P. Ultrasound-guided drainages and sclerotherapy. Eur Radiol. 2001;12(2):288–95.
15. Gerzof S, Robbins A, Johnson W, Birkett D, et al. Percutaneous catheter drainage of abdominal abscesses: a five-year experience. N Engl J Med. 1981;305(12):653–7.
16. Johnson W, Gerzof S, Robbins A, Nabseth D. Treatment of abdominal abscesses: comparative evaluation of operative drainage versus percutaneous catheter drainage guided by computed tomography or ultrasound. Ann Surg. 1981;194(4):510–20.
17. Lorenz J, Thomas J. Complications of percutaneous fluid drainage. Semin Interv Radiol. 2006;23(2):194–204.
18. Kassi F, Dohan A, Soyer P, et al. Predictive factors for failure of percutaneous drainage of postoperative abscess after abdominal surgery. Am J Surg. 2014;207(6):915–21.
19. Mandai K, Uno K, Yasuda K. Endoscopic ultrasound-guided drainage of postoperative intra-abdominal abscesses. World J Gastroenterol. 2015;21(11):3402–8.
20. Patel J, Siriwardana HP, Hammond T, et al. Successful ultrasound-guided drainage of an intra-abdominal collection in late pregnancy. Case Rep. 2017;2017:bcr-2017-219479.
21. Velasco JM, Hood K. Percutaneous ultrasound guidance techniques and procedures. In: Hagopian E, Machi J, editors. Abdominal ultrasound for surgeons. New York: Springer New York; 2014. p. 89–107.
22. Velasco JM, Vaince F. Abdominal wall anatomy, pathology, and intervention. In: Hagopian E, Machi J, editors. Abdominal ultrasound for surgeons. New York: Springer New York; 2014. p. 71–88.
23. D'Onofrio M, Beleù A, De Robertis R. Ultrasound-guided percutaneous procedures in pancreatic diseases: new techniques and applications. Eur Radiol Exp. 2019;3(1):2.

Ultrasound-Guided Peripheral Venous Access

12

Lori Stolz

Introduction

The placement of a peripheral intravenous (PIV) catheter is a routine procedure in most medical settings: inpatient, outpatient, clinics, emergency department, emergency medical services, etc. It is performed by many different kinds of healthcare professionals including nurses, paramedics, midlevel practitioners, and physicians. It is the one of the most common procedures performed in healthcare, especially in the emergent setting [1]. Despite being so commonly performed, PIV placement can be difficult to perform for a variety of reasons. Failed attempts during PIV placement are unfortunately very common, occurring in approximately 35% of patients who present to the emergency department [2].

Traditionally, PIVs are placed using landmarks to predict the usual course of peripheral veins and using visualization and palpation to locate and cannulate them. Risk factors for difficulty with traditional PIV placement include conditions that make it more difficult to locate peripheral veins by palpation or visualization or decrease the caliber and quantity of available peripheral veins. These conditions include but are not limited to obesity, edema, sickle cell disease, diabetes, dark skin, dehydration, intravenous (IV) drug use, chemotherapy, dialysis, and other chronic medical conditions [3].

Failure to obtain IV access quickly negatively affects patient care. It delays the delivery of necessary medications, IV fluids, blood products, and other treatments and hinders the ability of providers to perform laboratory and radiologic testing [2, 4]. Additionally, patient pain and perception of pain are directly related to multiple IV attempts [5, 6]. When PIV access cannot be obtained, alternative therapeutic options include central catheter placement, peripherally inserted central catheter placement, intraosseous line placement, and oral therapy. These alternatives all have distinct disadvantages over PIV placement, and the option with the greatest potential for patient harm, placement of a central line, is often the only recourse in emergent or urgent situations. Central lines, though relatively quick to place and utilitarian, can be complicated by hemothorax, pneumothorax, retroperitoneal bleed, hematoma, arteriovenous fistula, pseudoaneurysm, deep vein thrombosis, arterial puncture, local skin infection, and bloodstream infection. These complications and the time required to place a central line increase when dynamic ultrasound guidance is not utilized. Reducing central line-associated bloodstream infections by decreasing the use of central lines has become a top priority for several regulatory bodies, insurers, and providers [7–9].

L. Stolz (✉)
University of Cincinnati, Department of Emergency Medicine, Cincinnati, OH, USA
e-mail: stolzla@ucmail.uc.edu

S. Adhikari, M. Blaivas (eds.), *The Ultimate Guide to Point-of-Care Ultrasound-Guided Procedures*, https://doi.org/10.1007/978-3-030-28267-7_12

Using ultrasound guidance to place PIVs can allow a practitioner to successfully place a PIV in situations when traditional techniques fail. These ultrasound-guided PIVs have several advantages. Patient satisfaction is improved when ultrasound guidance is utilized in situations where there are known difficult IV access predictors [10]. In addition, the associated infection rate is the same [11]. Overall, there is a decrease in the number of needle sticks required to successfully obtain access and a decrease in procedure time [12–14]. Importantly, when ultrasound-guided PIVs become a routine and integrated within a practice, the central line placement rate decreases [15, 16].

Anatomy

Whereas traditional IVs are most commonly placed in the upper extremity in the antecubital space and in the forearm or hand, ultrasound-guided PIVs are more commonly placed in the upper arm. The principal veins used are the basilic vein, the cephalic vein, and the brachial vein (Fig. 12.1). The basilic vein courses along the ulnar aspect of the forearm. Several smaller veins join it in the antecubital fossa. In the upper arm, its path is along the medial aspect of biceps brachii muscle until it connects proximally with the brachial veins to form the axillary vein [17]. The basilic vein is ideal for ultrasound-guided PIVs as it is somewhat superficial and not paired with an artery. Nearby branches of the medial cutaneous nerve of the forearm may complicate IV access of this vein. The cephalic vein courses along the anterolateral aspect of the upper arm along the lateral aspect of the biceps brachii muscle. It reliably traverses the deltopectoral groove before joining the axillary vein proximally. This vein may be accessible to IV drug users and may be affected by all of the same conditions mentioned above that decrease vein caliber. It is therefore not always identifiable on ultrasonographic evaluation. The brachial vein is paired with the brachial artery. It forms in the antecubital fossa where the radial vein and ulnar vein join and courses along the medial aspect of the upper arm deep to the brachial vein. As it is adjacent to both the brachial artery and the median nerve, more advanced skill and careful technique are necessary to cannulate this vein while avoiding these sensitive structures.

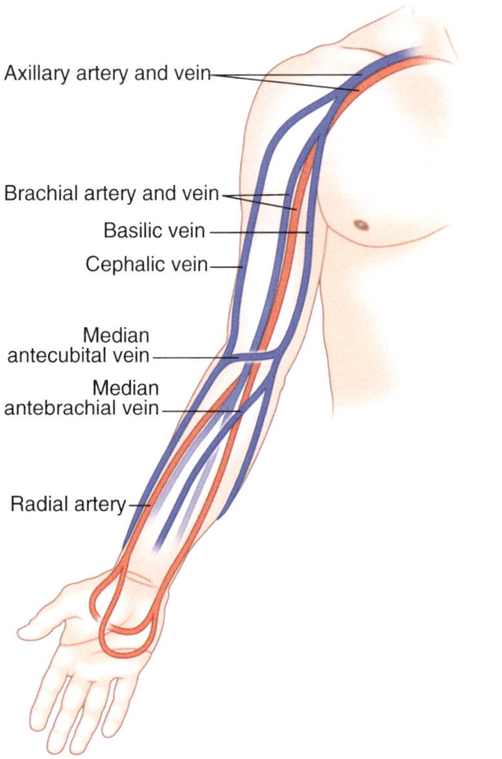

Fig. 12.1 Arterial and venous anatomy of the upper extremity

Though less common, the great saphenous vein can also be located with ultrasound in the lower extremity and offers an alternative to the upper extremities for cannulation. This vein courses along the medial aspect of the lower extremity from the anterior aspect of the medial malleolus, along the medial calf, posterior to the medial condyle of the femur, along the medial thigh. In the thigh it courses anteriorly where it joins the femoral vein in the groin (Fig. 12.2). It is often cannulated at the level of the ankle. Due to its superficial nature, ultrasound use during cannulation may be challenging secondary to venous compression.

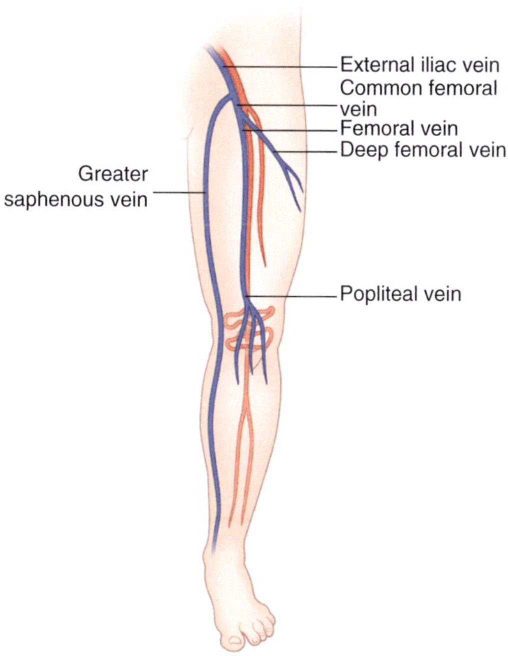

Fig. 12.2 Arterial and venous anatomy of the lower extremity

The external jugular vein is another viable alternative. Its course is along the lateral neck along the posterior border of the sternocleidomastoid muscle caudally. As it travels more proximally, it crosses anterior to the sternocleidomastoid muscle and enters the subclavian triangle to join the subclavian vein (Fig. 12.3). Though this vein often has good caliber and is easily accessible, it is easily compressible and use of a tourniquet is not possible in this area. Ultrasound can be used to cannulate an external jugular vein; however, adjustments need to be made to allow visualization. Patient positioning in reverse Trendelenburg can decrease the vein's compressibility, and the operator must be extremely cognizant of the amount of pressure applied with the probe.

A similar technique can be used when utilizing ultrasound guidance for accessing the radial artery for arterial line placement as is used for peripheral venous access. Ultrasound guidance for arterial access can be useful when arterial pulses are not

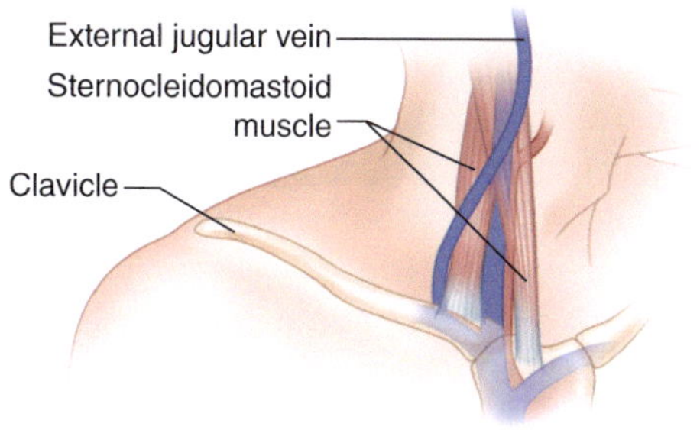

Fig. 12.3 Anatomy of the external jugular vein and surrounding structures

easily palpable (scar tissue, obesity, low blood pressure, etc.). The radial artery is very superficial in nature, coursing from the radial aspect of the wrist along the forearm to the antecubital fossa, where it joins the brachial artery. It is cannulated at the level of the wrist where it is found medial and proximal to the radial styloid and lateral to the flexor carpi radialis tendon.

Indications and Contraindications

The indications for ultrasound-guided PIV placement include any disease state or planned intervention which requires IV placement in patients who have proven or predicted difficult IV access. In situations where traditional methods of IV placement have failed or are predicted to fail, proceeding directly to ultrasound guidance is advised in most situations. Contraindications to ultrasound-guided PIV are similar to the contraindications for traditional IV placement including the presence of a dialysis fistula or catheter on the chosen limb, prior lymph node dissection of the affected limb, overlying infection or other overlying severe skin disease, known superficial thrombus in the target vein, or deep vein thrombosis in the ipsilateral limb. Relative contraindications include severe edema as the ability to detect extravasation is poor and use of the lower extremity veins in patients with diabetes as the ability to detect complications may be impaired by neuropathy.

Equipment

Necessary equipment for the procedure is listed in Table 12.1. The ultrasound machine utilized for the procedure is ideally a lightweight, sturdy, mobile unit with a user-friendly interface. A high-frequency (12-5 MHz) linear array transducer should be utilized as the target structures are very superficial. There are a variety of these transducers, including a traditional linear transducer, downsized linear transducers with smaller footprints, and the so-called hockey stick transducer.

The placement of a PIV is a clean/aseptic, but not sterile, procedure. Traditional, non-sterile examination gloves should be utilized and should be latex-free as necessary to protect the patient and provider. As with any procedure with the potential for blood-borne pathogen exposure, mask and eye protection are recommended. Sterile gel should be utilized to minimize the infection as the skin will be breached. To protect the equipment and the patient, a single-use barrier adhesive or a single-use sterile probe cover should be utilized. Additionally, disinfectant for the patient's skin should include chlorhexidine swabs or alcohol swabs for cleaning the skin prior to needle insertion.

A catheter of an appropriate gauge and length should be chosen. Standard length IV catheters (generally 24–44 mm) are usually not sufficient as the veins used for ultrasound-guided PIV placement are frequently deep. When longer catheters are utilized (generally >50 mm), there is a decreased failure rate of the catheter [18]. Appropriate choice of gauge should be determined by patient needs for rapid resuscitation or rapid administration of medications or blood products and by the chosen vein caliber.

An optional piece of equipment is the stand-off or gel pad which can be used to improve visualization of a very superficial vein. The decreased spatial resolution which is present in the first few millimeters of the near field on most ultrasound imaging can affect the ability of a practitioner to adequately visualize the most superficial veins. Using a fluid-filled stand-off between the patient and the ultrasound probe will increase the distance from the probe to the structure of interest, thereby increasing the spatial resolution of the structure. A small (100 ml) bag of saline can be used as well as a commercially available product (Fig. 12.4).

Another optional and recommended piece of equipment is a catheter stabilization device. There are several commercially available products. These are used to secure the device to the patient's skin. Given the increased depth at which these catheters are placed, there is greater potential for displacement of the catheter compared to traditionally placed IVs.

Table 12.1 Necessary equipment for the placement of an ultrasound-guided peripheral intravenous catheter

Ultrasound machine with an appropriate high-frequency transducer
Non-sterile gloves
Mask and eye protection for the provider
Sterile ultrasound gel packets
Ultrasound probe cover/barrier
Alcohol or other disinfectant for skin preparation
Appropriate length and gauge IV catheter
Device or tape to secure the catheter
Barrier dressing
Saline flush

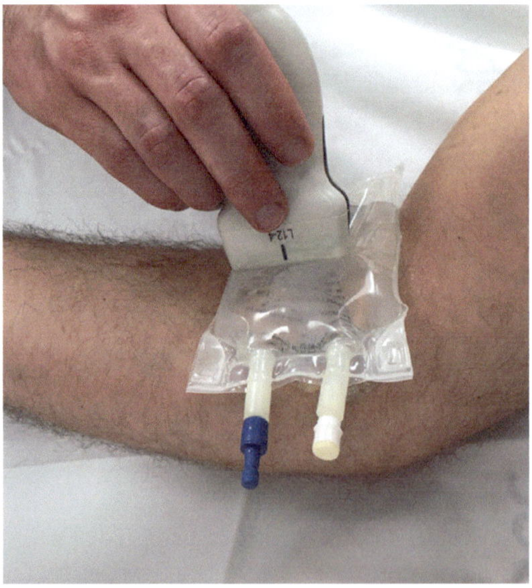

Fig. 12.4 Use of a saline bag as a stand-off for ultrasound imaging of superficial structures

Pre-procedural Evaluation

Patient should be consented and counseled prior to procedure performance. The risks of the procedure are similar to those for traditional IV placement including infection, phlebitis, bruising, infiltration, arterial puncture, nerve damage, pain, and bleeding. These complications do occur with less frequency with ultrasound-guided PIV placement than with traditional techniques, however.

The preferred limb should be chosen on each patient depending on patient factors, and the limb should be evaluated for an ideal vessel. Unpaired veins (those without a paired artery) are ideal but not always available. An ideal vessel is one that is superficial and of larger caliber and can be accessed without damaging other structures (arteries, nerves, tendons, etc.). Success rates in placing ultrasound-guided PIVs are improved when veins that are greater than 4 mm in size and are at a depth between 3 mm and 15 mm are utilized [19]. Size of the vessel is the most important predictor of success [20]. Additionally, when possible, the catheter should not be larger than 1/3 of the vessel diameter to decrease the possibility of vein thrombosis.

Peripheral veins can be distinguished sonographically from superficial arteries using several techniques. The first and easiest is to use compression. With B-mode imaging, the operator can visualize the compression of a peripheral vein using light pressure applied to the patient's skin with the ultrasound probe (Fig. 12.5a, b). Venous structures will compress and collapse with little pressure, and arteries compress less easily. A potential drawback to this technique is in hypotensive patients because the pressure required to compress an artery is less and it may be mistaken for a vein. In these situations, veins will still require less compression for complete collapse than an artery, and this must be distinguished by the operator. Another confounder is when venous congestion occurs due to patient factors or a very tight tourniquet. In these situations, the pressure required to compress a vein is greater and may approach the pressure required to compress an artery, decreasing the ability to distinguish the two.

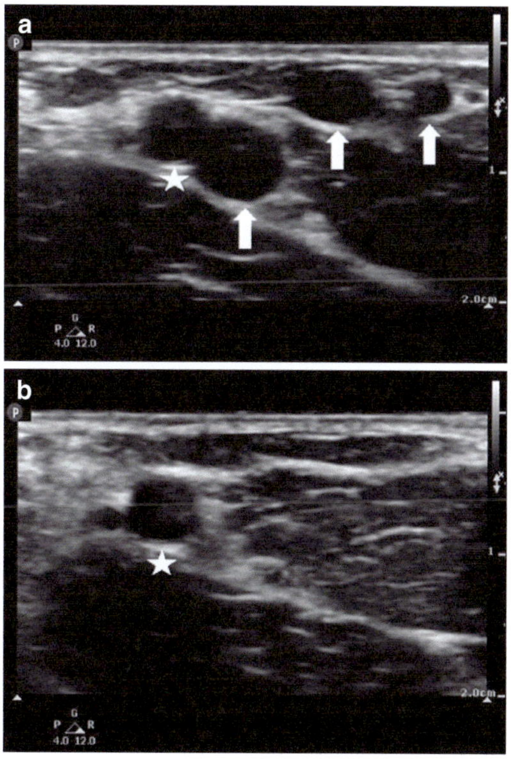

Fig. 12.5 (**a**) B-mode image of a peripheral vein and artery without compression. (**b**) The same vessels with compression applied with the ultrasound probe. Note the compression of the artery but not the vein

Doppler, either pulsed wave or color, can be used to distinguish peripheral veins from arteries. Using pulsed wave Doppler, the sample gate is placed over the vessel in question and a waveform obtained. A pulsatile waveform will confirm that the vessel is an artery (Fig. 12.6). A vein may have low continuous flow, intermittent low level flow, or none at all (Fig. 12.7). Augmentation, whereby the operator squeezes the limb distal to the transducer during the ultrasound examination, can be utilized. With augmentation, veins will demonstrate a sudden increase in return which will be visualized on the Doppler waveform (Fig. 12.8). Color Doppler is used similarly to pulsed wave Doppler. The color box is placed over the vessel in question. Pulsatile flow will confirm an artery, and low continuous flow, intermittent low level flow, or no flow can confirm that it is a vein. Vein augmentation can also be visual-

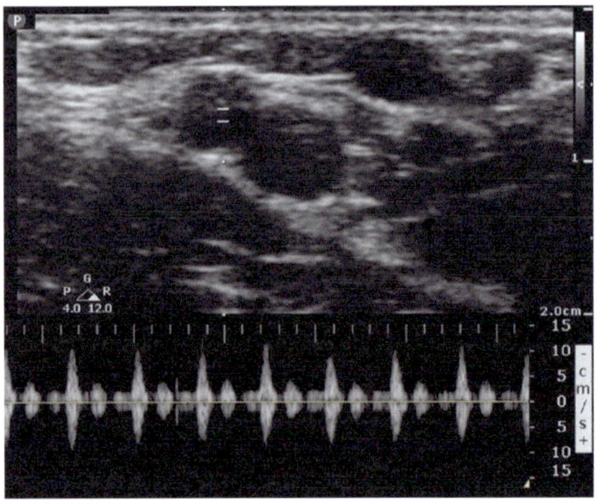

Fig. 12.6 Pulsed wave Doppler waveform of a peripheral artery

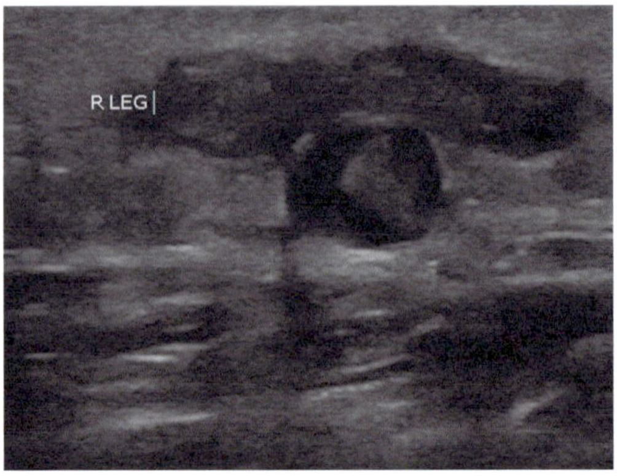

Fig. 12.9 B-mode image of a superficial venous thrombosis

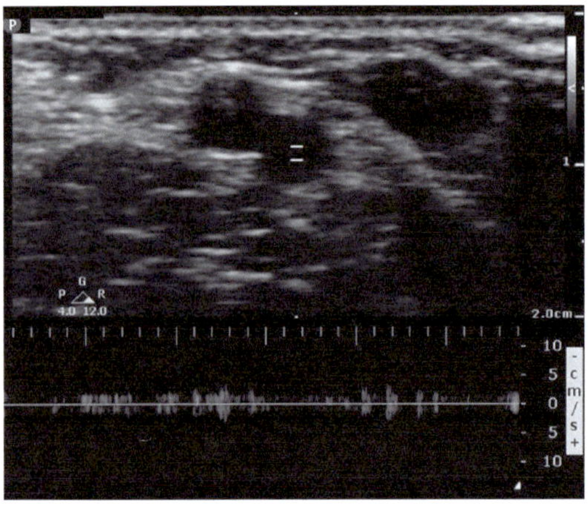

Fig. 12.7 Pulsed wave Doppler waveform of a peripheral vein demonstrating phasic flow

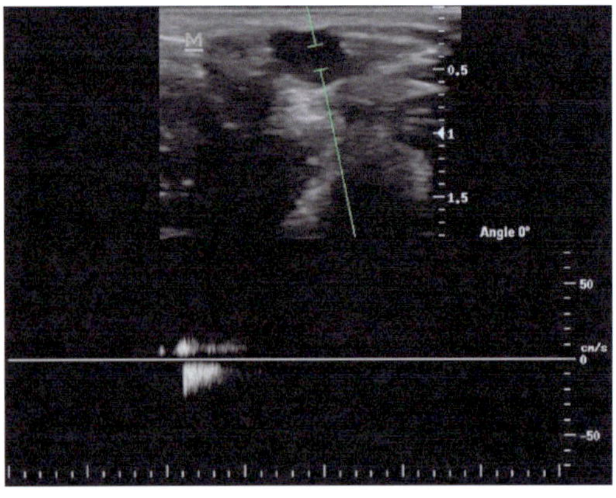

Fig. 12.8 Pulsed wave Doppler waveform of a peripheral vein with augmentation

ized as a sudden increase in flow within a vessel when distal compression is applied to the limb. One potential problem when using Doppler to distinguish arteries from veins can occur if the tourniquet is causing impedance of arterial flow. In this situation, the arterial waveforms may appear dampened or non-existent and may lead to misidentification of an artery as a vein.

The patency of the chosen vein should also be confirmed prior to procedure. A superficial thrombus may appear as an echogenic or isoechoic area within the vessel (Fig. 12.9). Alternatively, a thrombus can be anechoic, and the chosen vein should be confirmed to have full compression in B-mode imaging.

Performing the Procedure

Once the patient has been consented (as required by local policies), the procedure and the patient confirmed, the appropriate vessel evaluated and chosen, and all equipment ready, the patient and operator should be positioned properly. Procedural success is improved with good operator and patient positioning. The operator should be in a seated position with all equipment within arm's reach. It is ideal to have the ultrasound machine placed on the patient's contralateral side directly in the operator's field of view when

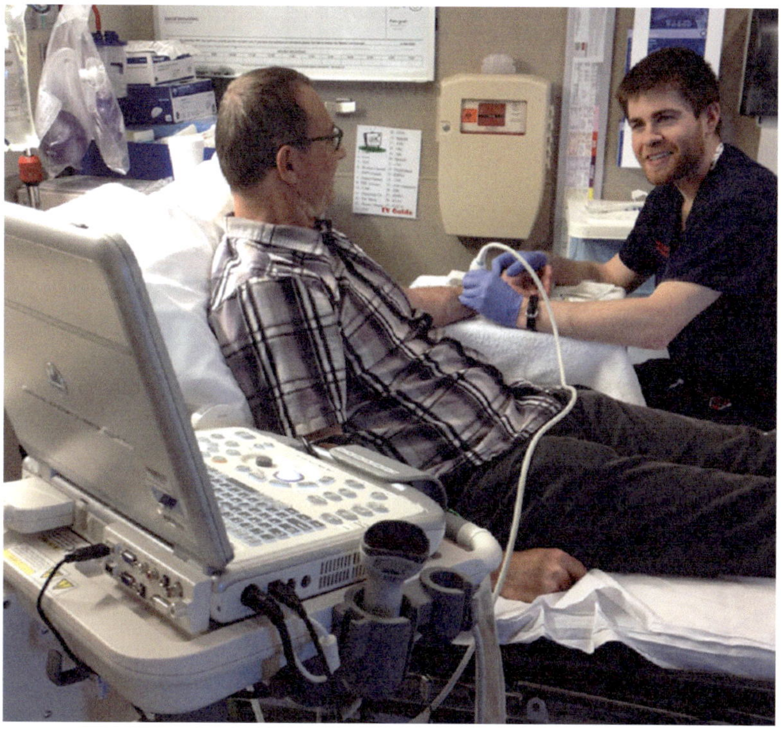

Fig. 12.10 Ideal positioning of the ultrasound machine and the operator with the ultrasound machine on the patient's contralateral side and in full view of the operator

performing the cannulation (Fig. 12.10). Any positioning which requires the operator to turn their head to look from their procedural field to the ultrasound machine should be avoided.

Real-time ultrasound guidance should be used to visualize the catheter entering the vein, and this is best facilitated using the in-plane approach. The use of the in-plane approach for real-time visualization of needle guidance allows the operator to continuously visualize the needle tip and improves visualization of the needle at the time of vessel puncture [21].

A tourniquet should be placed to distend the veins. The appropriate preset should be selected on the ultrasound machine and the chosen vein visualized. Once the appropriate vein is visualized and confirmed in the short axis, the probe should be turned into the longitudinal plane of the vein (Fig. 12.11a, b). The skin surface where the needle will enter the skin should be cleansed with a chlorhexidine swab or other disinfectant per institutional policy for PIV placement. A large transparent tegaderm can be applied to the footprint of the transducer which will prevent contamination of the transducer with blood. Care must be taken not to trap any air bubbles between the tegaderm and the transducer. The non-dominant hand of the operator should stabilize the probe with the hand firmly planted on the patient's extremity. With the dominant hand and the needle bevel facing up, the operator should puncture the skin with the needle using in-plane approach (Figs. 12.12 and 12.13). Care should be taken not to damage the probe surface with the needle tip. In order to enter the skin, the probe can be rocked, lifting the end closest to the needle using a "ski-lift maneuver" [22]. The needle tip should be visualized at all times as it is advancing, and if it cannot be visualized, it should not be advanced. Maintaining a shallow angle of approach will improve visualization of the needle because it will allow a more perpendicular angle between the ultrasound waves and the needle surface. Once the needle tip enters the vessel, the needle angle should be flattened and advanced to ensure that the entire catheter tip is within the vessel walls (Fig. 12.14).

At this point the operator can use a one-handed technique to advance the catheter over the needle without moving the needle while continuing to

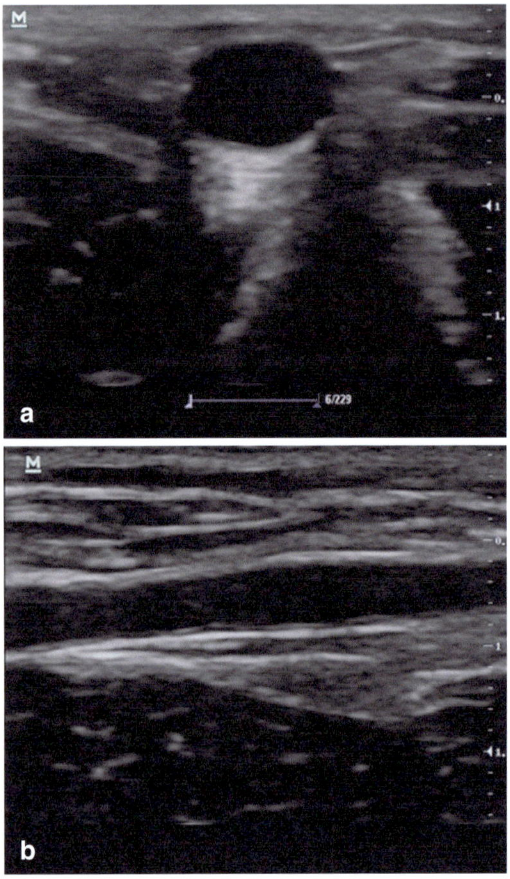

Fig. 12.11 B-mode image of vein in the short axis (**a**) and in the long axis (**b**)

visualizing this step with ultrasound guidance. As this one-handed technique requires a high level of manual dexterity, another option is for the operator to set the probe down, use two hands to advance the catheter and then return the probe to the skin to visualize the catheter in the vessel (Fig. 12.15).

Once the catheter is in the vessel, its patency should be confirmed. This can be done with several techniques. First, the operator can visualize the vein and catheter sonographically as the catheter is being gently flushed with normal saline. Microbubbles within the saline flush can be visualized sonographically (Fig. 12.16). Color or power Doppler can also be used to confirm the catheter placement in the vein while flushing the catheter (Fig. 12.17). Withdrawal of venous blood from the catheter also confirms its patency. The catheter should be securely affixed to the extremity with a catheter stabilization device and covered per institutional policy.

Complications

Extravasation, infiltration, or displacement of a ultrasound-guided PIV may be masked as the veins utilized are generally deeper than those utilized for traditional IVs. For this reason, the limb should be closely monitored for increase in circumference, patient pain at the site, and patency. As with other IVs, the IV should not be used if displacement is suspected. The location of symptoms may be distant from the insertion site, depending on catheter length.

Arterial puncture is a complication which can be avoided if careful evaluation of vessels is performed prior to the procedure and an ideal vein is chosen distant from an artery. Additionally, real-time ultrasound guidance in the in-plane approach will decrease the likelihood of this complication as the location of the needle tip in relation to the vein and any surrounding arteries will be known. If an arterial puncture is suspected, this can be confirmed by visualizing pulsatile blood from the catheter or by using ultrasound to visualize the catheter in the vessel and then evaluate the vessel as being venous or arterial with the techniques mentioned previously. If an artery is punctured, the operator should hold pressure at the location of the puncture for 10 minutes, longer if the patient has anti-coagulation or risk factors for bleeding. The affected limb or area should not be utilized again for venous or arterial access during that encounter.

Infection can be avoided through careful clean procedure technique and appropriate IV dressings and maintenance of the catheter. If an infection is suspected due to warmth, pain, or purulence at the site, the catheter should be removed immediately. Further treatment should be discussed with the treating clinicians.

Thrombophlebitis risk depends on several factors, namely, catheter size and patient fac-

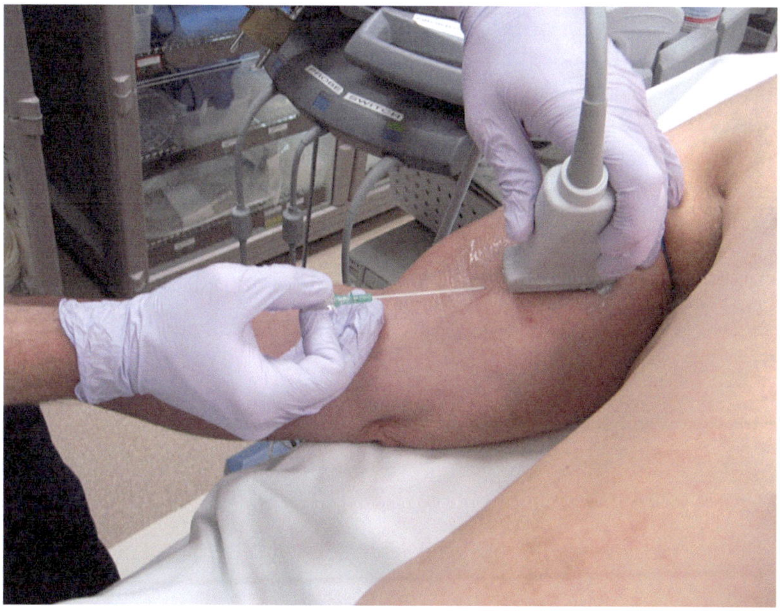

Fig. 12.12 In-plane approach. Long axis of the probe is parallel to long axis of the vein

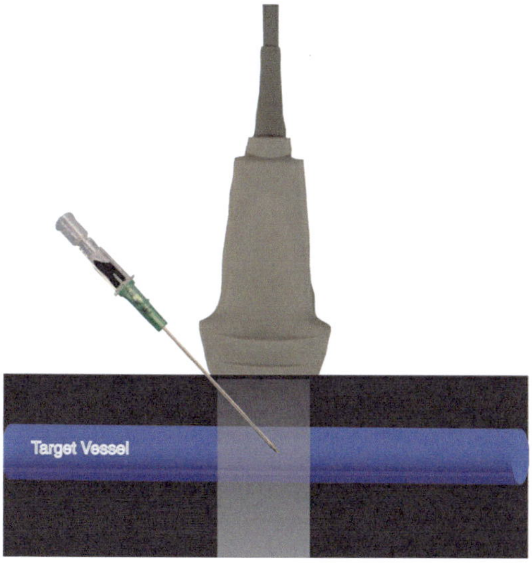

Fig. 12.13 In-plane approach. Needle insertion into the target vessel

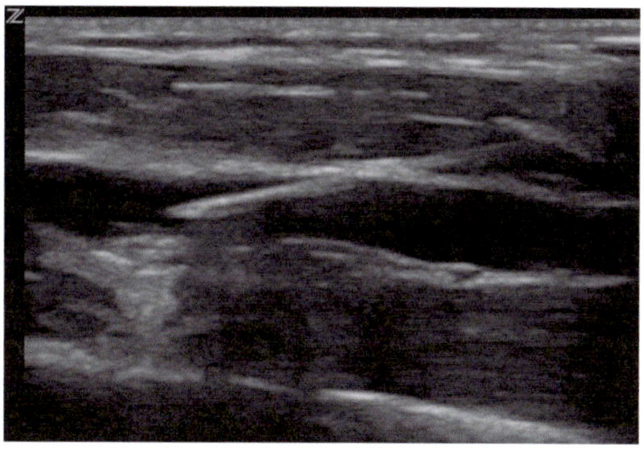

Fig. 12.14 B-mode image of a needle within a peripheral vein

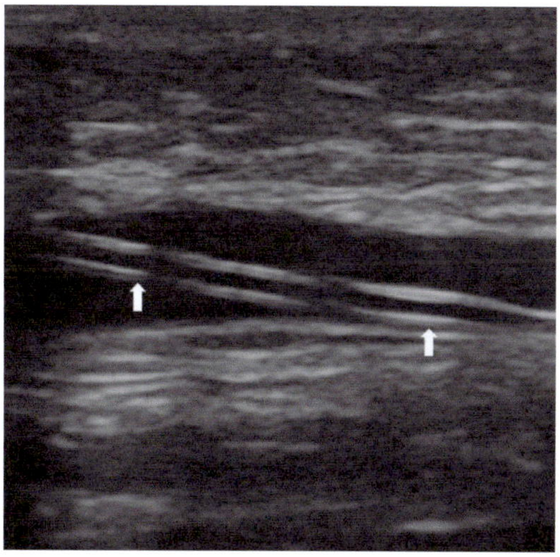

Fig. 12.15 A peripheral venous catheter (arrows) within a peripheral vein

tors. Catheters should be chosen to balance the need for fluid resuscitation and the size of the available catheter. A catheter that is greater than 1/3 of the vessel diameter should be avoided. Findings that should alert a healthcare provider to the presence of thrombophlebitis are redness, pain, and tenderness along the course of the vessel. The catheter should be immediately removed. Supportive care should be provided with warm compresses and NSAIDs as indicated.

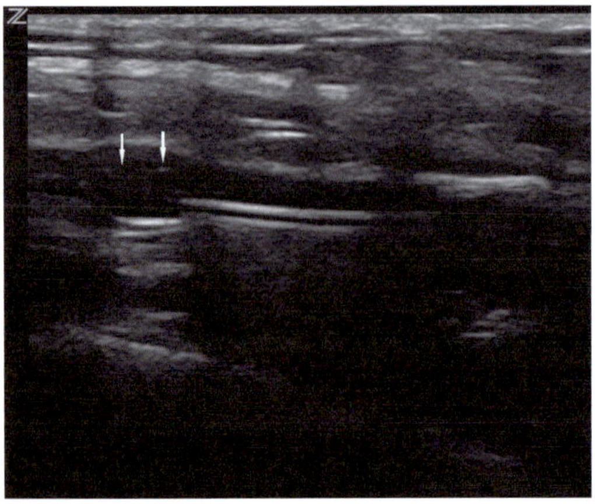

Fig. 12.16 Microbubbles seen within the vessel with saline flush (arrows)

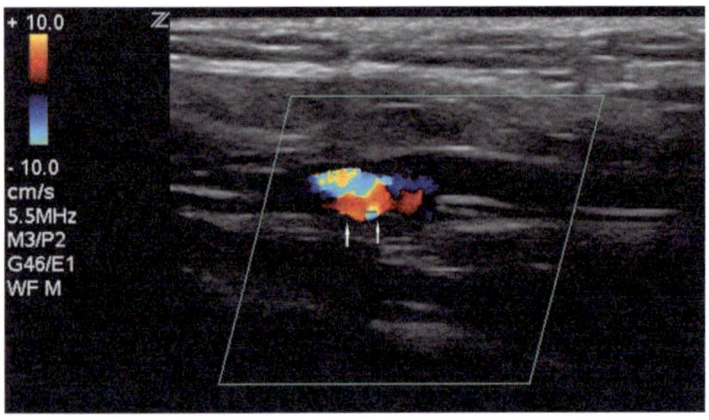

Fig. 12.17 Microbubbles seen on color Doppler while flushing the catheter (arrows)

Pearls and Pitfalls

Ultrasound-guided PIV placement success can be improved by adhering to several key principles. The operator should perform a thorough pre-procedural evaluation of patient sites and appropriate choice of an ideal vessel. Veins that are too deep or too small should be avoided. Veins that are close to arteries, nerves, or other sensitive anatomic structures should also be avoided if possible. Thorough sonographic evaluation of a vessel for venous or arterial characteristics will minimize the possibility of arterial puncture. The use of the in-plane approach for real-time ultrasonographic visualization throughout the procedure will also improve the operator's chances of a successful cannulation. Careful choice of catheters will decrease the possibility of thrombophlebitis, and watchful monitoring of the placement site will allow for early detection of catheter displacement or other complications. A catheter which takes up more than 50% of the diameter of a vein will increase the risk of thrombosis and vessel failure as a vascular access point at that location.

Integration into Clinical Practice

Adoption of ultrasound guidance for placement of PIVs is an easy procedure with a high clinical utility which can easily be integrated into clinical practice. All levels of practitioners that perform traditional IV placement can learn and succeed at ultrasound-guided PIV placement. Nurses, paramedics, and physicians in training have all been successfully taught how to perform the procedure with resulting improved rates of success compared to traditional techniques when used on patients with difficult IV access [4, 23–27]. Several nursing organizations support nurses who integrate the procedure into their clinical practice. And perhaps most importantly of all, patients stand to benefit greatly with wide adoption.

Evidence

The evidence is strong that ultrasound-guided PIVs increase success in obtaining IV access when there are difficult access predictors or when other techniques have failed. Several randomized controlled trials which have compared traditional IV placement to ultrasound-guided PIV placement have overwhelmingly found that the ultrasound-guided PIVs are safe and generally improved technique for obtaining IV access in patients with difficult access [28–34]. These studies have utilized several patient care settings (intensive care unit, emergency department, operative room) and several types of providers (emergency medicine technicians, physicians, nurses, etc.). Several meta-analyses have been published demonstrating improved success as well [12–14]. Other endpoints of improved patient care have been demonstrated in the literature on this topic. Central line rates and therefore the risk of central line-associated bloodstream infections decrease when robust programs to integrate ultrasound-guided PIV into clinical practice are implemented [15, 16]. Additionally, patient satisfaction is improved with the use of ultrasound guidance [10].

Key Points

- Ultrasound guidance improves the success rate of IV placement on patients with difficult venous access.
- The most common veins used for ultrasound-guided PIV placement are the cephalic vein, the brachial vein, and the basilic vein.
- Compression, color Doppler, and pulsed wave Doppler can be used to distinguish an artery from a vein sonographically.
- Operators should avoid veins paired with arteries, vessels that are too deep, and those that have a small diameter.
- Real-time, in-plane approach should be utilized while performing ultrasound-guided PIV placement.

References

1. Centers for Disease Control. National Hospital Ambulatory Medical Care Survey: 2010 Emergency Department summary tables. 2010. http://www.cdc.gov.ezproxy2.library.arizona.edu/nchs/data/ahcd/nhamcs_emergency/2010_ed_web_tables.pdf. Accessed 27th Jan 2015.
2. Witting MD. IV access difficulty: incidence and delays in an urban emergency department. J Emerg Med. 2012;42(4):483–7. https://doi.org/10.1016/j.jemermed.2011.07.030.
3. Sebbane M, Claret PG, Lefebvre S, Mercier G, Rubenovitch J, Jreige R, et al. Predicting peripheral venous access difficulty in the emergency department using body mass index and a clinical evaluation of venous accessibility. J Emerg Med. 2013;44(2):299–305. https://doi.org/10.1016/j.jemermed.2012.07.051.
4. Miles G, Salcedo A, Spear D. Implementation of a successful registered nurse peripheral ultrasound-guided intravenous catheter program in an emergency department. J Emerg Nurs: JEN. 2012;38(4):353–6. https://doi.org/10.1016/j.jen.2011.02.011.
5. Cummings EA, Reid GJ, Finley GA, McGrath PJ, Ritchie JA. Prevalence and source of pain in pediatric inpatients. Pain. 1996;68(1):25–31.
6. Fields JM, Piela NE, Ku BS. Association between multiple IV attempts and perceived pain levels in the emergency department. J Vasc Access. 2014;15(6):514–8. https://doi.org/10.5301/jva.5000282.
7. http://www.hhs.gov/ash/initiatives/hai/actionplan/Naptph-airmteDoHaHSws.
8. Liang SY, Marschall J. Update on emerging infections: news from the Centers for Disease Control and Prevention. Vital signs: central line-associated blood stream infections--United States, 2001, 2008, and 2009. Ann Emerg Med. 2011;58(5):447–51. https://doi.org/10.1016/j.annemergmed.2011.07.035.
9. O'Grady NP, Alexander M, Burns LA, Dellinger EP, Garland J, Heard SO, et al. Guidelines for the prevention of intravascular catheter-related infections. Clin Infect Dis. 2011;52(9):e162–93. https://doi.org/10.1093/cid/cir257.
10. Schoenfeld E, Shokoohi H, Boniface K. Ultrasound-guided peripheral intravenous access in the emergency department: patient-centered survey. West J Emerg Med. 2011;12(4):475–7. https://doi.org/10.5811/westjem.2011.3.1920.
11. Adhikari S, Blaivas M, Morrison D, Lander L. Comparison of infection rates among ultrasound-guided versus traditionally placed peripheral intravenous lines. J Ultrasound Med. 2010;29(5):741–7.
12. Egan G, Healy D, O'Neill H, Clarke-Moloney M, Grace PA, Walsh SR. Ultrasound guidance for difficult peripheral venous access: systematic review and meta-analysis. Emerg Med J. 2013;30(7):521–6. https://doi.org/10.1136/emermed-2012-201652.
13. Heinrichs J, Fritze Z, Vandermeer B, Klassen T, Curtis S. Ultrasonographically guided peripheral intravenous cannulation of children and adults: a systematic review and meta-analysis. Ann Emerg Med. 2013;61(4):444–54 e1. https://doi.org/10.1016/j.annemergmed.2012.11.014.
14. Stolz LA, Stolz U, Howe C, Farrell IJ, Adhikari S. Ultrasound-guided peripheral venous access: a meta-analysis and systematic review. J Vasc Access. 2015;0(0):0. https://doi.org/10.5301/jva.5000346.
15. Shokoohi H, Boniface K, McCarthy M, Khedir Al-tiae T, Sattarian M, Ding R, et al. Ultrasound-guided peripheral intravenous access program is associated with a marked reduction in central venous catheter use in noncritically ill emergency department patients. Ann Emerg Med. 2013;61(2):198–203. https://doi.org/10.1016/j.annemergmed.2012.09.016.
16. Au AK, Rotte MJ, Grzybowski RJ, Ku BS, Fields JM. Decrease in central venous catheter placement due to use of ultrasound guidance for peripheral intravenous catheters. Am J Emerg Med. 2012;30(9):1950–4. https://doi.org/10.1016/j.ajem.2012.04.016.
17. Netter FH. Atlas of human anatomy. 5th ed. Philadelphia: Saunders/Elsevier; 2011.
18. Elia F, Ferrari G, Molino P, Converso M, De Filippi G, Milan A, et al. Standard-length catheters vs long catheters in ultrasound-guided peripheral vein

cannulation. Am J Emerg Med. 2012;30(5):712–6. https://doi.org/10.1016/j.ajem.2011.04.019.
19. Witting MD, Schenkel SM, Lawner BJ, Euerle BD. Effects of vein width and depth on ultrasound-guided peripheral intravenous success rates. J Emerg Med. 2010;39(1):70–5. https://doi.org/10.1016/j.jemermed.2009.01.003.
20. Panebianco NL, Fredette JM, Szyld D, Sagalyn EB, Pines JM, Dean AJ. What you see (sonographically) is what you get: vein and patient characteristics associated with successful ultrasound-guided peripheral intravenous placement in patients with difficult access. Acad Emerg Med. 2009;16(12):1298–303. https://doi.org/10.1111/j.1553-2712.2009.00520.x.
21. Stone MB, Moon C, Sutijono D, Blaivas M. Needle tip visualization during ultrasound-guided vascular access: short-axis vs long-axis approach. Am J Emerg Med. 2010;28(3):343–7. https://doi.org/10.1016/j.ajem.2008.11.022.
22. Schofer JM, Nomura JT, Bauman MJ, Hyde R, Schmier C. The "Ski Lift": a technique to maximize needle visualization with the long-axis approach for ultrasound-guided vascular access. Acad Emerg Med. 2010;17(7):e83–e84. https://doi.org/10.1111/j.1553-2712.2010.00784.x.
23. Brannam L, Blaivas M, Lyon M, Flake M. Emergency nurses' utilization of ultrasound guidance for placement of peripheral intravenous lines in difficult-access patients. Acad Emerg Med. 2004;11(12):1361–3. https://doi.org/10.1197/j.aem.2004.08.027.
24. Walker E. Piloting a nurse-led ultrasound cannulation scheme. Br J Nurs (Mark Allen Publishing). 2009;18(14):854, 6, 8–9.
25. Weiner SG, Sarff AR, Esener DE, Shroff SD, Budhram GR, Switkowski KM, et al. Single-operator ultrasound-guided intravenous line placement by emergency nurses reduces the need for physician intervention in patients with difficult-to-establish intravenous access. J Emerg Med. 2013;44(3):653–60. https://doi.org/10.1016/j.jemermed.2012.08.021.
26. Bauman M, Braude D, Crandall C. Ultrasound-guidance vs. standard technique in difficult vascular access patients by ED technicians. Am J Emerg Med. 2009;27(2):135–40. https://doi.org/10.1016/j.ajem.2008.02.005.
27. Schoenfeld E, Boniface K, Shokoohi H. ED technicians can successfully place ultrasound-guided intravenous catheters in patients with poor vascular access. Am J Emerg Med. 2011;29(5):496–501. https://doi.org/10.1016/j.ajem.2009.11.021.
28. Aponte H, Acosta S, Rigamonti D, Sylvia B, Austin P, Samolitis T. The use of ultrasound for placement of intravenous catheters. AANA J. 2007;75(3):212–6.
29. Benkhadra M, Collignon M, Fournel I, Oeuvrard C, Rollin P, Perrin M, et al. Ultrasound guidance allows faster peripheral IV cannulation in children under 3 years of age with difficult venous access: a prospective randomized study. Paediatr Anaesth. 2012;22(5):449–54. https://doi.org/10.1111/j.1460-9592.2012.03830.x.
30. Costantino TG, Kirtz JF, Satz WA. Ultrasound-guided peripheral venous access vs. the external jugular vein as the initial approach to the patient with difficult vascular access. J Emerg Med. 2010;39(4):462–7. https://doi.org/10.1016/j.jemermed.2009.02.004.
31. Costantino TG, Parikh AK, Satz WA, Fojtik JP. Ultrasonography-guided peripheral intravenous access versus traditional approaches in patients with difficult intravenous access. Ann Emerg Med. 2005;46(5):456–61.
32. Doniger SJ, Ishimine P, Fox JC, Kanegaye JT. Randomized controlled trial of ultrasound-guided peripheral intravenous catheter placement versus traditional techniques in difficult-access pediatric patients. Pediatr Emerg Care. 2009;25(3):154–9. https://doi.org/10.1097/PEC.0b013e31819a8946.
33. Kerforne T, Petitpas F, Frasca D, Goudet V, Robert R, Mimoz O. Ultrasound-guided peripheral venous access in severely ill patients with suspected difficult vascular puncture. Chest. 2012;141(1):279–80. https://doi.org/10.1378/chest.11-2054.
34. Stein J, George B, River G, Hebig A, McDermott D. Ultrasonographically guided peripheral intravenous cannulation in emergency department patients with difficult intravenous access: a randomized trial. Ann Emerg Med. 2009;54(1):33–40. https://doi.org/10.1016/j.annemergmed.2008.07.048.

Ultrasound-Guided Spinal Procedures

13

Maged A. Guirguis, Samita S. Das, William K. White, and Matthew E. Patterson

Introduction

Neuraxial procedures are those procedures pertaining to the neuraxis, which include spinal anesthesia and epidural anesthesia/analgesia. These procedures are commonly used to provide surgical anesthesia and/or postoperative analgesia. They are differentiated by the location of drug injection: spinal anesthesia occurring in the subarachnoid space and epidural anesthesia occurring in the epidural space. Injection of local anesthetics into the subarachnoid space blocks spinal nerve roots, allowing this to be used as the primary anesthetic or combined with general anesthesia for various surgical procedures involving the abdomen and lower extremities. Epidural anesthesia can be accomplished with a single injection or through insertion of an epidural catheter. The principal site of action of local anesthetics during epidural blocks is the spinal nerve roots within the epidural space and diffusion across the dura. Commonly, a catheter is inserted into the epidural space to allow intermittent boluses or continuous infusion of local anesthetic. Epidural techniques are widely used to provide obstetric anesthesia/analgesia, surgical anesthesia, and postoperative or post-traumatic (e.g., rib fractures) analgesia. In areas where general anesthesia is less relied upon, these blocks can be exceedingly helpful for completely managing pain during an entire procedure.

M. A. Guirguis (✉)
Department of Interventional Pain Management, Ochsner Health System, New Orleans, LA, USA
e-mail: mguirguis@ochsner.org

S. S. Das · W. K. White · M. E. Patterson
Department of Anesthesiology & Critical Care Medicine, Ochsner Health System, New Orleans, LA, USA

Advantages of Ultrasound Guidance

Some of the advantages of ultrasound guidance include identifying correct vertebral level and the midline and assessing the depth of various structures (spinous processes, lamina, epidural and subarachnoid spaces), the optimal interspace, and, lastly, any anatomical abnormalities (scoliosis, prior laminectomy and instrumentation). Altogether, ultrasound can be beneficial in all patients, but it is particularly useful in patients with poorly identifiable surface landmarks, morbid obesity, scoliosis, or ankylosing spondylitis and patients on anticoagulation and previous lumbar spinal instrumentation.

S. Adhikari, M. Blaivas (eds.), *The Ultimate Guide to Point-of-Care Ultrasound-Guided Procedures*, https://doi.org/10.1007/978-3-030-28267-7_13

Anatomy

Neuraxial procedures, which include spinal anesthesia and epidural anesthesia/analgesia, involve the neuraxis. The spinal cord consists of white and gray matter similar to the brain. There are essentially four surfaces to the spinal cord, two lateral and an anterior and a posterior one. The gray matter in the spinal cord is located centrally and is butterfly-like in shape when viewed in cross section, containing lateral, posterior, and anterior horns. The gray matter is surrounded by neuronal axons, which make up the white matter. The spinal cord itself and the spinal nerve roots are covered by three separate layers of meninges. The dura mater is the outermost layer and the pia mater is the deepest layer. Between them resides the arachnoid mater. Two layers can be discerned in the dura mater, the periosteal and meningeal, between which lies the epidural space. The subarachnoid space lies between the arachnoid and pia mater and contains cerebrospinal fluid. Branches of the segmental and vertebral arteries supply the spinal cord. Anterior and posterior spinal arteries arise from the vertebral artery. Veins, which share their names with the arteries, run adjacent to them.

Spinal anesthesia involves the subarachnoid space, and epidural anesthesia involves the epidural space. Spinal anesthesia targets the same anatomic area accessed during lumbar puncture for the collection of cerebral spinal fluid (CSF). The principal site of action of local anesthetics during epidural blocks is the spinal nerve roots within the epidural space and diffusion across the dura. A catheter can be inserted into the epidural space to allow intermittent boluses or continuous infusion of local anesthetic. The sacroiliac joint is composed of ear-shaped auricular surfaces of the ilium and sacrum, and the joint lies in a vertical and anterolateral orientation. The joint configuration is complex with the posterosuperior compartment more fibrous in nature than the synovial anteroinferior compartment [1]. Facet joints are an important target in interventional pain management. These diarthrodial joints are formed from the superior articular process of one vertebra articulating with the inferior articular process of the vertebrae above, at the level of the junction of the pedicle and the lamina. The joint has a fibrous capsule and is lined by a synovial membrane, and itself contains adipose and fibrous tissue. Along with the intervertebral disc, the facet joint helps to alleviate the axial compressive load on the spine and contributes to shear strength of the spine. Lumbar facet joint compression or capsular ligament strain can produce lower back pain after injury. Furthermore, the joint and capsule have been shown to contain nociceptive factors, which independently may generate pain. Facet joint degeneration, commonly seen in the older patient population, is a significant and common pathogenesis of lower back pain.

The epidural space extends from the base of the skull to the sacral hiatus. It is demarcated posteriorly by the ligamentum flavum, anteriorly by the dura mater, and laterally by the pedicles and the intervertebral foramina. The epidural space contains epidural fat and veins, which exit laterally through the neural foramen and become peripheral nerves. The paravertebral space begins at the cervical spine and terminates at the sacrum. The paravertebral space is a wedge-shaped compartment adjacent to the vertebrae that encases the spinal nerve roots as they emerge from the intervertebral foramen. The vertebral bodies and intervertebral disc make up the medial boundary of the paravertebral space. The parietal pleura of the lung define the anterior boundary. The superior costotransverse ligament and transverse processes form the posterior border. The internal intercostal membrane is continuous with the superior costotransverse ligament.

Indications

Neuraxial anesthesia is useful as an adjunctive anesthetic with general anesthesia or as a primary anesthetic in both major and minor surgeries. This type of anesthetic is commonly used to provide surgical anesthesia and/or postoperative analgesia. Injection of local anesthetics in the subarachnoid space blocks spinal nerve roots, allowing this to be used as the primary anesthetic or combined with general anesthesia for various surgical procedures involving the abdomen and lower extremities. Epidural anesthesia can be a useful alternative to general anesthesia in surgeries of the thorax, abdomen, or lower extremities, particularly in patients with cardiac or pulmonary comorbidities, who have a higher risk associated with undergoing general anesthesia. In particular, lumbar epidural anesthesia is ubiquitously employed for labor pain in the parturient. Thoracic epidural anesthesia is useful for postoperative pain management after thoracic procedures such as thoracotomies.

Paravertebral blocks result in ipsilateral motor, sensory, and sympathetic blockade and are most commonly used to provide analgesia to the chest and abdomen in cases of acute or chronic pain but may also be used as a primary anesthetic. Thoracic paravertebral blocks are most commonly used for analgesia after thoracic surgery or surgery on the chest wall including breast surgery, while lumbar paravertebral blocks are useful in the setting of abdominal surgeries, such as cholecystectomies and nephrectomies.

Lumbar facet nerve blocks, or medial branch blocks, are used to diagnose and briefly alleviate facet joint-mediated pain. After identification of the involved zygapophyseal joint, a radiofrequency neurotomy can be performed to damage the nerve for sustained pain relief. Ultrasound is a consistent and accurate technique to visualize the lumbar paravertebral anatomy and inject small volumes of local anesthetic. A posterior paravertebral parasagittal ultrasound image is obtained to localize the spinal levels involved. The transverse process is identified in the paravertebral region as a hyperechoic line with dropout noted underneath. Transverse plane imaging at each level will delineate the spinous and transverse processes, zygapophyseal articulations, inferior and superior facets, and the lamina of the vertebral arch.

An epidural blood patch is indicated for postdural puncture headache, typically when conservative management has failed. A blood patch procedure consists of injecting autologous blood into the epidural space, usually at the same level where the lumbar puncture was performed.

Contraindications

Absolute contraindications to neuraxial anesthesia include refusal by the patient, bleeding disorders or active anticoagulation, elevated intracranial pressure (pseudotumor cerebri being the only exception), infection at or around the injection site, severe hypovolemia, allergy to the anesthetic, and indeterminate neurological disease. Several other disease processes such as severe aortic or mitral stenosis or left ventricular outflow obstruction are relative contraindications. Particularly with spinal anesthesia, or rapidly achieved epidural anesthesia, sudden, severe hypotension may result. In the setting of underlying heart disease, it can lead to cardiac ischemia. Venodilation secondary to sympathetic blockade leads to venous pooling and ultimately decreased preload. Contraindications to a blood patch include coagulopathy, sepsis, puncture site infection, active neurological disease, hematologic malignancy, and patient refusal. Albeit infrequent, the more common complications of a blood patch include pain at the injection site, dural puncture, and radicular pain. Serious complications are rare, but incidences of cauda equina syndrome, sinus thrombosis, and aseptic arachnoiditis have been reported in the literature [2]. While an infection in itself is not an absolute contraindication to neuraxial blockade, it is recommended to exercise caution in these patients.

Contraindications to paravertebral blocks include local infection at site of injection, severe coagulopathy or use of concurrent anticoagulants or antiplatelet agents, severe respiratory disease, allergy to local anesthetics, and patient refusal.

Equipment/Probe Selection

Neuraxial procedures carry potential risk and should ideally be performed in facilities where emergency equipment and qualified personnel are readily available. Adequate intravenous access is necessary prior to beginning the procedure. ASA "Standards for Basic Anesthetic Monitoring" requires that every patient receiving regional anesthesia have continuous electrocardiogram monitoring as well as arterial blood pressure and heart rate evaluation at least every 5 minutes in anesthesiology settings. An ultrasound machine with a low-frequency curvilinear probe (5–2 MHz) as well as high-frequency curvilinear (9–2 MHz) and linear array (12–5 MHz) probes should be available in order to accommodate different anatomic regions and patient sizes. Standard monitoring should be available, as dictated by facility policy, such as noninvasive blood pressure (NIBP) and pulse oximeter. Appropriate procedure kit for epidural, spinal, or lumbar puncture, including sterile drapes and gloves, should be located in a separate cart for easy access. Standard local anesthetic medications for spinal or epidural anesthesia should be readily available in the procedure room [3].

Preparation/Pre-procedural Evaluation

Preparation for neuraxial anesthesia should begin with informed consent. After discussing the risks and benefits and obtaining consent, the clinician should then obtain a detailed yet concise pertinent history. Questions concerning prior anesthetic complications, history of difficult epidural or spinal anesthesia placement and of spinal disorders (i.e., scoliosis) or surgeries, thrombocytopenia, coagulopathies, and anticoagulant use can help avoid complications and improve the overall chances of success. The discussion concerning potential risks and benefits associated with neuraxial blockade should include both the rare but serious complications such as bleeding, infection, or temporary nerve damage and more common but less severe risks such as mild pain and post-dural puncture headache.

Lumbar neuraxial anesthesia may be performed with no, minimal, or deep sedation. While deep sedation/general anesthesia has the benefits of patient comfort and minimal patient movement, it is controversial as the patient is unable to verbalize pain or paresthesias during injection. These symptoms are associated with intraneural injection, which can lead to postoperative neurological deficits. This becomes particularly important when performing thoracic or cervical epidurals and spinal injections. Pediatric patients are an exception to this, as the majority of patients are unable to tolerate the procedure and require general anesthesia.

Premedication with midazolam and fentanyl is often beneficial particularly in patients with significant anxiety. In pregnant patients receiving labor epidural anesthesia, premedication is avoided, so it is often beneficial to discuss expectations and verbally guide the patient through the procedure.

Patient Positioning

Positioning is important in any neuraxial procedure. The three positions outlined below are the most common. The one chosen will depend on the patient, the procedure being performed, and what the clinician is comfortable with. Regardless of the position chosen, the ultimate goal in any neuraxial procedure is spinal flexion and the separation of adjacent spinous processes and interlaminar foramen.

Sitting

This position is typically well tolerated by most patients and clinician alike and is the most common for spinal and epidural anesthesia. The patient is typically seated with their legs hanging off the edge of the bed and their hips square. Ask the patient to press their chin to their chest and their buttocks into the bed. The resulting flexion helps to open up the interlaminar foramen and press the spinous processes toward the skin surface. Maintaining alignment of the patient's hips, shoulders, and head allows for midline to be easily recognized in this position, which is particularly beneficial in obese or otherwise difficult patients.

Lateral Decubitus

The lateral decubitus position is typically performed in patients who have difficulty sitting up or supporting themselves either due to sedation, weakness, or debility. It is also the position required for an accurate opening pressure in a diagnostic lumbar puncture. The patient is placed in the lateral decubitus position, with their hips perpendicular to the plane of the bed. Ask the patient to curl forward bringing their chin and their knees to their chest. This allows for flexion of the spine similar to the sitting position described above.

Prone

This position is most typical of neuraxial procedures performed under the guidance of fluoroscopy. The patient is usually under general anesthesia for these procedures. In this position, it is more difficult to appreciate midline surface landmarks, as the patient is unable to flex the spine similar to what was shape described above. In addition, because the instrumentation is above the patient, the CSF pressure is usually not high enough to overcome gravity, requiring aspiration of the CSF for subarachnoid injections [4].

Procedure

Lumbar Puncture

The patient should be placed in the position that the procedure will be performed, either sitting or lateral decubitus. There are two basic approaches to scanning the lumbar spine, a transverse (short axis) and sagittal (long axis) views. When utilizing the transverse imaging plane, place the transducer on the approximate center of the patient's back as shown in Fig. 13.1 and identify the dropout (acoustic shadow) of the spinous process with its characteristic acoustic outline (Fig. 13.2). Slide the probe cephalad or caudal to obtain a transverse interspinous view (Fig. 13.3). The acoustic shadow of the spinous process will give way to an echogenic interspinous ligament. A slight cephalad tilt of the probe may be necessary. The ligamentum flavum is visualized as a horizontal hyperechoic line running between the

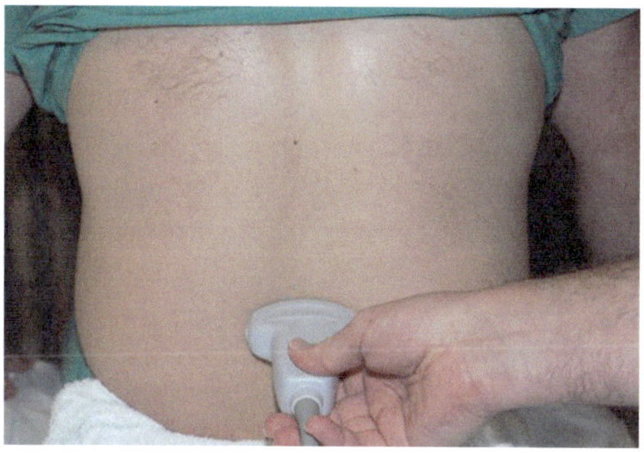

Fig. 13.1 Probe in the transverse plane approximately in the center of the patient's back

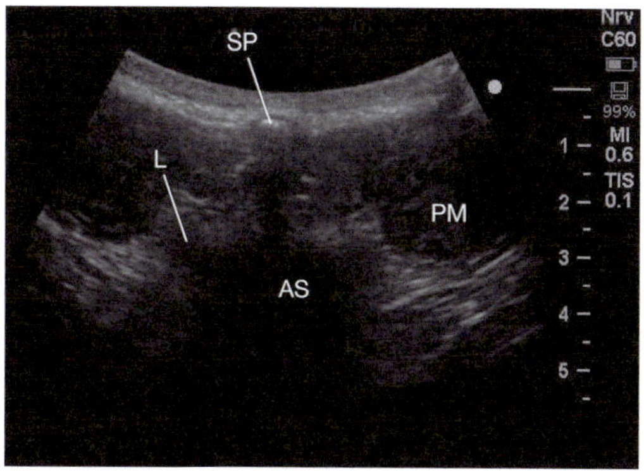

Fig. 13.2 Midline transverse probe placement: spinous view (SP spinous process, AS acoustic shadow behind spinous process and laminae, PM paraspinous muscle, L lamina)

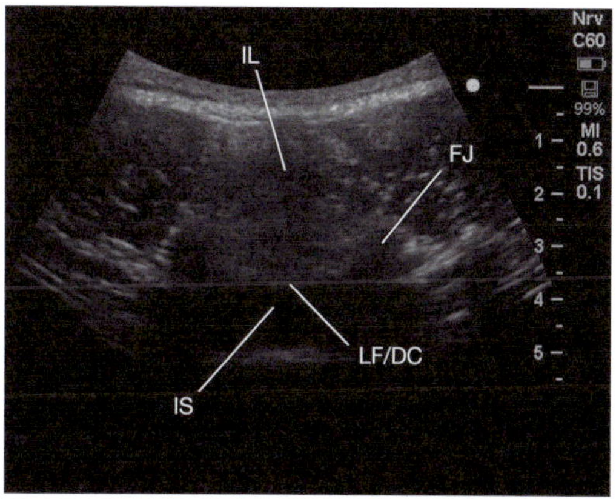

Fig. 13.3 Midline transverse probe placement: interspinous view (IL interspinous ligament, FJ facet joint, LF/DC ligamentum flavum/dura complex, IS intrathecal space)

articular processes and facet joints. It is common to see a single hyperechoic line representing the ligamentum flavum/dura complex (Fig. 13.4). Deep to this is the hypoechoic intrathecal space that appears gray or black due to its weaker spectral reflection. The anterior dura, posterior longitudinal ligament, and the posterior aspect of the vertebral disc are visualized using ultrasonography collectively as a single linear hyperechoic structure, which is named the anterior complex [5]. Visualizing the anterior complex ensures you have an appropriate acoustic window for the interspinous view.

When utilizing a longitudinal approach, place the transducer in a paramedian sagittal plane 2–3 cm from the midline (Fig. 13.5), and tilt the probe medially to obtain a paramedian sagittal oblique view. The lamina/articular processes of each vertebral level can be visualized as hyperechoic humps, which form a sawtooth pattern. The hyperechoic line of the ligamentum flavum can be visualized in the paramedian interlaminar spaces. It is helpful to identify the L5–S1 junction, and from that point, the provider can count up to the desired level.

First, identify the L5–S1 junction by visualizing the sacrum, which will appear as a hyperechoic curvilinear structure. Scanning in a cephalad direction from the sacrum, the lamina/articular processes of each vertebral level can be visualized as hyperechoic humps which form a sawtooth pattern. Continue to slide the probe until the appropriate level has been identified. Once the chosen level is positioned in the center of the ultrasound image, a mark on the patient's skin is made in the center of the probe (Fig. 13.6). Obtain a short axis view by rotating the probe 90° at the desired spinal level with the ultrasound probe in a transverse plane on the midline. Slide the probe cephalad or caudad to obtain a transverse interspinous view of the desired interspace. A slight cephalad tilt of the probe may be necessary to visualize the ligamentum flavum, and this angle should be noted as this is the same angle your needle will need to be inserted. Mark on the patient's skin at the midpoint of the probe's long and short sides. The needle insertion site should be the intersection of these two marks (Fig. 13.7).

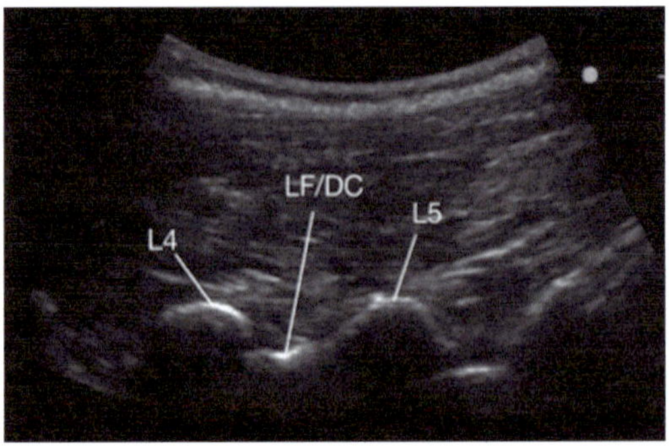

Fig. 13.4 B-mode image of the ligamentum at L4–L5 interspace (L4 and L5 lumbar vertebrae, LF/DC ligamentum flavum/dura complex)

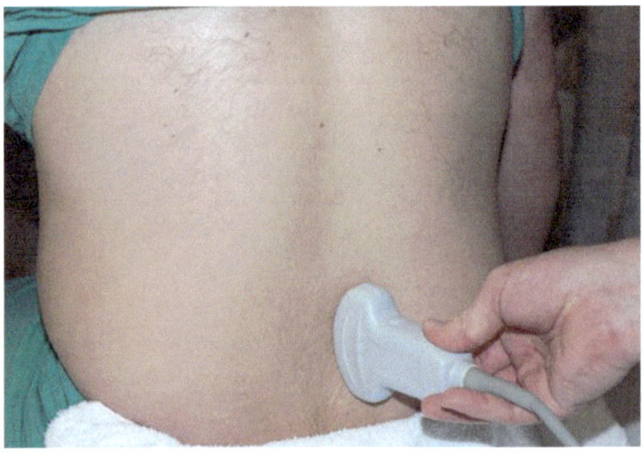

Fig. 13.5 Paramedian sagittal probe orientation

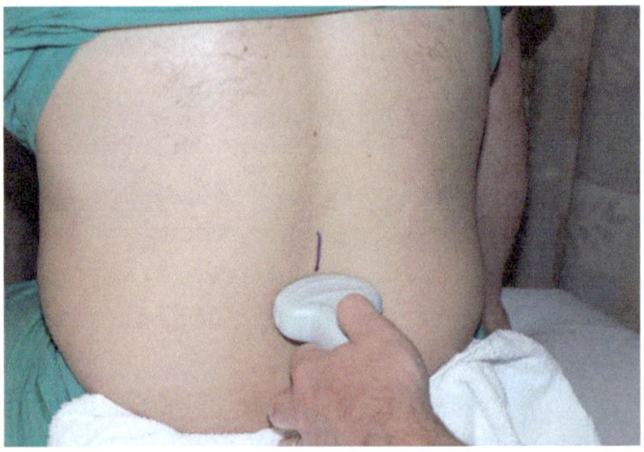

Fig. 13.6 The center of the ultrasound image is aligned over the spinous process, and a mark is made on the patient's skin in the center of the probe

At this point, it is beneficial to freeze the ultrasound image. The ultrasound machine's electronic calipers can be used to measure the depth from the skin to the ligamentum flavum to provide the expected depth of needle insertion

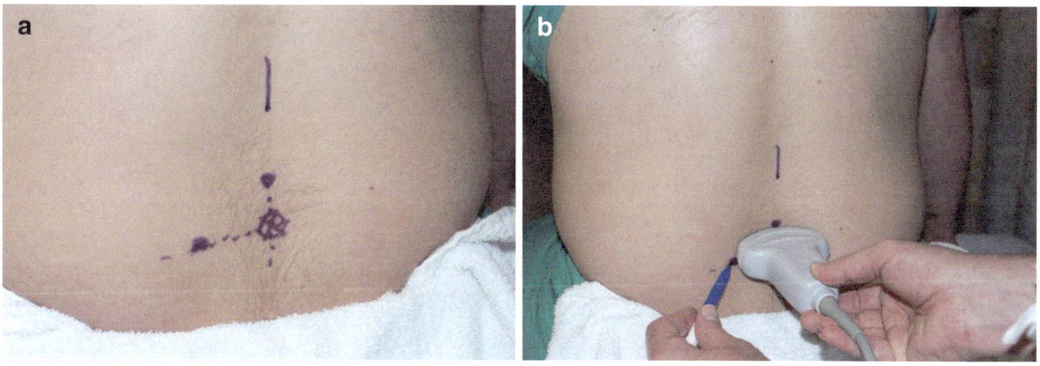

Fig. 13.7 (**a**) Marks indicating midline of long and short probe axes. (**b**) Needle insertion should be at the intersection of these two dots

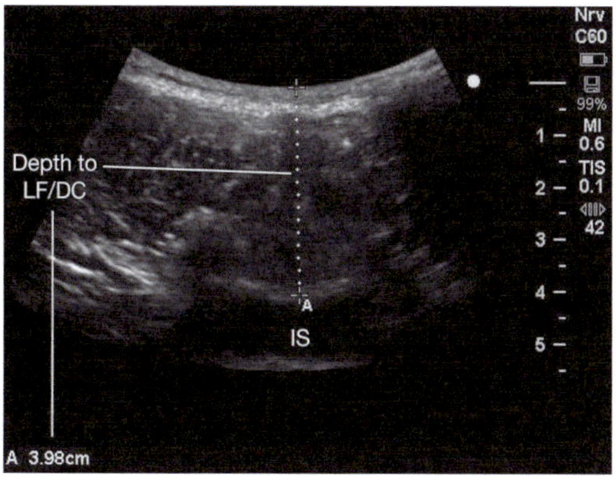

Fig. 13.8 The ultrasound machine's electronic caliper function measures the depth from the skin to the ligamentum flavum to provide the expected depth of needle insertion (IS intrathecal space, LF/DC ligamentum flavum/dura complex)

(Fig. 13.8). Be careful not to use excessive pressure with the ultrasound probe, as this will depress the patient's skin and subcutaneous tissue, which could predict a falsely lower estimated depth of needle insertion.

After the above landmarks have been identified as described above, the area should be prepped and draped in a sterile fashion to comply with facility guidelines and policies. The spinal needle should be inserted at the respective mark on the skin, and the initial angle should attempt to reproduce the cephalad angulation used with the ultrasound probe needed to obtain the interspinous view. When a "pop" is perceived as the spinal needle passes the dura mater, the stylet should be removed to observe the flow of cerebral spinal fluid from the needle hub. Measurement of the skin to ligamentum flavum obtained above will predict the expected depth of needle insertion.

Blood Patch

The epidural space can be identified by the procedure described in detail above with a loss of resistance technique. With a blood patch, a second operator can facilitate the procedure by obtaining approximately 15–20 ml of the patient's blood from a peripheral site in a sterile fashion. The blood is injected into the epidural space under real-time ultrasound scanning. Post injection, an increase in space between the ligamentum flavum and posterior dura and the posterior longitudinal ligament and anterior dura can be noted on ultrasound. The use of real-time ultrasound-guided placement of a blood patch is limited albeit it can reliably confirm placement of injectate into the epidural space [6].

Epidural Block

An ultrasound-guided epidural block is approached similarly to a lumbar puncture by initially using the midline transverse probe placement to obtain spinous and interspinous views. Again, a mark on the patient's skin is made at the midpoint of the probe's long and short sides. The epidural needle should be inserted at the respective mark on the skin, and the initial angle should attempt to reproduce the cephalad angulation used with the ultrasound probe needed to obtain the interspinous view. A loss of resistance to air or saline technique, indicating penetration through the ligamentum flavum, should be employed for epidural procedures to confirm entry into the epidural space and to avoid dural puncture. Once the epidural space is identified by employing a loss of resistance or hanging drop technique, a catheter may be advanced through the Tuohy needle for continuous or re-dosable analgesia through a bolus or a continuous infusion. Typically, 4–5 cm is added to the depth of the Tuohy needle to ensure that the catheter remains in the epidural space. After placement, the catheter should be aspirated for blood or CSF to detect intravascular or intrathecal placement, respectively. A test dose of lidocaine with epinephrine should be administered after a negative aspiration to confirm an extravascular and epidural catheter placement. It should be noted that an intravascular injection of epinephrine would produce clinical signs such as tachycardia, and lidocaine can elicit a metallic taste in the mouth, dizziness, or tinnitus. An intrathecal injection could produce motor blockade of the lower extremities [7]. Once proper placement is confirmed, adequate analgesia can be reached by intermittent bolus or continuous infusion dependent upon the patient's clinical picture.

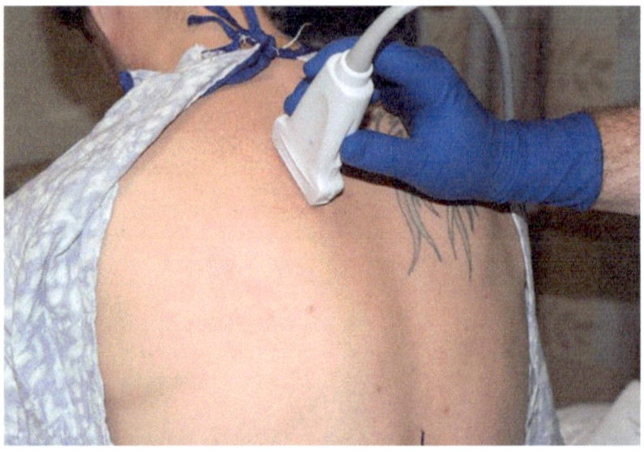

Fig. 13.9 Probe orientation for identifying appropriate spinal level

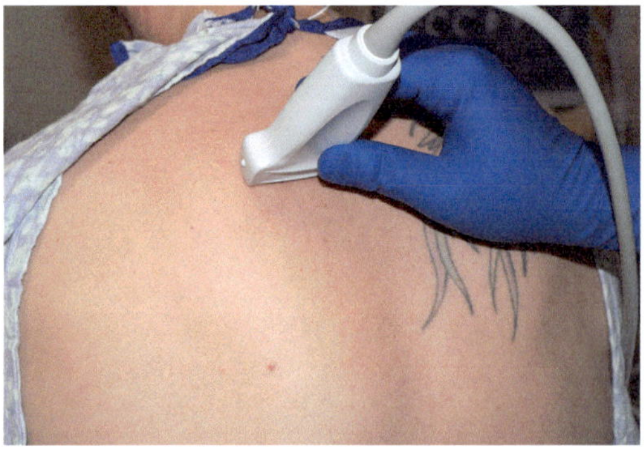

Fig. 13.10 After identifying the appropriate spinal level, the ultrasound transducer has been rotated so that it is oriented parallel to the ribs and perpendicular to the spine

Paravertebral Block

Identify the appropriate spinal level by holding the ultrasound probe perpendicular to the ribs (Fig. 13.9) approximately 5 cm lateral to midline. The appropriate level can be located by counting ribs from the 1st rib and counting down or counting up from the 12th rib. After identifying the appropriate spinal level, rotate the ultrasound probe so that it is oriented parallel to the ribs and perpendicular to the spine (Fig. 13.10). Identify the rib by sliding the probe cephalad or caudad. The rib will appear as a bright hyperechoic (white) line with ultrasound dropout below (black). Medially the rib articulates with the transverse process, which is often identified with a slight depression at the point of articulation. While remaining parallel to the rib, slide the probe caudally. The transverse process will remain in view, but the intercostal muscles will come into view and will have a gray appearance. The internal intercostal membrane is contiguous with the costotransverse ligament and may be visualized as a thin hyperechoic (white) line extending from the transverse process. Deep to the intercostal muscles will be a bright hyperechoic line; this is the pleura of the lung. This will appear different to the rib as the ultrasound waves can penetrate to the deeper lung tissue, which can appear to shimmer and move with patient respirations (Fig. 13.11). The needle is inserted in-plane to the ultrasound probe from a lateral to medial direction (Fig. 13.12). It is important to not advance the needle medial to the transverse process, because this will increase

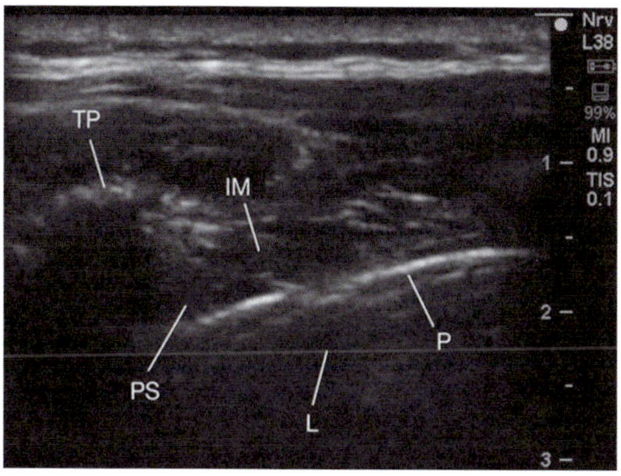

Fig. 13.11 Transverse lateral ultrasound view: TP transverse process, PS posterior shadowing, P pleura, IM intercostal muscle, L lung

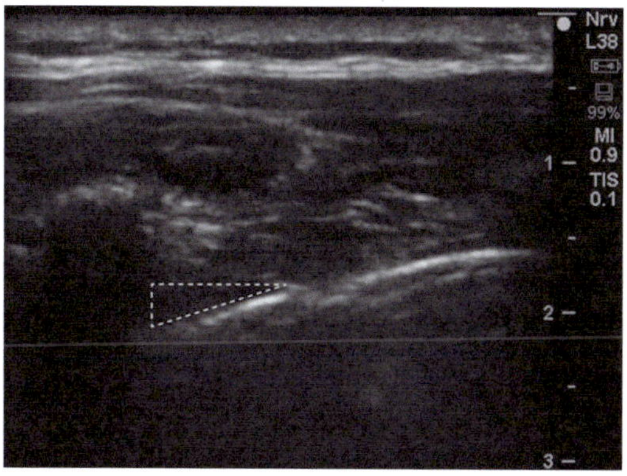

Fig. 13.13 Needle target outlined by triangle

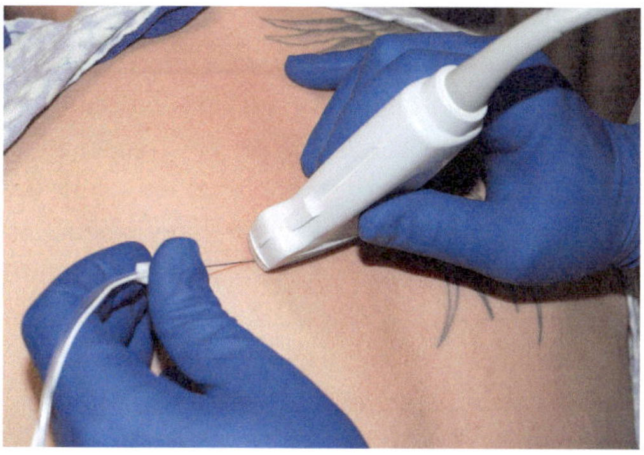

Fig. 13.12 Needle insertion from the lateral to medial direction

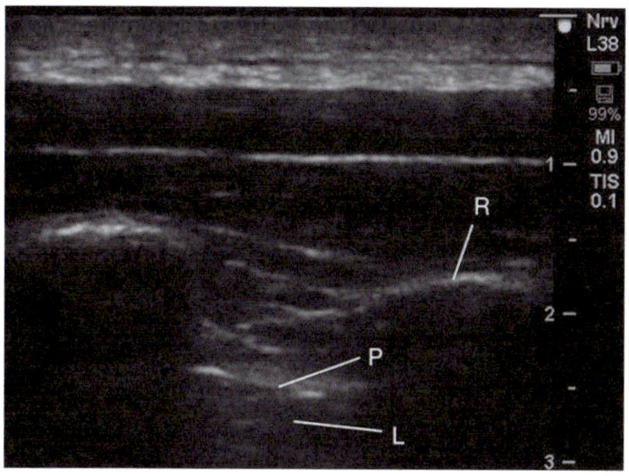

Fig. 13.14 Ribs seen on ultrasound: R rib, P pleura, L lung

the risk of entering the spinal or epidural space. The goal is to advance the needle through the internal intercostal membrane deep to the transverse process just above the pleura (Fig. 13.13). It is essential to be aware of the position of the needle tip at all times to avoid complications such as pneumothorax and spinal or epidural injections. After aspiration of the needle, local anesthetic can be incrementally injected. An anterior displacement of the pleura is typically observed. Hydrodissection with preservative-free normal saline may help accurately identify needle tip position prior to local anesthetic injection. This also assures proper placement of the local anesthetic. This procedure can be repeated at each desired level.

When utilizing a paramedian sagittal approach, identify the appropriate spinal level as described above with the probe in a paramedian sagittal orientation (probe is perpendicular to the ribs and parallel to the spine) approximately 5 cm lateral to midline. At the desired level, slide the probe medially to visualize the transverse process and the paravertebral space. Ribs typically appear to be more superficial and rounded (Fig. 13.14) compared to transverse process, which are typically slightly deeper and square in appearance (Fig. 13.15). The hyperechoic line of the parietal pleura can be identified running deep to the adjacent transverse processes (Fig. 13.15). The needle can be inserted out-of-plane to the ultrasound probe until contact is made with the transverse process. Walk off the transverse process and advance the needle 1 cm deeper. Alternatively, the needle can be inserted in-plane to the ultrasound probe in a cephalad orientation and enter

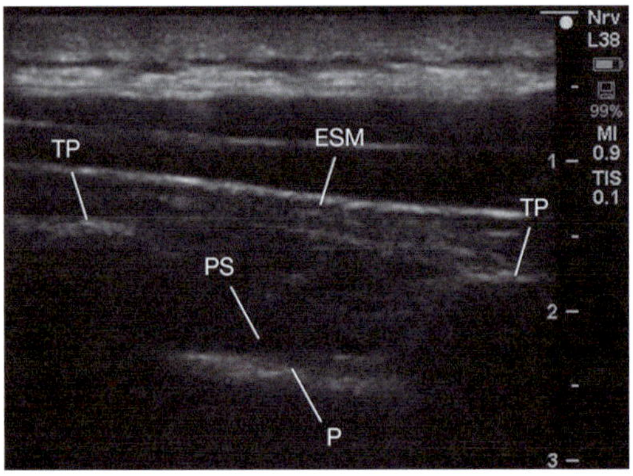

Fig. 13.15 Transverse process seen on ultrasound: TP transverse process, P pleura, PS posterior shadowing, Erector spinae muscle (ESM)

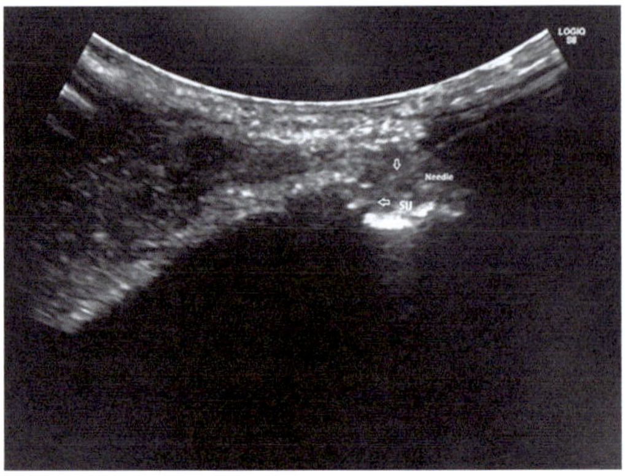

Fig. 13.16 An ultrasound image showing a needle approaching the sacroiliac joint (SIJ). The needle should be angulated slightly from medial to lateral and parallel to the joint

the paravertebral space midway between 2 adjacent transverse processes. In either case the tip of the needle is advanced until it pierces the costotransverse ligament. If the costotransverse ligament is not easily seen, the needle is advanced until it is directly above the pleura.

For the in-plane technique, a steep angle is often required which often leads to difficult visualization of the needle. Whether you use an out-of-plane or in-plane approach, it is useful to intermittently inject small boluses of preservative-free normal saline to confirm the position of the needle tip. When the needle tip has pierced the costotransverse ligament and is immediately above the pleura, injection of normal saline will result in anterior displacement of the pleura. Once this correct needle position is confirmed and after a negative aspiration, local anesthetic can be incrementally injected. An anterior displacement of the pleura should be observed. This procedure can be repeated at each desired level.

Sacroiliac Joint Injection

A high-frequency transducer can be used in children and smaller adults. For the procedure, the patient is placed in the prone position with a pillow placed under the abdomen to straight the lumbar lordosis [8]. The patient is then cleaned with antiseptic solution and draped appropriately. The ultrasound transducer is placed in a transverse orientation to initially identify the sacral hiatus and sacral cornua. The transducer is moved laterally until the lateral edge of the sacrum is seen. Next, the transversely positioned transducer is moved in a cephalad fashion until the bony contour of the ileum is identified. The posterior aspect of the SI joint is the hypoechoic cleft between the bony contours of the ileum and the sacrum. The lower third of the sacroiliac joint can be identified in this position with a caudal tilt. It is recommended to inject directly into the synovial portion with a vertically oriented needle position (Fig. 13.16). Altogether, the lower third of the sacroiliac joint is a preferred target of the injection secondary to its synovial component, more vertical orientation, and relative superficial location in non-obese patients. A medial to lateral injection technique is recommended for ultrasound-guided sacroiliac joint injections [9].

The upper level of the sacroiliac joint can also be targeted as an appropriate alternative if lower-level access is difficult (i.e., bone spurs). For orientation, the posterior superior iliac spine should be visualized laterally and the fifth lumbar spinous process medially. The transducer should be moved in a caudal fashion to bring the dorsal surface of the sacrum, the medial and lateral sacral crest, the gluteal surface of the ilium, and the posterior sacral foramen into view. The needle is then inserted into the hypoechoic cleft between the surface of the sacrum and the bony contour of the ileum. The needle should be angulated slightly from medial to lateral for insertion parallel to the joint [1].

Lumbar Facet Joint Injection

For the ultrasound-guided zygapophyseal joint block, the patient should be positioned in a prone position with an underlying pillow to straighten the lumbar lordosis. A linear array, high-frequency probe or a curvilinear, low-frequency probe (6–2 MHz) should be used for visualization. The probe is oriented in the longitudinal axis in the paravertebral to identify the vertebral levels, which can be identified by counting the transverse processes upward from the sacrum. The probe should then be rotated 90° to identify the site for injection. In this view, the spinous and transverse processes, erector spinae muscle, and superior articular process should be identified. The target for the tip of the needle should be the junction between the superior articular process and the transverse process.

Complications

An inadvertent complication may arise secondary to inexact positioning of the needle during the block with spread of local anesthetic into the intervertebral foramen, epidural space, or subarachnoid space, which may render a false-positive result or more disastrously produce spinal anesthesia [1]. General complications of neuraxial anesthetics include post-dural puncture headache, intravascular injection, local anesthetic toxicity, infection, epidural hematoma, nerve injury, hypotension, total spinal anesthesia, and urinary retention. Injection of local anesthetic in 3–5 ml aliquots with intermittent aspirations to observe for the presence of blood is important to avoid intravascular injection, as well as the use of an epinephrine containing test dose during the placement of epidural catheters.

Complications associated with thoracic paravertebral blocks include infection, inadvertent vascular puncture, hematoma, hypotension, nerve injury, epidural or intrathecal spread, pleural puncture, and pneumothorax. Epidural and intrathecal spread is best avoided by minimizing medial angulation of the needle, aspiration before injection to detect cerebrospinal fluid, and avoiding forceful injection of the local anesthetic. Pleural puncture is a potential risk and may be reduced using ultrasound guidance by allowing visualization of the needle tip, but it is also important not to advance more than 1–1.5 cm deep to the transverse process. Additionally, sharp (non-Tuohy) smaller-gauge needles (22 gauge) have been associated with some reported cases of total spinal anesthesia and neurological injury [10].

Pearls/Pitfalls

- Hypotension is more common when bilateral blocks are performed.
- A lower-frequency curvilinear probe may be necessary in patients with deeper structures.
- Familiarity with the bony anatomy of the spine is essential to understand the sonoanatomy.
- In morbidly obese patients where structures are very deep, the ability to at least identify midline and the approximate interspace levels can improve the success of the neuraxial procedure.
- When measuring various depths, it is important to be aware of the pressure you are applying with the ultrasound probe as this will falsely decrease the depths of structures you may be measuring.
- The angle of the ultrasound probe that obtains the optimal image will predict the angle needed upon insertion of the needle.
- Failure of a successful injection or complications can occur when sonoanatomical landmarks are not well visualized.

Integration into Clinical Practice

Spinal anesthesia and paravertebral blocks and their benefits have become more accessible than ever to clinicians in various specialties with the use of ultrasound guidance. Providers who see patients in pain or perform procedures, which would benefit from ultrasound-guided blocks, should analyze how their use might improve workflow and patient satisfaction and decrease complications. Control of patient discomfort without the use of opioid agents can result in significant benefit to patients.

Evidence

The use of regional and neuraxial anesthesia has demonstrated to significantly improve patient outcome. The largest meta-analysis (CORTRA) of randomized controlled trials comparing intraoperative neuraxial versus general anesthesia demonstrated a significant decrease in mortality and morbidity in the neuraxial group [11]. Evidence supports that regional anesthesia may improve outcomes by decreasing cardiac, pulmonary, and gastrointestinal complications [12–14]. Furthermore, evidence demonstrates superior pain control with epidural and continuous peripheral nerve blockade in comparison with systemic opioids [15, 16].

Several publications have described the process and benefits of ultrasound-guided neuraxial blocks. The majority of the literature has focused on pre-procedural ultrasound examination to aid in the successful insertion of a spinal or epidural needle. The use of ultrasound has been shown to improve efficiency, by decreasing the number of needle insertions or passes, including patients with difficult surface anatomy [17–19]. Studies support that ultrasound guidance assists in identifying the correct lumbar intervertebral level and the required needle insertion depth [20, 21]. It is common for even trained providers to be one or more levels off from the intended vertebral space, and therefore ultrasound guidance can assist in more accurately identifying the desired spinal level. This may be important in patients with known pathology or hardware present.

Paravertebral blocks have gained much attention in the setting of breast surgery for breast cancer. Paravertebral blocks provide better postoperative pain control and may reduce the risk of chronic pain after breast cancer surgery [22, 23]. The evidence supporting the use of ultrasound guidance while performing paravertebral blocks mostly focuses on techniques and the feasibility studies [24]. However, it is reasonable that the use of ultrasound guidance is a safe and effective way to facilitate correct needle placement and observe the spread of local anesthetic for paravertebral nerve blocks. Additionally, the use of ultrasound guidance may be a useful aid in patients with difficult surface anatomy.

Key Points

- Use appropriate ultrasound and adjunct equipment.
- Know the gross and sonographic anatomy.
- Infection control is important.
- Be aware of needle tip at all times and inject anesthetic in small aliquots.
- Pre-scan target area prior to initiating procedure preparation.
- Ultrasound is an adjunct to the procedure, which is little changed from its blind version.

References

1. Klauser A, De Zordo T, Feuchtner G, Sogner P, Schirmer M, Gruber J, Sepp N, Moriggl B. Feasibility of ultrasound-guided sacroiliac joint injection considering sonoanatomic landmarks at two different levels in cadavers and patients. Arthritis Rheum. 2008;59(11):1618–24.
2. Turnbull DK, Shepherd DB. Post-dural puncture headache: pathogenesis, prevention and treatment. Br J Anaesth. 2003;91:718–29.
3. Standards for Basic Anesthetic Monitoring (amended by ASA House of Delegates Oct 25, 2015). https://www.asahq.org/~/media/Sites/ASAHQ/Files/Public/Resources/standards-guidelines/standards-for-basic-anesthetic-monitoring.pdf.

4. Brull R, Macfarlane A, Chan V. Spinal, epidural and caudal anesthesia. In: Millers anesthesia. 8th ed. Philadelphia: Elsevier Saunders; 2015. p. 1684–720.
5. Karmakar MK. Ultrasound for central neuraxial blocks. Tech Reg Anesth Pain Manag. 2009;13:161–70.
6. Khayata I, Lichtor JL, Amelin PA. Ultrasound-guided epidural blood patch. Anesthesiology. 2011;114(6):1453.
7. Gruber EM, et al. The effects of thoracic epidural analgesia with bupivacaine 0.25% on ventilatory mechanics in patients with severe chronic obstructive pulmonary disease. Anesth Analg. 2001;92(4):1015–9.
8. Seib RK, Peng PWH. Ultrasound-guided peripheral nerve block in chronic pain management. Tech Reg Anesth Pain Manag. 2009;13(3):110–6.
9. Chang WH, Lew HL, Chen C. Ultrasound guided sacroiliac joint injection technique. Am J Phys Med Rehabil. 2013;92(3):278–9.
10. Boezaart AP, Lucas SD, Elliott CE. Paravertebral block: cervical, thoracic, lumbar, and sacral. Curr Opin Anaesthesiol. 2009;22(5):637–43.
11. Rodgers A, Walker N, Schug S, McKee A, Kehlet H, Van Zundert A, Sage D, Futter M, Saville G, Clark T, MacMahon S. Reduction of postoperative mortality and morbidity with epidural or spinal anesthesia: results from overview of randomized trials. BMJ. 2000;321(7275):1493.
12. Beattie WS, Badner NH, Choi P. Epidural analgesia reduces postoperative myo- cardial infarction: a meta-analysis. Anesth Analg. 2001;93:853–8.
13. Ballantyne JC, Carr DB, deFerranti S, et al. The comparative effects of postop- erative analgesic therapies on pulmonary outcome: cumulative meta-analyses of randomized, controlled trials. Anesth Analg. 1998;86:598–612.
14. Marret E, Remy C, Bonnet F, Postoperative Pain Forum Group. Meta-analysis of epidural analgesia versus parenteral opioid analgesia after colorectal surgery. Br J Surg. 2007;94(6):665–73.
15. Wu CL, Cohen SR, Richman JM, et al. Efficacy of postoperative patient-controlled and continuous infusion epidural analgesia versus intravenous patient-controlled analgesia with opioids: a meta-analysis. Anesthesiology. 2005;103:1079–88.
16. Richman JM, Liu SS, Courpas G, et al. Does continuous peripheral nerve block provide superior pain control to opioids? A meta-analysis. Anesth Analg. 2006;102:248–57.
17. Grau T, Leipold RW, Conradi R, Martin E, Motsch J. Efficacy of ultrasound imaging in obstetric epidural anesthesia. J Clin Anesth. 2002;14(3):169–75.
18. Arzola C, Davies S, Rofaeel A, Carvalho JC. Ultrasound using the transverse approach to the lumbar spine provides reliable landmarks for labor epidurals. Anesth Analg. 2007;104(5):1188–92.
19. Chin KJ, Perlas A, Chan V, Brown-Shreves D, Koshkin A, Vaishnav V. Ultrasound imaging facilitates spinal anesthesia in adults with difficult surface anatomic landmarks. Anesthesiology. 2011;115(1):94–101.
20. Perlas A, Chaparro LE, Chin KJ. Lumbar neuraxial ultrasound for spinal and epidural anesthesia: a systematic review and meta-analysis. Reg Anesth Pain Med. 2016;36:126–7.
21. Perlas A. Evidence for the use of ultrasound in neuraxial blocks. Reg Anesth Pain Med. 2010;35:S43–6.
22. Schnabel A, Reichl SU, Kranke P, Pogatzki-Zahn EM, Zahn PK. Efficacy and safety of paravertebral blocks in breast surgery: a meta-analysis of randomized controlled trials. Br J Anaesth. 2010;105(6):842–52.
23. Andraea MH, Andreae DA. Regional anesthesia to prevent chronic pain after surgery: a Cochrane systematic review and meta-analysis. Br J Anaesth. 2013;111(5):711–20.
24. Neal JM, Brull R, Chan VW, Grant SA, Horn JL, Liu SS, McCartney CJ, Narouze SN, Perlas A, Salinas FV, Sites BD, Tsui BC. The ASRA evidence-based medicine assessment of ultrasound-guided regional anesthesia and pain medicine: executive summary. Reg Anesth Pain Med. 2010;35(2 Suppl):S1–9.

Ultrasound-Guided Thoracic Procedures

14

Kay Odashima, Samuel Blake Kluger, Pete Keenan, and Eitan Dickman

Thoracentesis

Introduction

Pleural effusions are a common problem affecting 1.5 million patients presenting to inpatient units and emergency departments every year in the United States. Patients with symptomatic pleural effusions often complain of shortness of breath, chest pain, cough, or weakness, and large pleural effusions can cause respiratory distress and hypoxia. Thoracentesis, the drainage of pleural fluid with a needle or catheter, is performed 200,000 times annually in the United States [1, 2].

Lung ultrasound, which has been utilized for decades in the diagnosis of pleural effusions, has been shown to have superior accuracy when compared to radiography [3, 4]. Lung ultrasound can be performed at the bedside, can be completed rapidly, and has been demonstrated to lead to changes in management decisions [5].

K. Odashima · E. Dickman (✉)
Department of Emergency Medicine, Maimonides Medical Center, Brooklyn, NY, USA
e-mail: edickman@maimonidesmed.org

S. B. Kluger
Ultrasound Faculty, Emergency Care Specialists, Grand Rapids, MI, USA

P. Keenan
Lakewood Regional Medical Center, Lakewood, CA, USA

Los Alamitos Medical Center, Los Alamitos, CA, USA

Advantages of Ultrasound Guidance

In addition to the advantages listed above, ultrasound can be used to estimate the volume of pleural fluid and can aid in differentiating transudates from exudates prior to thoracentesis [6, 7]. Ultrasound-guided thoracentesis (USGT) is associated with a decreased rate of hemothorax and pneumothorax compared with an anatomic landmark-based approach, leading to decreased health-care costs and hospital length of stay [8–11]. Previous studies have demonstrated that the use of point-of-care ultrasound for diagnosis and drainage of pleural effusions is a readily acquired skill [12–14].

Anatomy

A pleural effusion is a gravitationally dependent fluid collection between the visceral and parietal pleura. Intercostal arteries, veins, and nerves run inferior to each rib, supplying the superficial structures, ribs, intercostal muscles, and parietal pleura. In spontaneously breathing patients, an upright patient position is recommended when performing thoracentesis, using a posterior approach above the 9th rib to avoid entering the abdominal or retroperi-

S. Adhikari, M. Blaivas (eds.), *The Ultimate Guide to Point-of-Care Ultrasound-Guided Procedures*, https://doi.org/10.1007/978-3-030-28267-7_14

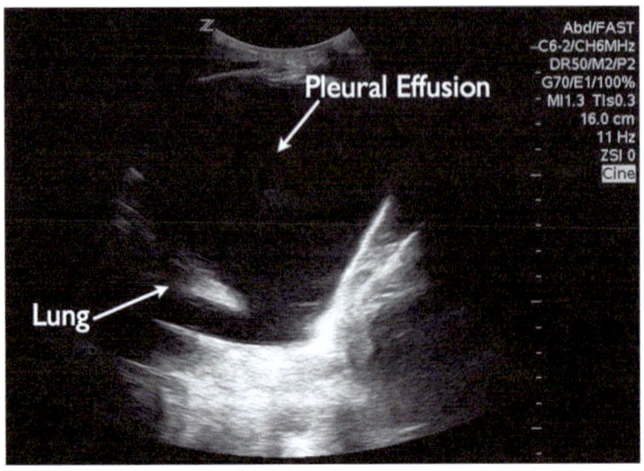

Fig. 14.1 Coronal view of pleural effusion with ultrasound transducer placed on the patient's left lateral chest

toneal cavities. In supine, mechanically ventilated patients, fluid will tend to collect more posteriorly, and the lateral approach to needle entry is utilized. With the ultrasound transducer held in a sagittal or coronal orientation, the pleura is identified deep to the ribs. A pleural effusion appears as an anechoic or echogenic fluid collection between the pleura (Fig. 14.1). The thin echogenic diaphragm can be used as a landmark to confirm that the fluid collection is within the thoracic cavity. The exact site of needle entry should be chosen based on the location of the largest fluid collection and the absence of the lung, diaphragm, or other organs.

Indications

Thoracentesis may be performed for therapeutic or diagnostic purposes. Therapeutic thoracentesis is performed in the setting of a moderate to large symptomatic pleural effusion. Patients with an underlying pleural effusion who develop hypoxia or respiratory distress and do not respond to conservative therapy may be good candidates for thoracentesis. Diagnostic thoracentesis is indicated for new pleural effusions with an unclear etiology. Conversely, patients with small bilateral pleural effusions and a clear cause such as underlying congestive heart failure are less likely to benefit from thoracentesis.

Contraindications

Abnormal coagulation parameters are commonly cited as a contraindication to thoracentesis, with cutoff values of international normalized ratio (INR) greater than 1.6 or fewer than 50,000 platelets per microliter [15]. However, retrospective evidence demonstrates that USGT is not associated with significantly increased bleeding even in the setting of abnormal coagulation parameters [15, 16]. Regardless, the risk of the procedure should be weighed against the benefit in all patients, particularly those who are coagulopathic.

Skin puncture through areas of overlying cellulitis or herpes zoster is contraindicated. Care must be used when performing thoracentesis among mechanically ventilated patients due to the increased risk of pneumothorax in the setting of positive-pressure ventilation. However, the incidence of pneumothorax among mechanically ventilated patients undergoing USGT has been shown to be low, and many likely occur secondary to injury from re-expansion or trapping rather than needle penetration [12].

Equipment/Probe Selection

Equipment required for USGT is shown in Fig. 14.2. The choice of ultrasound transducer depends on operator preference and the patient's body habitus. A low-frequency curvilinear or phased array transducer allows for deeper penetration and a wider picture of the anatomic area, whereas a high-frequency linear transducer offers increased resolution of superficial structures. The procedure should be performed using sterile technique including a sterile probe sheath.

Preparation/Pre-procedural Evaluation

Prior to the procedure, informed consent should be obtained after discussing risks and benefits. Complications of USGT are listed in Table 14.1. The procedure can be performed with the patient in either the seated upright or supine position depending on clinical conditions and patient comfort. Following any changes in patient positioning, the ultrasound should be repeated due to possible changes in fluid location.

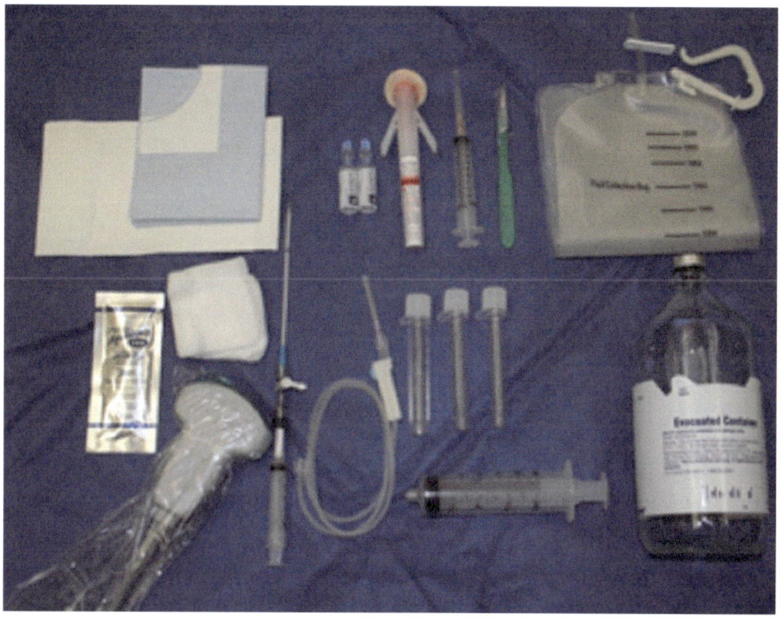

Fig. 14.2 Equipment required for ultrasound-guided thoracentesis. From top left: fenestrated and non-fenestrated drapes; local anesthetic; chlorhexidine; 10 cc syringe with 25 gauge needle; scalpel; collection bag and evacuated container; 60 cc syringe; sample collection tubes; thoracentesis needle, catheter, syringe, and tubing; ultrasound probe with sterile gel and sheath; and sterile gauze

Table 14.1 Complications associated with thoracentesis

Pneumothorax
Bleeding
Re-expansion pulmonary edema
Infection
Solid organ injury
Pain
Cough

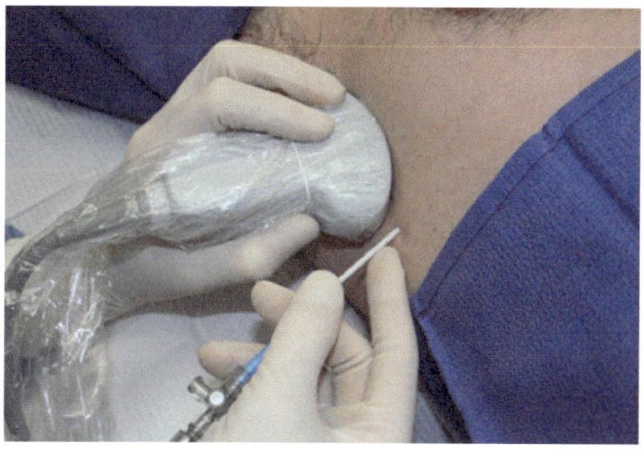

Fig. 14.3 Ultrasound-guided thoracentesis using an in-plane approach

Procedure

Following patient positioning, a safe area for needle entry is identified using ultrasound, and the skin is marked. The remainder of the procedure should be performed using sterile technique to avoid introducing infection. The skin is prepped using a chlorhexidine- or iodine-based solution, and a sterile drape is placed on the patient. Next, the skin, subcutaneous tissues, and pleura are anesthetized using a local anesthetic such as 1% lidocaine. The ultrasound probe is then covered with a sterile sheath and placed on the previously marked spot. Using an in-plane technique, the thoracentesis needle is then used to puncture through the skin using care to avoid the neurovascular bundle running below the rib (Fig. 14.3). The needle should be visualized penetrating through the parietal pleura and into the fluid collection in the thorax (Fig. 14.4). Once the needle has been placed into the pleural effusion, the cath-

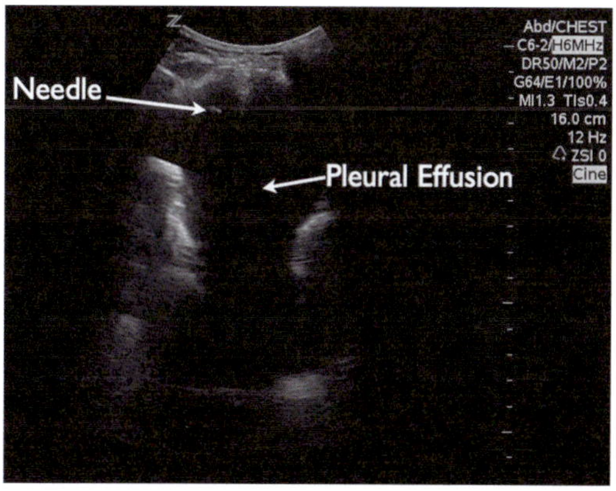

Fig. 14.4 Ultrasound-guided thoracentesis using an in-plane approach

eter is advanced over the needle as the needle is removed. The thoracentesis tubing is then connected to the catheter at one end and to the drainage device at the other end. At this time, a three-way stopcock can be used to collect fluid for laboratory analysis, if desired. The drainage of the effusion can be observed in real time using ultrasound. Following drainage of the fluid, the catheter is removed, and a sterile dressing is placed.

Complications

Complications associated with thoracentesis include pneumothorax, hemothorax, re-expansion pulmonary edema, and laceration to surrounding structures including the liver, spleen, heart, diaphragm, bowel, and kidneys. The use of ultrasound has been shown to decrease the incidence of complications associated with thoracentesis [10–13]. There is a lower risk of pneumothorax when thoracentesis volume is less than 1.2 L [17–19]. The incidence of pneumothorax during USGT is between 1% and 5% [10, 12, 13], and the incidence of significant bleeding is also low when USGT is performed by experienced operators. In one study of 1009 patients, the incidence of hemorrhagic complication was 0.4% overall and 1.3% among patients with abnormal coagulation parameters [15]. In another study of 1076 patients, no hemorrhagic complications were identified despite 17% of patients having a pre-procedure INR greater than 2.0% and 6% of patients having a pre-procedure platelet count less than 50,000 per microliter [16].

Re-expansion pulmonary edema is a rare complication of thoracentesis, but has a mortality as high as 20% and usually occurs when the volume of fluid removed is greater than 1500 mL [20]. In one prospective study of 941 patients undergoing thoracentesis, the incidence of re-expansion pulmonary edema was 0.2% of patients overall and 0.5% of patients with greater than 1 L of fluid removed [19]. Symptoms include dyspnea, chest pain, and increased sputum production. Treatment is supportive and includes lateral decubitus positioning with the affected side up and positive-pressure ventilation.

Pearls/Pitfalls

Failure to properly align the needle in-plane with the ultrasound transducer will impede needle visualization during dynamic USGT. To minimize the risk of procedural complications, the needle should be visualized throughout the procedure. Not having good control of the needle and using excess force to puncture through the chest wall can lead to inadvertent excessive needle length insertion into the thorax and could result in lung penetration. Good needle control and measured movements/force applied will minimize this risk. In addition, removal of large volumes of fluid can increase the risk of complications.

Integration into Clinical Practice

The use of ultrasound can be integrated into the clinical practice of providers who are qualified to perform thoracentesis. It has been shown that the technique is readily learned and can decrease complication rates [12–14].

Evidence

Authors of a large study from 2013 analyzed 61,261 thoracenteses occurring over a two-year period using a hospital database and determined that USGT was associated with a 19% decrease in the risk of post-procedure pneumothorax compared to landmark-based thoracentesis. The overall incidence of pneumothorax associated with thoracentesis was 2.7% (n = 1670). In this study, patients with a post-procedural pneumothorax had an increased cost of hospitalization of $2801 and increased duration of hospitalization of 1.5 days when compared to patients who did not suffer this complication [11].

A meta-analysis of 24 studies found a 4.0% incidence of pneumothorax for USGT compared with 9.3% for landmark-based thoracentesis ($p < 0.001$) [7]. Moreover, a prospective study of 211 patients undergoing 232 separate USGT while mechanically ventilated found a 1.3% (3/232) incidence of pneumothorax [12].

In addition, a prospective study of 59 emergency department patients with suspicion for pleural effusion found that US changed management in 41% of patients. Ultrasound was completed in approximately 2 minutes and significantly altered the provider's suspicion of pleural effusion ($p < 0.05$) [5].

Key Points

- Lung ultrasonography allows the clinician to rapidly and accurately assess for the presence of a pleural effusion.
- In patients who require a thoracentesis, sonographic guidance allows this procedure to be performed safely and efficiently. USGT is easily learned, decreases complication rates, and lowers hospitalization cost and length of stay.
- Either a high- or low-frequency transducer can be utilized depending on patient body habitus and operator comfort.
- The needle should be visualized penetrating through the parietal pleura and into the fluid collection in the thorax under ultrasound guidance using an in-plane technique.
- Limiting the volume of fluid removed to 1 L is associated with decreased rates of pneumothorax and re-expansion pulmonary edema.

Needle Aspiration of Primary Spontaneous Pneumothorax

Introduction

A pneumothorax is an emergent medical condition that requires rapid and accurate evaluation and treatment. There are multiple etiologies of a pneumothorax, including a ruptured bleb within the lung, pneumothorax secondary to traumatic injury, or a spontaneous pneumothorax. If not treated appropriately, a pneumothorax can lead to respiratory and cardiovascular compromise.

Though a pneumothorax can occur by various mechanisms, this section will focus primarily on primary spontaneous pneumothorax (PSP) which is defined as a pneumothorax occurring without inciting trauma or the presence of clinically apparent lung disease [21–23]. Data on the age-adjusted incidence of PSP ranges from 7.4 to 24/100,000 per year in males and 1.2 to 9.8/100,000 per year in females [24–26].

Management options for a PSP include tube thoracostomy, small-bore pleural catheter, needle aspiration, and observation, but international guidelines and standard practice are variable [21]. The American College of Chest Physicians (ACCP) recommends tube thoracostomy or a pleural catheter as the first-line treatment of symptomatic pneumothorax and endorses the use of needle aspiration only for stable patients with small pneumothoraces [27]. In contrast, the British Thoracic Society (BTS) guidelines recommend that needle aspiration be the first-line management for stable patients less than 50 years old with a PSP [23, 28, 29]. Traumatic pneumothorax is not addressed in the BTS or ACCP guidelines.

While no consensus exists on the management of pneumothorax, there is a growing body of evidence supporting needle aspiration of pneumothorax in patients with uncomplicated first-time PSP [30, 31]. Several prospective studies have shown promising results for needle aspiration [22, 29, 30, 32–35]. Compared to tube thoracostomy, needle aspiration has been shown to have similar clinical outcomes [33, 34], is less invasive and painful, leads to decreased admission rates and hospital length of stay, and has similar 1-year recurrence rates of pneumothorax [29, 30, 35].

Advantages of Ultrasound Guidance

Lung ultrasound has demonstrated better sensitivity (89% vs. 52%) and comparable specificity (98% vs. 99%) in detecting pneumothorax when compared to chest x-ray [36–38] and has also been shown to be superior in detecting residual pneumothoraces after chest tube insertion [39].

Anatomy

The anterior chest wall is delineated by the clavicle superiorly, the diaphragm inferiorly, by the sternum medially, and the mid-axillary line laterally [40]. In general, air will rise to the least dependent portion of the hemithorax, which in a supine patient is at the anteromedial portion of the chest. However, in patients with a high degree of suspicion for pneumothorax, there is utility in sonographically evaluating a larger area.

To sonographically evaluate for pneumothorax, a high-frequency probe is placed in a longitudinal axis over the anterior chest wall between two ribs. Posterior shadowing will be noted deep to the ribs. The pleural interface appears as a hyperechoic line between the two rib shadows. This view has been described by Lichtenstein as the "bat sign" [38] (Fig. 14.5). Normal pleura exhibits a characteristic shimmering appearance that is synchronized with respirations [40]. In addition, M-mode can demonstrate the presence of normal lung sliding by generating a "seashore sign," which appears as a granular pattern below the pleural line (Fig. 14.6). In the absence of lung sliding, M-mode will demonstrate a "stratosphere sign" (also known as "barcode sign"), in which the granular pattern is replaced by horizontal lines [38] as shown in Fig. 14.7. Alternatively, the "power slide" uses power Doppler to detect movement at the pleural line (Fig. 14.8) [41]. M-mode and power Doppler both have the advantage over B-mode imaging of being able to capture the presence of lung sliding in a static ultrasound image.

Ultrasonographic diagnosis of pneumothorax depends on three sonographic findings: (1) absence of lung sliding, (2) the A-line sign, and (3) the lung point [40, 42, 43]. The absence of

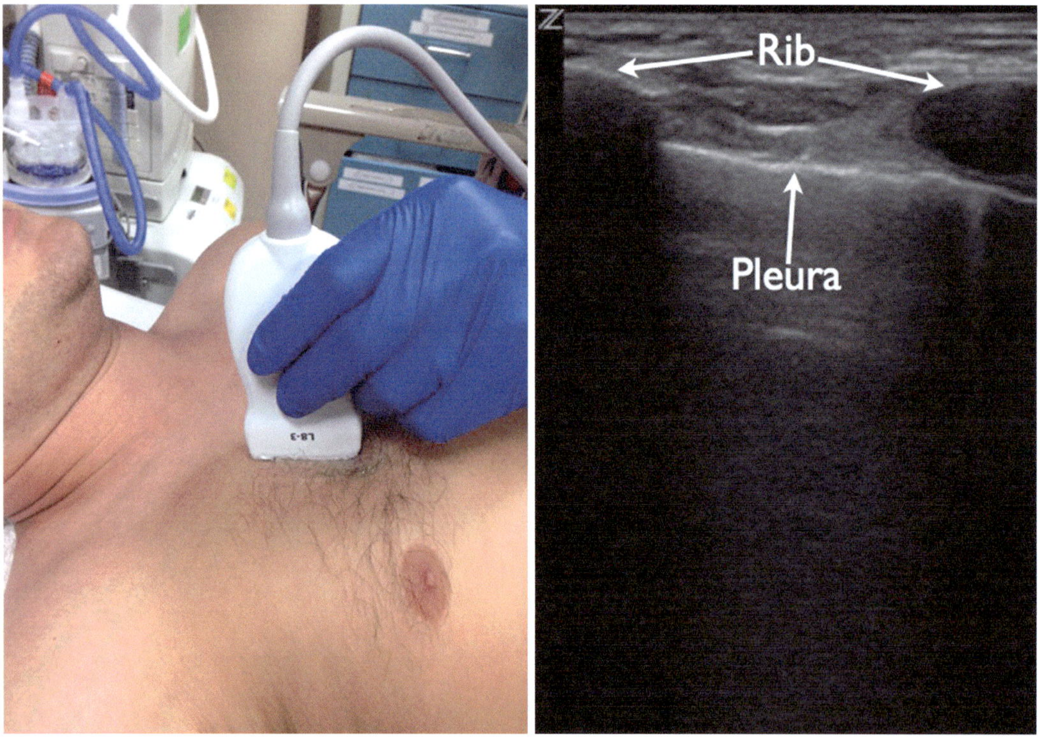

Fig. 14.5 The "bat sign" describes the sonographic image in which the pleural interface appears as a hyperechoic line flanked by two rib shadows. This image is obtained by placing the linear probe in a sagittal plane between two ribs

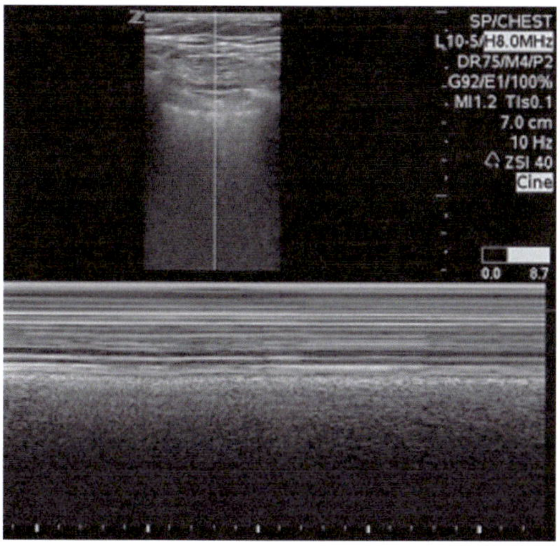

Fig. 14.6 The presence of a "seashore sign," which appears as a granular pattern below the pleural line in M-Mode, demonstrates normal lung sliding

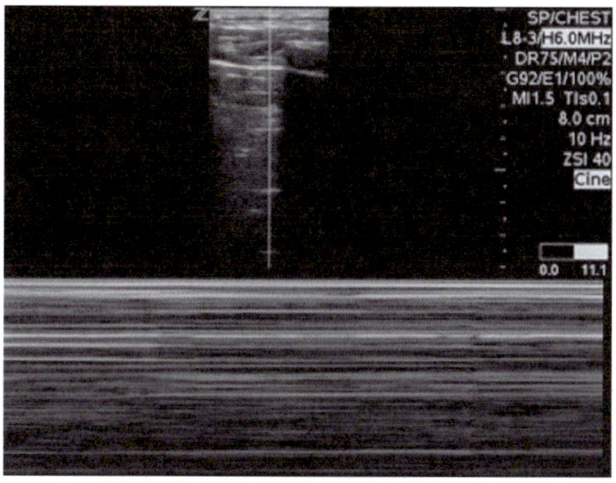

Fig. 14.7 The "barcode sign" or "stratosphere sign," in which the normal granular pattern below the pleural line is replaced by horizontal lines, indicates the absence of lung sliding

lung sliding represents air within the thoracic cavity which has caused the normally apposed visceral and parietal pleura to separate. The A-line sign (the presence of A-lines without B-lines) in conjunction with absent lung sliding is 96.5% specific for the presence of pneumothorax [40]. Finally, the lung point represents the transition point between normal lung sliding and adjacent pneumothorax (Fig. 14.9). While the lung point is not always visualized, its presence has been shown to be 100% specific for pneumothorax [38, 43].

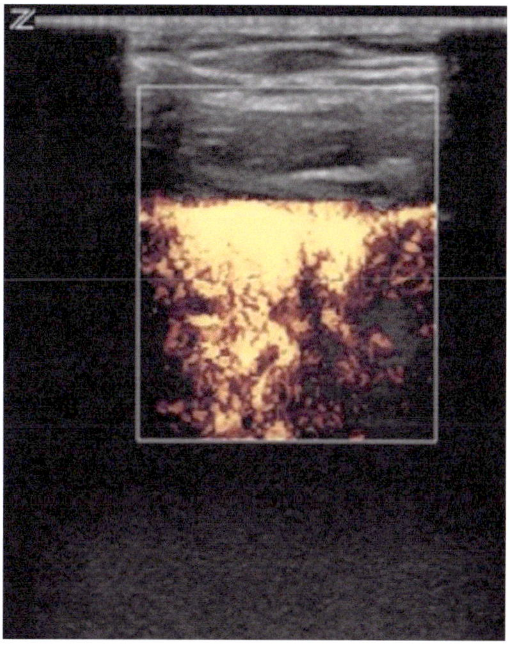

Fig. 14.8 Power slide. Power Doppler may be used as an alternative to M-Mode to demonstrate the presence of lung sliding in a static image

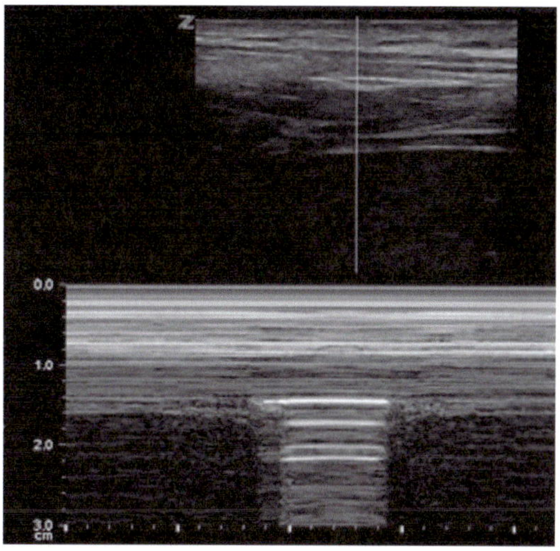

Fig. 14.9 Lung point. The alternating granular and linear patterns below the pleural line demonstrate the precise transition point between normal lung sliding and pneumothorax

Existing guidelines recommend drainage of large pneumothoraces even if the patient appears clinically well, making estimation of pneumothorax size an important aspect of assessing a patient prior to performing an aspiration. However definitions for a "large" pneumothorax differ [23, 27, 44]. While computed tomography (CT) of the chest is the most accurate method of measuring pneumothorax volume, it is not always an indicated or available imaging modality. Several methods have been suggested for estimating pneumothorax volume on chest radiograph [23]. According to ACCP guidelines, a distance greater than 3 cm from the lung cupola to the apex of the thoracic cavity represents a "large" pneumothorax [27]. BTS guidelines define a "large" pneumothorax as a rim of air greater than 2 cm at the level of the hilum on chest radiograph [28]. The Belgian Society of Pulmonology (BSP) defines a "large" pneumothorax as one that extends along the entire length of the lateral chest wall [44]. However, there is poor agreement among the size classification methods described by the AACP, BTS, and BSP, and in one retrospective study, the use of these different methods resulted in agreement in only 47% of cases [45].

Point-of-care ultrasound may be a useful method to estimate the size of pneumothoraces. In a prospective study of 58 patients who had a CT diagnosis of pneumothorax, sonography reliably predicted larger pneumothorax volumes. A lung point located anterior to the mid-axillary line, at the mid-axillary line, and posterior to the mid-axillary line were predictive of a pneumothorax size of less than 10%, between 11% and 30%, and greater than 30%, respectively [46].

Indications

According to the BTS Guidelines, needle aspiration of pneumothorax is indicated in stable patients less than 50 years of age with a symptomatic PSP measuring greater than 2 cm at the level of the hilum on chest x-ray or a PSP of any size from which the patient is symptomatic [23].

Contraindications

Patients who are over the age of 50 with a smoking history or evidence of underlying lung disease based on physical examination, history, or chest x-ray are not suitable candidates for aspiration. Other contraindications include patients with unstable vital signs, tension or bilateral pneumothoraces, or associated pleural effusions (hydropneumothorax). In addition, as mentioned above, skin with overlying areas of cellulitis or herpes zoster should not be pierced. Recurrent pneumothorax is a relative contraindication as such cases are likely to require more aggressive interventions such as chest tube drainage, pleurodesis, or VATS (video-assisted thoracoscopic surgery) [47–50]. Finally, repeat needle aspiration following a failed attempt is not recommended as it is unlikely to be successful in the absence of a technical issue such as a blocked or kinked catheter [23].

Though, some experts recommend chest tube or small-bore catheter placement for pneumothoraces that are 40% or larger [51, 52], BTS guidelines suggest PSP of all sizes can be drained by needle aspiration.

Equipment/Probe Selection

The equipment necessary for this procedure is depicted in Fig. 14.10. A high-frequency linear probe is ideal for the detection of pneumothorax using the previously described methods.

Preparation/Pre-procedural Evaluation

For this procedure, place the patient in a supine position with the arm ipsilateral to the pneumothorax raised above the patient's head. In this position, inter-pleural air will preferentially collect in the nondependent anteromedial portion of the patient's chest. Using tactile and visual landmarks, identify and mark the second intercostal space in the midclavicular line. This location is where the needle aspiration will be performed. Using a high-frequency linear probe oriented in the sagittal plane and starting at the marked needle aspiration site, locate the lung point by sliding the transducer laterally. Mark the skin with a

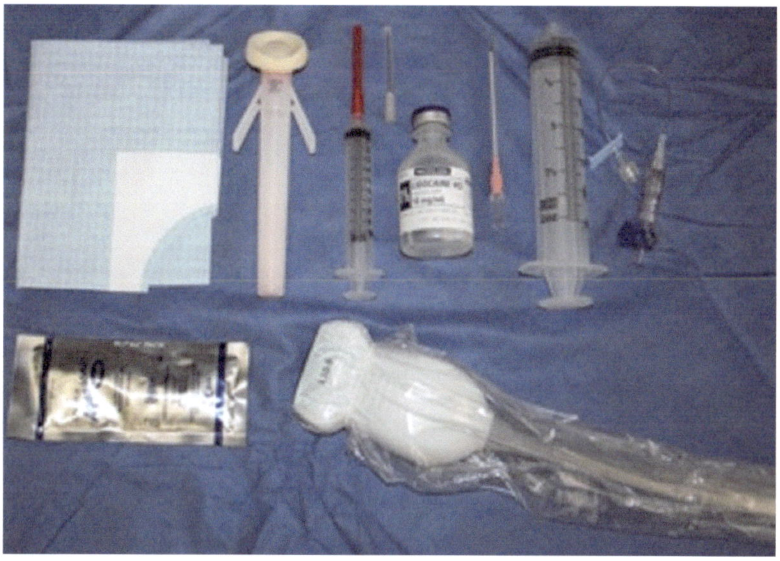

Fig. 14.10 Equipment required for ultrasound-guided needle aspiration of a primary spontaneous pneumothorax. From top left: fenestrated drape, chlorhexidine, 10 cc syringe with 18-gauge blunt needle, 27 gauge needle, local anesthetic, catheter over a needle, 60 cc syringe, IV tubing attached to a three-way stopcock, ultrasound probe with sterile sheath, and sterile gel

surgical marker at the lung point so that it can be readily located later [53–55].

Procedure

This procedure requires two individuals, one person performing the aspiration while the other sonographically tracking the lung point. Alternatively, if there is a single operator, the location of the lung point can be checked intermittently throughout the procedure.

In addition to standard sterile patient preparation, the transducer is covered with the sterile probe cover and placed onto the field. At the previously identified location at the second intercostal space in the midclavicular line, the soft tissue should be anesthetized along the superior margin of the third rib in order to avoid the neurovascular bundle that lies just below the second rib. The needle is advanced until bubbles are seen in the syringe, which should still contain lidocaine. These bubbles indicate that the pleural space has been entered. While the needle is slowly withdrawn, lidocaine is instilled into the tissues between the pleura and the skin surface. Next, while applying continuous negative pressure on the plunger, insert the 16 g catheter over a needle attached to a 10 mL syringe filled with 3–5 mL of sterile saline or lidocaine. As soon as bubbles are seen in the syringe, advance the needle a few millimeters further to ensure that the catheter tip is fully within the pleural space (Fig. 14.11). Have the patient cough or exhale while removing the

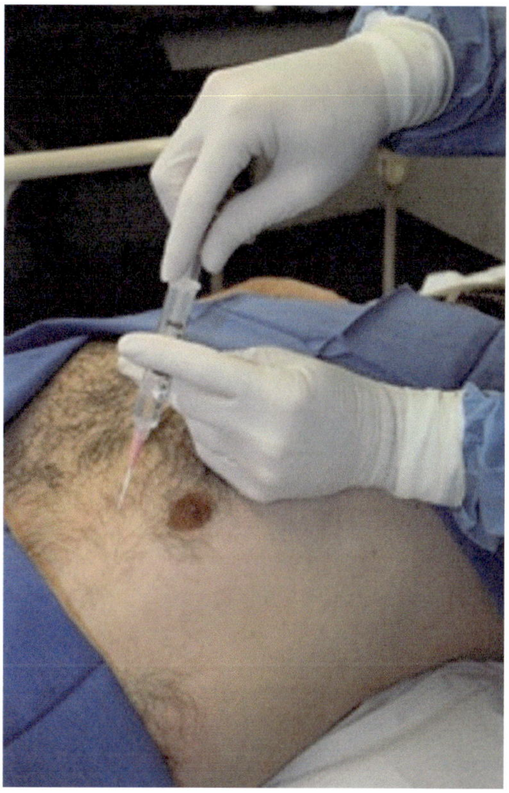

Fig. 14.11 Insertion of the catheter over a needle

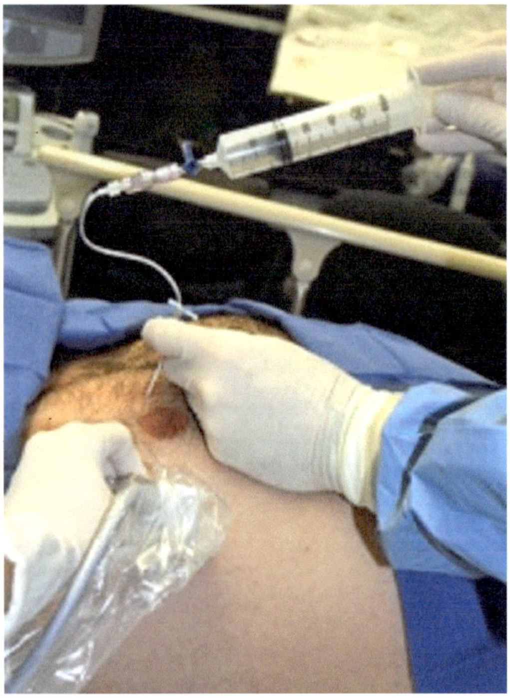

Fig. 14.12 Tracking the lung point in real time as the lung re-expands during aspiration

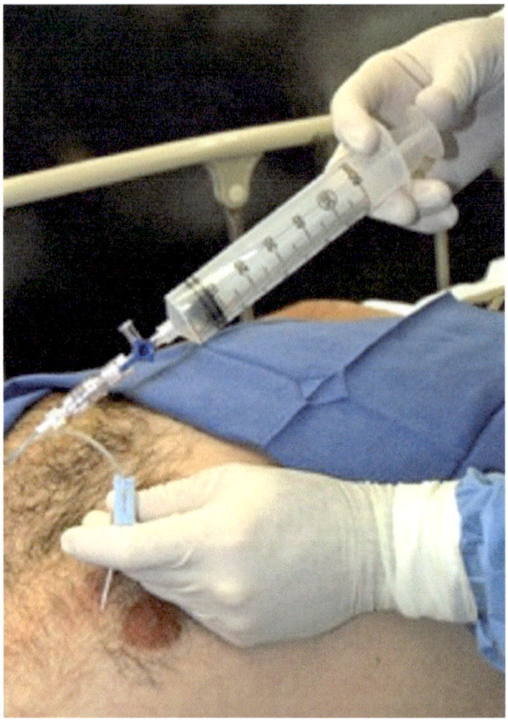

Fig. 14.13 Evacuation of aspirated air

needle and syringe, and simultaneously advance the catheter. Immediately occlude the catheter opening to prevent additional air from entering the pleural space. Attach the preassembled tubing, three-way stopcock, and 60 mL syringe to the end of the catheter. It is critical to ensure that the stopcock is never open between the patient and the ambient air as this will worsen the pneumothorax. Locate the lung point with the linear transducer, and with the stopcock closed to ambient air, begin aspirating the pneumothorax into the syringe. As the lung re-expands, the lung point will move anteriorly and medially. While aspirating, have a second operator track the lung point in real time as it moves toward the catheter insertion site (Fig. 14.12). Once the syringe is full, evacuate it to ambient air by closing the stopcock to the patient (Fig. 14.13). Repeat the process of aspirating air from the patient's chest and evacuating it until the lung point reaches the catheter site or no more air can be drawn into the syringe. Keep track of the total volume aspirated by counting the number of times the syringe is filled. If air continues to be aspirated after evacuating 2.5 L, the procedure should be stopped as it may indicate an air leak [23]. At the completion of the procedure, remove the catheter and place a sterile occlusive dressing on the chest at the needle insertion site [54, 55].

Evidence for discharge criteria after simple aspiration of pneumothorax is lacking, and BTS guidelines simply state that the patient should be clinically stable prior to discharge without providing a specific time frame for observation [23, 56]. After confirming successful lung re-expansion, some experts suggest a protocol of observing the patient for 6 hours and confirming sustained re-expansion prior to discharging the patient home [32]. The patient must have reliable follow-up and understand strict return precautions for recurrent symptoms prior to being released. Recommendations from the ACCP consensus statement include follow-up and repeat chest x-ray within 48 hours of discharge for patients treated with a small-bore chest tube, and these can reasonably be applied to patients who were treated with needle aspiration [27, 56]. Although alternative sites to needle aspiration including a lateral and posterior approach have been described in the literature [28, 57], only the anterior approach has been described as an ultrasound-assisted procedure [53].

Complications

After the procedure has been completed, the patient can be monitored for recurrence of the pneumothorax with serial ultrasound examinations. Recurrence is a concern if the lung point migrates away from the point of aspiration [53]. Furthermore, ultrasound has the added benefit of being able to detect post-procedural hemothorax [52, 53, 58].

Possible complications of needle aspiration include bleeding, infection, vasovagal reaction, subcutaneous emphysema, persistent pneumothorax, and tension pneumothorax [56]. However, in a literature review of 9 studies with a combined total of more than 300 cases, there were only 3 cases of reported hemothorax and 1 case of pneumonia [52], indicating that complication rates with simple aspiration are low. Re-expansion pulmonary edema is a rare albeit potentially serious complication associated with treatment of pneumothorax [59–61].

Patients should be advised to return immediately for recurrent or worsening breathlessness and should be followed up by a respiratory physician until full resolution of the pneumothorax. While there is no evidence to suggest that physical exertion is linked to recurrence of pneumothorax, the BTS guidelines recommend that patients refrain from extreme physical exertion until complete resolution of symptoms. The risk of air travel and diving should also be discussed with patients as the possibility of recurrence of pneumothorax only significantly decreases after 1 year [23].

Pearls/Pitfalls

Detection of a pneumothorax under sonographic guidance is particularly challenging in patients with subcutaneous emphysema, pleural calcifications or adhesions, atelectasis, acute respiratory distress syndrome, pleural blebs, and mainstem intubation that may prevent normal lung sliding [39, 40].

Integration into Clinical Practice

Point-of-care ultrasound can be used to diagnose pneumothorax, estimate the size of a pneumothorax, visualize intra-procedural lung re-expansion, and monitor for recurrence of pneumothorax and post-procedural complications such as hemothorax.

Evidence

As previously discussed, the medical literature supporting needle aspiration for PSP is growing. However, research on ultrasound-guided needle aspiration is lacking and has only been described in case reports and case series [53, 62].

Key Points

Needle aspiration is indicated in stable patients less than 50 years old without evidence of underlying lung disease, who have a large PSP or symptomatic PSP of any size. Needle aspiration offers advantages over tube thoracostomy in that it reduces patient pain scores, hospital admission rates, and duration of hospital admission with comparable recurrence rates. Ultrasonography can be used to diagnose pneumothoraces, visualize resolution of a pneumothorax in real time, and detect residual or recurrent post-procedure pneumothorax.

Pigtail Thoracostomy for Treatment of Pneumothorax

Introduction

Patients with pneumothorax require intervention in order to treat their symptoms and to prevent progression of the disease. Recently, there has been increased utilization of small-bore (pigtail) catheters. Small-bore chest tubes cause less pain than their larger counterparts [63] while having similar clinical outcomes [64, 65]. Even in patients with traumatic pneumothoraces, one study was able to demonstrate a shorter length of chest tube duration as well as a shorter length of hospital stay in stable patients who had small-bore chest tubes placed when compared to large-bore chest tubes.

Advantages of Ultrasound Guidance

The advantages of ultrasonography for the diagnosis of pneumothorax are described above in the aspiration of pneumothorax section.

Anatomy

The relevant anatomy when evaluating a patient for the presence of a pneumothorax is described above in the aspiration of pneumothorax section.

Indications

Thoracostomy in the setting of a pneumothorax is indicated in patients with a large PSP, mechanically ventilated patients with pneumothorax, secondary spontaneous pneumothorax, hemodynamically unstable patients with pneumothorax, persistent pneumothorax, tension pneumothorax, and traumatic pneumothorax [66]. Spontaneous and traumatic pneumothoraces are indications for pigtail thoracostomy with small-bore (6–16 French) catheters as long as there is no concurrent hemothorax for which a larger-bore catheter is typically used. Research has shown that treatment with pigtail thoracostomy compared with large-bore tube thoracostomy has similar successful outcomes but with less complications and infections [67] and the added benefit of a less invasive and less painful procedure [64, 68]. Pigtail thoracostomy has also been proven to be as successful in the treatment of pneumothorax as tube thoracostomy in pediatric patients [69].

Contraindications

There are no absolute contraindications to pigtail placement. Relative contraindications for pigtail thoracostomy include current use of anticoagulation medications, coagulopathy, and thrombocytopenia. The specific clinical scenario will dictate whether the benefits of the procedure outweigh the risks. Areas of overlying cellulitis or zoster should be avoided when placing a pigtail catheter.

Equipment

The equipment required for a pigtail thoracostomy is shown in Fig. 14.14. The choice of ultrasound transducers is based on user preference and body habitus. Typically, a linear transducer optimizes the detection of a pneumothorax as described previously. The procedure should be performed under sterile conditions with a sterile probe cover over the transducer.

Preparation

In the setting of trauma, this procedure likely requires the patient to be supine. However, the lateral recumbent position is also acceptable in the setting of spontaneous pneumothorax. Traditionally, a tube thoracostomy is placed at the level of the fifth intercostal space at the anterior axillary line. This space typically corresponds to the nipple line in men and the inframammary fold in women. An alternative location when using a pigtail catheter is the anterior second intercostal space at the midclavicular line.

Procedure

Utilize the same techniques to locate a pneumothorax as were described in the needle aspiration section. After correctly positioning the patient, mark the catheter entry site. Raising the patient's arm above the head on the affected side increases the space between the ribs, which facilitates both

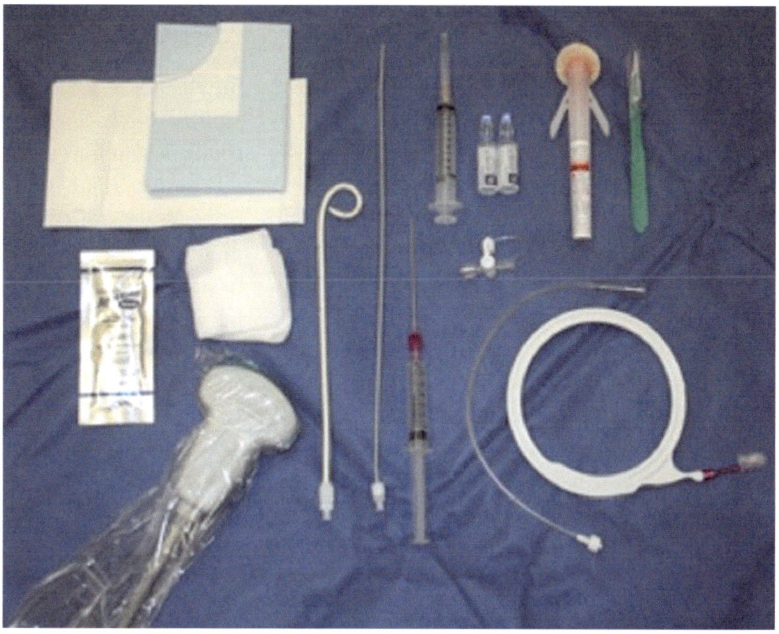

Fig. 14.14 Equipment required for ultrasound-guided pigtail thoracostomy. From top left: fenestrated and non-fenestrated drapes, 10 cc syringe with 25 gauge needle, local anesthetic, chlorhexidine, scalpel, ultrasound gel, sterile gauze, pigtail catheter, catheter-straightening obturator, finder needle with syringe, three-way stopcock, connection tubing, guidewire, ultrasound probe with sterile sheath

image acquisition and tube placement. Maintain sterile technique throughout the procedure to decrease the chance of infection. Clean the area with an antiseptic solution, such as chlorhexidine, and drape in the normal sterile fashion. At this point, cover the ultrasound probe with a sterile probe sheath. Anesthetize the skin at the entry point followed by the deep tissues including the parietal pleura just above the rib in order to avoid the neurovascular structures underneath the rib. Insert the finder needle above the rib into the pleura while applying negative pressure on the plunger (Fig. 14.15). When the needle passes into the pleura, the resistance should change, and air should be aspirated. Placing a small amount of sterile saline in the syringe can help confirm placement as bubbles will develop once the pleural cavity is entered. Using the Seldinger technique, remove the syringe and thread the guidewire into the pleural space. Remove the finder needle. Make a small incision with a scalpel adjacent to the guidewire. Use the dilator to create a tract which can accommodate the pigtail catheter. Pass the pigtail catheter over the guidewire and into the pleural space directing it anteriorly toward the apex of the chest cavity, ensuring that the last hole on the catheter is within the pleural space. In pre-made kits, the pigtail catheter may include a trocar that helps guide the catheter into the pleural space. Remove the guidewire and trocar, and suture the pigtail catheter in place. Once secured, connect the catheter to a water-seal suction device.

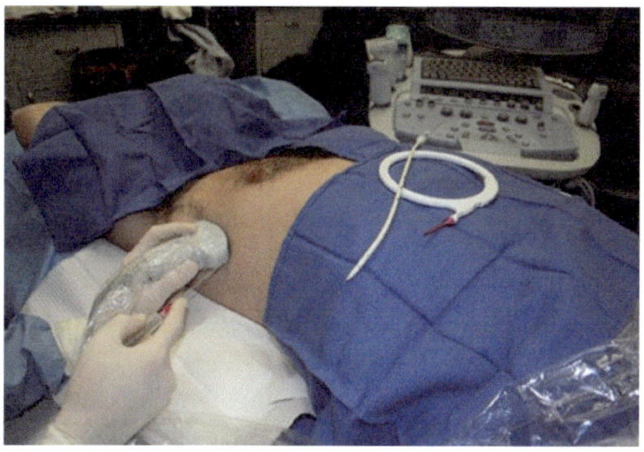

Fig. 14.15 Insertion of the finder needle using ultrasound guidance in the placement of a pigtail catheter

Complications

Complications from pigtail thoracostomy include recurrent pneumothorax, infection, and perforation of the lung, liver, spleen, diaphragm, or heart. The tube could become displaced if not secured properly. Complication rates were lower when small-bore chest tubes were used when compared to large-bore chest tubes [63].

Re-expansion pulmonary edema is another possible complication after tube thoracostomy. It occurs when a lung rapidly expands after treatment of a pneumothorax. The exact pathophysiology of the pulmonary edema is not completely understood. However, in the setting of a spontaneous pneumothorax, the incidence is as high as 16% [59]. Risk factors for developing re-expansion pulmonary edema include large pneumothoraces, prolonged duration of the pneumothorax, and a history of diabetes mellitus [59–61]. Treatment is mainly supportive with oxygen and positive-pressure ventilation if necessary. As aforementioned, mortality rates have been described as high as 20% [20]. No previous studies have assessed rates of re-expansion pulmonary edema when patients were treated with pigtail thoracostomy as compared to tube thoracostomy.

Pearls/Pitfalls

The lung point is the only sonographic sign for pneumothorax which is 100% specific. Multiple other pathologies may cause the lack of lung sliding on ultrasound including a tumor, bleb, pneumonia, pleural adhesions, previous pleurodesis, and right mainstem intubation which leads to left-sided atelectasis; this can lead to a misdiagnosis of pneumothorax. The ultrasound findings must be correlated to the history and clinical presentation.

Integration into Clinical Practice

POCUS can be used for the rapid and accurate diagnosis of a pneumothorax. Ultrasonography can then be utilized to facilitate placement of a pigtail thoracostomy tube in both traumatic and nontraumatic pneumothoraces. Specific clinical scenarios and operator comfort will also play a role in determining which of these tubes will be used or whether aspiration of the pneumothorax is more appropriate.

Evidence

Small-bore catheters have been shown to have similar clinical outcomes when compared to traditional tube thoracostomy, with less patient discomfort and potentially fewer complications. A prospective study of 405 patient with a pleural infection showed no difference in death, thoracic surgery, length of hospital stay, and pulmonary function at 3 months when comparing pigtail and chest tube placement of varying sizes (<10 F vs. 10–14 F vs. 15–19 F vs. >20 F). However, pain scores were significantly lower when comparing small-bore (pigtail) to large-bore chest tubes in 128 of these patients [63]. In the setting of trauma requiring non-emergent thoracostomy, small-bore catheter thoracostomy duration was shown to be significantly shorter than large-bore tube thoracostomy, with significantly reduced incidence of fibrothorax. There was no significant difference between rates of recurrent pneumothoraces [64]. Another retrospective study in the setting of trauma specifically comparing pigtail catheter to chest tube in the setting of pneumothorax demonstrated no significant difference in tube duration, need for mechanical ventilation, or complications [68]. Furthermore, when compared with large-bore tube thoracostomy, small-bore pigtail thoracostomy had no significant difference in length of hospital stay, extubation time, recurrence rates, or complications in 91 patients with their first episode of a secondary spontaneous pneumothorax [65]. Likewise, another study looking at 49 spontaneous pneumothoraces found no significant difference in drainage success or duration. However, large-bore tubes had significantly higher incidence of complications, particularly related infections [67]. Even a study in pediatric patients with a primary spontaneous pneumothorax showed no difference in hospital duration but reduced duration of tube insertion [69]. No studies, however, have directly compared pigtail catheter placement under US guidance to a landmark-based technique.

Key Points
Ultrasonography is a sensitive and specific imaging modality for diagnosing pneumothorax. Pigtail thoracostomy for treatment of pneumothorax is as effective as chest tube thoracostomy with reduced duration of treatment and is better tolerated by patients.

Ultrasound-Guided Tube Thoracostomy

Introduction

A hemothorax is an emergent medical condition caused by blunt or penetrating trauma, occurring roughly 300,000 times per year in the United States [70]. Hemothoraces require prompt drainage to prevent immediate complications including respiratory failure and cardiovascular collapse and delayed sequelae such as empyema and pleural adhesions. A tube thoracostomy is the initial approach to treatment and helps determine if the patient requires immediate operative intervention. If the chest tube output is greater than 1500 mL initially or over 200 mL per hour for 3 hours, surgical thoracotomy is indicated [71].

Advantages of Ultrasound Guidance

Ultrasonography is often utilized to rapidly diagnose hemothorax. The sensitivity and specificity of this imaging modality are 96% and 100%, respectively [72]. Ultrasound of the chest is used in the primary assessment of trauma patients as part of the E-FAST examination (extended focused assessment with sonography in trauma). Ultrasonography is highly sensitive for the detection of a hemothorax, with as little as 20 mL visible by ultrasonography, as compared to a minimum 175 mL needed to detect a hemothorax on a chest x-ray in a supine patient [72]. Once a hemothorax or hemopneumothorax has been identified, a tube thoracostomy is indicated to drain the blood and air. Ultrasonography can be used to decrease complications while performing tube thoracostomy.

Anatomy

A traumatic injury of the chest can lead to bleeding within the potential space between the parietal and visceral pleura, which can ultimately cause compression of the lung parenchyma. If the pleura is violated, both superficial chest wall and lung injuries can lead to hemothorax.

Indications

Tube thoracostomy is indicated for the treatment of a hemothorax or hemopneumothorax in the setting of blunt or penetrating trauma.

Contraindications

There are no absolute contraindications to chest tube placement. Relative contraindications are the same as those listed for pigtail thoracostomy. The risks and benefits should be carefully weighed when performing this procedure.

Equipment

The equipment required for a tube thoracostomy is included in Fig. 14.16. A curvilinear or phased array transducer is used for viewing the fluid collection within the chest cavity. When performing the tube thoracostomy with sonographic guidance, the procedure should be performed under sterile conditions, including the use of a sterile probe cover.

Preparation

Tube thoracostomy can be performed in the supine, upright, or lateral decubitus positions. Because of the potential for spinal injuries,

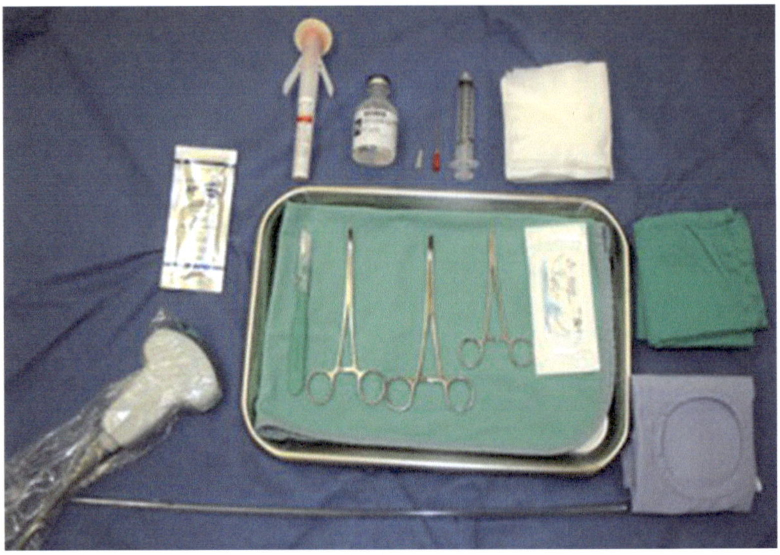

Fig. 14.16 Equipment required for ultrasound-guided tube thoracostomy. From top left: chlorhexidine, local anesthetic, needle and syringe, sterile gauze, ultrasound gel, scalpel, Kelly clamp × 2, needle driver, suture material (such as 0 nonabsorbable suture), sterile drapes, ultrasound probe with sterile sheath, and large-bore chest tube

trauma patients are typically positioned supine. Traditionally, a tube thoracostomy is placed at the level of the fifth intercostal space between the mid-axillary and anterior axillary lines. This space typically corresponds to the nipple line in men and the inframammary fold in women. To find the most appropriate location to place the chest tube, the ultrasound probe should be placed in this general area using a coronal orientation; the transducer is moved both cephalad and caudad as well as anteriorly and posteriorly over the chest wall to assess the size of the hemothorax. The proposed location of entry should be confirmed to be superior to the diaphragm and correspond to the largest fluid collection.

Procedure

In order to view a hemothorax using ultrasound, locate the diaphragm, which appears as a hyperechoic line overlying the liver and spleen. A hemothorax will manifest as a fluid collection superior to the diaphragm. The hemothorax may be anechoic, or may contain internal echoes, which represents clotted blood. The internal echoes can be used to help differentiate a hemothorax from a simple pleural effusion. Extension of the spinal stripe is a sensitive and specific finding for free fluid in the chest [73].

After correctly positioning the patient, locate the largest area of fluid using ultrasound, and mark the skin. The patient's arm is raised above the head in order to increase the space between the ribs. Maintain sterile technique throughout the procedure in order to minimize the chance of infection. Clean the area with an antiseptic solution, and then drape in the normal sterile fashion. Cover the ultrasound probe with a sterile probe sheath. Anesthetize the skin and deeper tissues including the parietal pleura starting approximately 2 cm below the rib interspace entry point. Use a scalpel to incise the skin at this location. Tunnel through the intercostal muscles and over the rib with a large Kelly clamp while avoiding the vascular bundle underneath the rib. Typically, in the case of a hemopneumothorax, a burst of air or blood is heard or seen as the pleural space is entered. Widen the hole in the pleural space to approximately 2 cm. Insert a gloved finger into the hole, and sweep to ensure that the lung is not adherent to the pleura; care should be taken to avoid injury on a fractured rib. Once in the pleural space, direct the chest tube into the correct location using a finger as a guide. A larger chest tube (32–40 French) is preferred in the setting of a hemothorax in order to adequately drain the fluid (Fig. 14.17). Advance the tube posterolaterally until the last hole for drainage is clearly within the chest cavity. Once inserted, attach the chest tube to a water-seal suc-

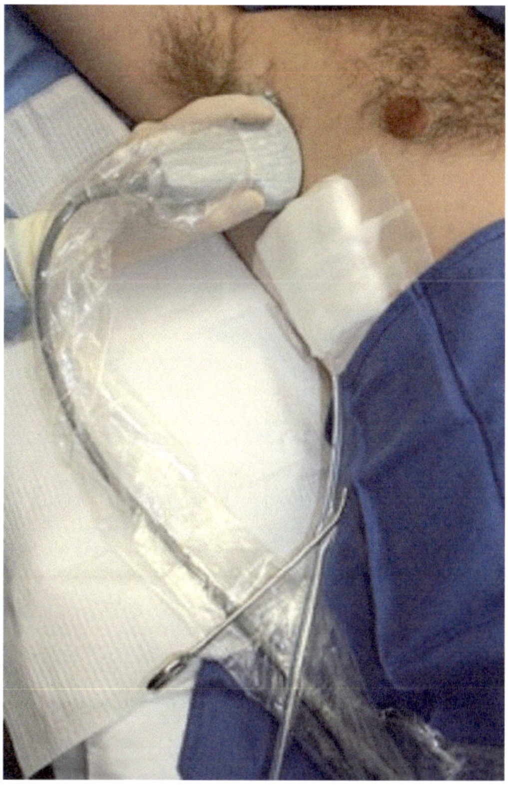

Fig. 14.17 Tube thoracostomy placement using ultrasound guidance

tion device. Secure the chest tube with sutures, and apply a sterile occlusive dressing.

Typically, a chest radiograph is obtained to confirm proper placement. However, ultrasound can be used to confirm that the chest tube is in an adequate location. The method starts by using a linear 10–5 MHz transducer and scanning in both the longitudinal and transverse planes from the skin insertion site until the chest tube passes through the pleural line. Once deep to the pleural line, the tube disappears from view unless surrounded by fluid. A tube which is improperly placed and remains in the extrathoracic space is visualized throughout its length. This protocol has been successfully utilized with both large-bore and small-bore (pigtail) thoracostomy tubes [74, 75].

Complications

Complications from tube thoracostomy include recurrent pneumothorax, infection, and perforation of the lung, liver, spleen, diaphragm, heart, and other organs. The tube can be malpositioned or become displaced. Malposition includes the possibility of the chest tube within the lung parenchyma or in the subcutaneous tissue. Studies have shown reduced complication rates in ultrasound-guided thoracentesis as compared to an anatomic landmark-based technique [8–11]. To date, there are no specific studies comparing tube thoracostomy performed with and without sonographic guidance.

Pearls/Pitfalls

Ultrasound-guided tube thoracostomy may help reduce complications from the procedure. Chest tube placement is not performed using real-time sonographic guidance. Rather, the hemothorax is localized, and the tube location can then be confirmed after placement.

Integration into Clinical Practice

Ultrasound is a useful bedside tool that can assist in the diagnosis of a hemothorax. Once diagnosed, US can then be used to confirm tube thoracostomy placement.

Evidence

There is a paucity of evidence specifically comparing ultrasound-guided thoracostomy with anatomic landmark-based chest tube placement. The data has largely been extrapolated from landmark- versus ultrasound-guided thoracentesis, as the procedure is similar in nature for both diagnostics and intervention. Recent literature has shown that ultrasound is highly sensitive (100%) and specific (100%) in confirming proper placement of chest tubes in cadaver models [74]. Furthermore, in a proof-of-concept study, one group was able to confirm thoracostomy tube location in all of their patients (21/21 insertion sites) [75]. In light of data indicating a significant complication rate (37%) for landmark-based tube thoracostomy placement, further research into sonographic guidance of this procedure is warranted [76].

Key Points
Ultrasonography is both sensitive and specific for the detection of hemothorax. Ultrasound has the potential to confirm appropriate tube thoracostomy placement, but more research is needed.

References

1. Feller-Kopman D. Ultrasound-guided thoracentesis. Chest. 2006;129(6):1709–14.
2. Sachdeva A, Shepherd RW, Lee HJ. Thoracentesis and thoracic ultrasound: state of the art in 2013. Clin Chest Med. 2013;34(1):1–9.
3. Joyner CR Jr, Herman RJ, Reid JM. Reflected ultrasound in the detection and localization of pleural effusion. JAMA. 1967;200(5):399–402.
4. Gryminski J, Krakowka P, Lypacewicz G. The diagnosis of pleural effusion by ultrasonic and radiologic techniques. Chest. 1976;70(1):33–7.
5. Tayal VS, Nicks BA, Norton HJ. Emergency ultrasound evaluation of symptomatic nontraumatic pleural effusions. Am J Emerg Med. 2006;24(7):782–6.
6. Balik M, Plasil P, Waldauf P, et al. Ultrasound estimation of volume of pleural fluid in mechanically ventilated patients. Intensive Care Med. 2006;32(2):318–21.
7. Vignon P, Chastagner C, Berkane V, et al. Quantitative assessment of pleural effusion in critically ill patients by means of ultrasonography. Crit Care Med. 2005;33(8):1757–63.
8. Patel PA, Ernst FR, Gunnarsson CL. Ultrasonography guidance reduces complications and costs associated with thoracentesis procedures. J Clin Ultrasound: JCU. 2012;40(3):135–41.
9. Gordon CE, Feller-Kopman D, Balk EM, Smetana GW. Pneumothorax following thoracentesis: a systematic review and meta-analysis. Arch Intern Med. 2010;170(4):332–9.
10. Barnes TW, Morgenthaler TI, Olson EJ, Hesley GK, Decker PA, Ryu JH. Sonographically guided thoracentesis and rate of pneumothorax. J Clin Ultrasound: JCU. 2005;33(9):442–6.
11. Mercaldi CJ, Lanes SF. Ultrasound guidance decreases complications and improves the cost of care among patients undergoing thoracentesis and paracentesis. Chest. 2013;143(2):532–8.
12. Mayo PH, Goltz HR, Tafreshi M, Doelken P. Safety of ultrasound-guided thoracentesis in patients receiving mechanical ventilation. Chest. 2004;125(3):1059–62.
13. Duncan DR, Morgenthaler TI, Ryu JH, Daniels CE. Reducing iatrogenic risk in thoracentesis: establishing best practice via experiential training in a zero-risk environment. Chest. 2009;135(5):1315–20.
14. Begot E, Grumann A, Duvoid T, et al. Ultrasonographic identification and semiquantitative assessment of unloculated pleural effusions in critically ill patients by residents after a focused training. Intensive Care Med. 2014;40(10):1475–80.
15. Hibbert RM, Atwell TD, Lekah A, et al. Safety of ultrasound-guided thoracentesis in patients with abnormal preprocedural coagulation parameters. Chest. 2013;144(2):456–63.
16. Patel MD, Joshi SD. Abnormal preprocedural international normalized ratio and platelet counts are not associated with increased bleeding complications after ultrasound-guided thoracentesis. AJR: Am J Roentgenol. 2011;197(1):W164–8.
17. Josephson T, Nordenskjold CA, Larsson J, Rosenberg LU, Kaijser M. Amount drained at ultrasound-guided thoracentesis and risk of pneumothorax. Acta Radiol. 2009;50(1):42–7.
18. Heidecker J, Huggins JT, Sahn SA, Doelken P. Pathophysiology of pneumothorax following ultrasound-guided thoracentesis. Chest. 2006;130(4):1173–84.
19. Jones PW, Moyers JP, Rogers JT, Rodriguez RM, Lee YC, Light RW. Ultrasound-guided thoracentesis: is it a safer method? Chest. 2003;123(2):418–23.
20. Trachiotis GD, Vricella LA, Aaron BL, Hix WR. As originally published in 1988: re-expansion pulmonary edema. Updated in 1997. Ann Thorac Surg. 1997;63(4):1206–7.
21. Baumann M. The clinician's perspective on pneumothorax management. Chest. 1997;112(3):822.
22. Wakai A, O'Sullivan R, McCabe G. Simple aspiration versus intercostal tube drainage for primary spontaneous pneumothorax in adults (review). Cochrane Collab. 2011;(1):1–8.
23. MacDuff A, Arnold A, Harvey J. Management of spontaneous pneumothorax: British Thoracic Society pleural disease guideline 2010. Thorax. 2010;65(Suppl 2):ii18–31.
24. Gupta D, Hansell A, Nichols T, Duong T, Ayres JG, Strachen S. Epidemiology of pneumothorax in England. Thorax. 2000;55:666–71.
25. Noppen M, DeKeukeleire T. Pneumothorax. Respiration. 2008;76(2):121–7.
26. Melton LJ, Heper NG, Offord KP. Incidence of spontaneous pneumothorax in Olmstead County, Minnesota. Am Rev Respir Dis. 1979;120(6):1379–82.
27. Baumann MH. Management of spontaneous pneumothorax∗. Chest. 2001;119(2):590.
28. Henry M. BTS guidelines for the management of spontaneous pneumothorax. Thorax. 2003;58(90002):39ii–52.
29. Harvey J, Prescott R. Simple aspiration versus intercostal tube drainage for spontaneous pneumothorax in patients with normal lungs. BMJ. 1994;309(6965):1338–3139.

30. Parlak M, Uil S, van den Berg J. A prospective, randomised trial of pneumothorax therapy: manual aspiration versus conventional chest tube drainage. Respir Med. 2012;106(11):1600–5.
31. Miller AC, Harvey JE. Guidelines for the management of spontaneous pneumothorax. Standards of Care Committee, British Thoracic Society. BMJ. 1993;307(6896):114–6.
32. Ho K, Ong M, Koh M, Wong E, Raghuram J. A randomized controlled trial comparing minichest tube and needle aspiration in outpatient management of primary spontaneous pneumothorax. Am J Emerg Med. 2011;29(9):1152–7.
33. Ayed A. Aspiration versus tube drainage in primary spontaneous pneumothorax: a randomised study. Eur Respir J. 2006;27(3):477–82.
34. Devanand A, Koh M, Ong T, et al. Simple aspiration versus chest-tube insertion in the management of primary spontaneous pneumothorax: a systematic review. Respir Med. 2004;98(7):579–90.
35. Noppen M, Alexander P, Driesen P, Slabbynck H, Verstraeten A. Manual aspiration versus chest tube drainage in first episodes of primary spontaneous pneumothorax. Am J Respir Crit Care Med. 2002;165(9):1240–4.
36. Alrajhi K. Test characteristics of ultrasonography for the detection of pneumothorax. Chest. 2012;141(3):703.
37. Ding W. Diagnosis of pneumothorax by radiography and ultrasonography. Chest. 2011;140(4):859.
38. Lichtenstein D, Mezière G, Lascols N, Biderman P, Courret J, Gepner A, Goldstein I, Tenoudji-Cohen M. Ultrasound diagnosis of occult pneumothorax*. Crit Care Med. 2005;33(6):1231–8.
39. Galbois A. Pleural ultrasound compared with chest radiographic detection of pneumothorax resolution after drainage. Chest. 2010;138(3):648.
40. Lichtenstein D, Mezière G, Biderman P, Gepner A. The comet-tail artifact: an ultrasound sign ruling out pneumothorax. Intensive Care Med. 1999;25(4):383–8.
41. Cunningham J, Kirkpatrick A, Nicolaou S, Liu D, Hamilton D, Lawless B, Lee M, Brown D, Simons R. Enhanced recognition of "lung sliding" with power color Doppler imaging in the diagnosis of pneumothorax. J Trauma: Inj Infect Crit Care. 2002;52(4):769–71.
42. Lichtenstein DA, Menu Y. A bedside ultrasound sign ruling out pneumothorax in the critically ill. Lung sliding. Chest. 1995;108(5):1345–8.
43. Lichtenstein D, Mezière G, Biderman P, Gepner A. The "lung point": an ultrasound sign specific to pneumothorax. Intensive Care Med. 2000;26(10):1434–40.
44. De Leyn P. Guidelines Belgian Society of Pulmonology. Guidelines on the management of spontaneous pneumothorax. Acta Chir Belg. 2005;105:265–7.
45. Kelly A, Druda D. Comparison of size classification of primary spontaneous pneumothorax by three international guidelines: a case for international consensus? Respir Med. 2008;102(12):1830–2.
46. Volpicelli G, Boero E, Sverzellati N, et al. Semi-quantification of pneumothorax volume by lung ultrasound. Intensive Care Med. 2014;40(10):1460–7.
47. Sahn SA, Heffner JE. Primary care: spontaneous pneumothorax. N Engl J Med. 2000;342:868–74.
48. Baumann M, Noppen M. Pneumothorax. Respirology. 2004;9(2):157–64.
49. Noppen M, Baumann M. Pathogenesis and treatment of primary spontaneous pneumothorax: an overview. Respiration. 2003;70(4):431–8.
50. Baumann MH. Management of spontaneous pneumothorax. Clin Chest Med. 2006;27(2):369–81.
51. Chan S, Lam PKW. Simple aspiration as initial treatment for primary spontaneous pneumothorax: results of 91 consecutive cases. J Emerg Med. 2005;28:133–8.
52. Chan SSW. The role of simple aspiration in the management of primary spontaneous pneumothorax. J Emerg Med. 2008;34(2):131–8.
53. Ng C, Tsung J. Point of care ultrasound for assisting in needle aspiration of spontaneous pneumothorax in the pediatric emergency department: a case series. Crit Ultrasound J. 2014;6(Suppl 1):A23.
54. Pasquier M, Hugli O, Carron P. Needle aspiration of primary spontaneous pneumothorax. New Engl J Med. 2013;368(19):e24.
55. Needle aspiration of primary spontaneous pneumothorax. N Engl J Med. 2013. [video] Available at: http://www.nejm.org/doi/full/10.1056/NEJMvcm1111468. Accessed 4 Jan 2015.
56. Repanshek Z, Ufberg J, Vilke G, Chan T, Harrigan R. Alternative treatments of pneumothorax. J Emerg Med. 2013;44(2):457–66.
57. Archer G, Hamilton A, Upadhyay R, Finlay M, Grace P. Results of simple aspiration of pneumothoraces. Br J Dis Chest. 1985;79:177–82.
58. Rawlins R. Life threatening haemorrhage after anterior needle aspiration of pneumothoraces. A role for lateral needle aspiration in emergency decompression of spontaneous pneumothorax. Emerg Med J. 2003;20(4):383–4.
59. Yoon JS, Suh JH, Choi SY, Kwon JB, Lee BY, Lee SH, Kim CK, Park CB. Risk factors for the development of reexpansion pulmonary edema in patients with spontaneous pneumothorax. J Cardiothorac Surg. 2013;8:164.
60. Haga T, Kurihara M, Kataoka H. The risk for pulmonary edema following spontaneous pneumothorax. Surg Today. 2014;44(10):1823–7.
61. Morioka H, Takada K, Matsumoto S, Kjima E, Iwata S, Okachi S. Re-expansion pulmonary edema: evaluation of risk factors in 173 episodes of spontaneous pneumothorax. Respir Investig. 2013;51(1):35–9.
62. Park J, Kim Y, Jeong S, Moon D. Ultrasound-guided aspiration of the iatrogenic pneumothorax caused by paravertebral block -a case report. Korean J Pain. 2012;25(1):33.

63. Rahman NM, Maskell NA, Davies CW, Hedley EL, Nunn AJ, Gleeson FV, Davies RJ. The relationship between chest tube size and clinical outcome in pleural infection. Chest. 2010;137(3):536–43.
64. Rivera L, O'Reilly EB, Sise MJ, et al. Small catheter tube thoracostomy: effective in managing chest trauma in stable patients. J Trauma. 2009;66(2):393–9.
65. Tsai WK, Chen W, Lee JC, Cheng WE, Chen CH, Hsu WH, Shih CM. Pigtail catheters vs large-bore chest tubes for management of secondary spontaneous pneumothoraces in adults. Am J Emerg Med. 2006;24(7):795–800.
66. Hogg JR, Caccavale M, Gillen B, McKenzie G, Vlaminck J, Fleming CJ, Stockland A, Friese JL. Tube thoracostomy: a review for the interventional radiologist. Semin Interv Radiol. 2011;28(1):39–47.
67. Benton IJ, Benfield GF. Comparison of large and small-calibre tube drain for managing spontaneous pneumothoraces. Respir Med. 2009;103(10):1436–40.
68. Kulvatunyou N, Vijayasekaran A, Hansen A, et al. Two-year experience of using pigtail catheters to treat traumatic pneumothorax: a changing trend. J Trauma. 2011;71(5):1104–7.
69. Kuo HC, et al. Small-bore pigtail catheters for the treatment of primary spontaneous pneumothorax in young adolescents. Emerg Med J. 2013;30(3):e17.
70. Richardson JD, Miller FB, Carrillo EH, Spain DA. Complex thoracic injuries. Surg Clin North Am. 1996;76(4):725–48.
71. De Lesquen H, et al. Surgical management for the first 48 h following blunt chest trauma: state of the art (excluding vascular injuries). Interact Cardiovasc Thorac Surg. 2015;20(3):399–408.
72. Ma OJ, Mateer J. Trauma ultrasound examination versus chest radiography in the detection of hemothorax. Ann Emerg Med. 1997;29(3):312–6.
73. Ahmed AA, Martin JA, Saul T, et al. The thoracic spine sign in bedside ultrasound. Three cases report. Med Ultrason. 2014;16(2):179–81.
74. Salz TO, Wilson SR, Liebmann O, Price DD. An initial description of a sonographic sign that verifies intrathoracic chest tube placement. Am J Emerg Med. 2010;28(5):626–30.
75. Jenkins JA, Gharahbghian L, Doniger SJ, Bradley S, Crandall S, Spain DA, Williams SR. Sonographic identification of tube thoracostomy study (SITTS): confirmation of intrathoracic placement. West J Emerg Med. 2012;13(4):305–11.
76. Sethuraman KN, Duong D, Mehta S, Director T, Crawford D, St George J, Rathlev NK. Complications of tube thoracostomy placement in the emergency department. J Emerg Med. 2011;40(1):14–20.

Ultrasound-Guided Vascular Procedures

15

Brian Burke and Srikar Adhikari

Introduction

Percutaneous vascular procedures are performed in a variety of clinical settings. While such procedures can be traditionally performed without imaging guidance, such as using anatomic landmarks, the use of ultrasound guidance can improve success rates and decrease procedure-related complications [1–3]. This translates into significantly decreased length of stay and reduced hospital costs. Use of ultrasound before and real-time image guidance during the procedure permits demonstration of regional vascular anatomy and luminal patency. Direct needle visualization results in successful vessel entry with fewer needle passes and less risk of injury to adjacent vital structures [4, 5].

Multiple published studies have demonstrated the clinical utility of ultrasound guidance [6–10]. Additionally, real-time ultrasound guidance increases operator confidence, patient safety, and satisfaction. Achieving maximal clinical benefit from the use of ultrasound guidance will depend on the training and experience of the operator. Knowledge of sonographic anatomy, understanding of fundamentals of needle guidance, and hand-eye coordination techniques are crucial to perform ultrasound-guided vascular procedures.

Advantages of Ultrasound Guidance

There is abundant evidence that use of ultrasound guidance increases overall success rates for vascular procedures. The benefit of ultrasound guidance is especially marked in difficult patients, including those who are of unfavorable body habitus, are uncooperative, or are on mechanical ventilation [11, 12]. Both pre-procedure sonographic survey to determine the optimal entry site and dynamic guidance of needle placement contribute to lower complication rates. This improved safety profile can be related to the increased rate of first-pass success, decreased number of needle passes, and overall decreased procedure time. Fewer needle passes through the skin result in less bacterial contamination at the catheter insertion site. Lower incidence of hematoma and venous thrombus decreases the substrate from which infection can arise.

Percutaneous Thrombin Injection for Pseudoaneurysm Treatment

Pseudoaneurysm of the femoral artery is a well-recognized complication following diagnostic and interventional procedures. Prior studies

B. Burke (✉)
Department of Radiology, North Shore University Hospital, Manhasset, NY, USA
e-mail: bburke@northwell.edu

S. Adhikari
Department of Emergency Medicine, University of Arizona, Tucson, AZ, USA

S. Adhikari, M. Blaivas (eds.), *The Ultimate Guide to Point-of-Care Ultrasound-Guided Procedures*, https://doi.org/10.1007/978-3-030-28267-7_15

reported incidence rates of up to 0.2% of diagnostic procedures and 8% of interventional procedures [13, 14]. Cardiac catheterization is one of the most common causes of femoral pseudoaneurysm formation [15]. The treatment options for femoral pseudoaneurysms include ultrasound-guided compression, percutaneous thrombin injection, and surgical repair. In the recent years, ultrasound-guided percutaneous injection of thrombin has become the treatment of choice in most institutions [16, 17]. Thrombin is a potent, naturally occurring enzyme that converts fibrinogen into stable cross-linked fibrin. This technique is relatively simple to perform for any clinician with ultrasound skills and is usually done at the patient's bedside, using a portable ultrasound device. This section highlights the procedure and provides step-by-step guidance for clinicians who are involved in treating the femoral pseudoaneurysms.

Anatomy

The common femoral artery is the continuation of the external iliac artery and lies lateral to the common femoral vein and inferior to the inguinal ligament. It is found just medial to the midpoint of the inguinal ligament, approximately halfway between the anterior superior iliac spine and pubic tubercle. The femoral vein and common femoral artery both emerge within the femoral sheath. The femoral nerve lies lateral to the common femoral artery but outside the femoral sheath. The common femoral artery bifurcates into the superficial femoral artery and profunda femoris artery in the proximal thigh (Fig. 15.1). Sonographically the common femoral artery looks tubular with an anechoic lumen, thicker wall, and visible pulsations. It is not easily compressible when compared to the common femoral vein. Color and spectral Doppler can be used to distinguish common femoral artery from common femoral vein by virtue of flow direction and pulsatility (Figs. 15.2, 15.3, and 15.4).

A pseudoaneurysm or a false aneurysm is a collection of blood between one or two outer layers of an artery (media or adventitia), whereas true aneurysm is an outpouching with all three layers of the arterial wall. Femoral pseudoaneurysm is typically seen as a round sac adjacent to, and often with, a connecting cylindrical neck from the native common femoral artery. Depending on the degree of thrombosis, the internal appearance of the pseudoaneurysm varies. Partial rupture of the pseudoaneurysm may result in a complex, multilobed pattern with multiple communicating sacs, whereas complete rupture may lead to a more diffusely infiltrative hematoma. Ultrasound is the most rapid and best imaging modality for the evaluation of pseudoaneurysm. On B-mode imaging, a pulsatile anechoic saccular lesion is visualized in the soft tissue with variable echogenicity. When there is no intraluminal thrombus, it appears anechoic with swirling blood; when there is a thrombus, the echogenicity varies according to the age of the thrombus (Figs. 15.5 and 15.6). It may be difficult to differentiate a completely thrombosed pseudoaneurysm from a hematoma. On color Doppler a characteristic yin-yang sign may be visualized due to bidirectional swirling turbulent blood flow in the sac (Fig. 15.7). On pulsed-wave Doppler, a "To and Fro" Doppler pattern (blood entering the sac during systole and leaving during diastole) is found in the neck of pseudoaneurysm with preserved native arterial flow distal to the neck of the sac (Figs. 15.8 and 15.9) [18].

Indications

The size of the pseudoaneurysm is used as a guide to determine the treatment option. A conservative approach is generally adopted for a small-diameter (<3.0 cm) femoral artery pseudoaneurysms since they may thrombose spontaneously. With a favorable risk/benefit ratio, the indications for direct percutaneous thrombin injection are broad and involve almost all patients except those with rare contraindications. However, it is particularly indicated if the femoral pseudoaneurysms are painful, growing, and affecting ambulation.

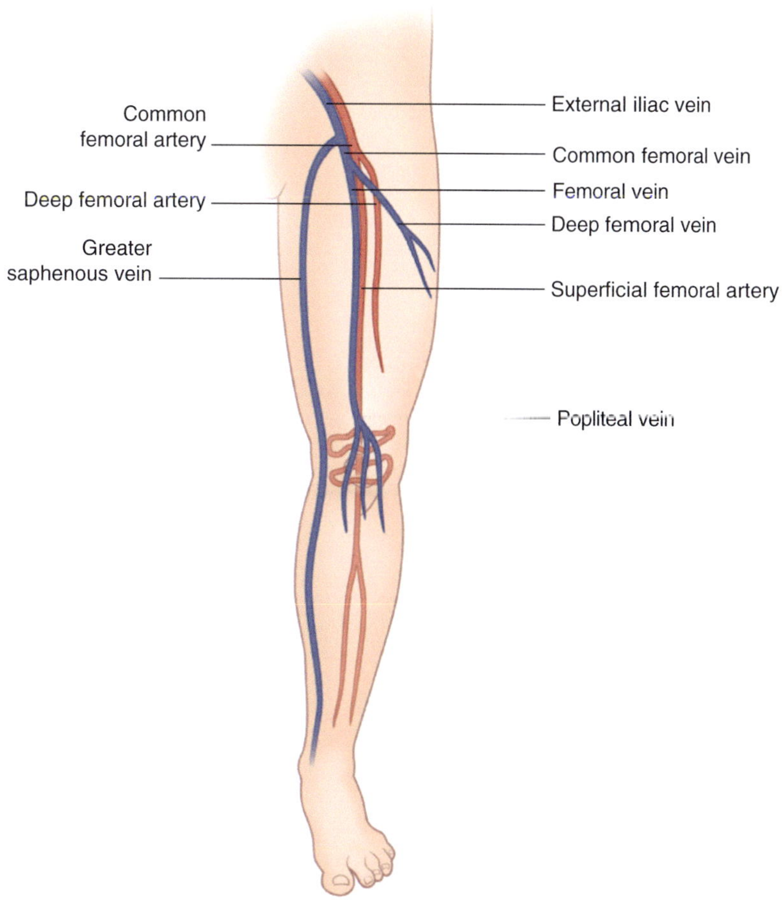

Fig. 15.1 Arterial and venous anatomy of the lower extremity

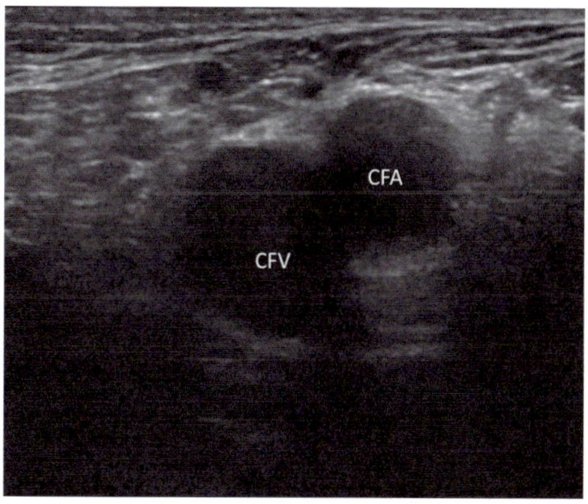

Fig. 15.2 B-mode image of transverse view of left common femoral artery (CFA) and common femoral vein (CFV)

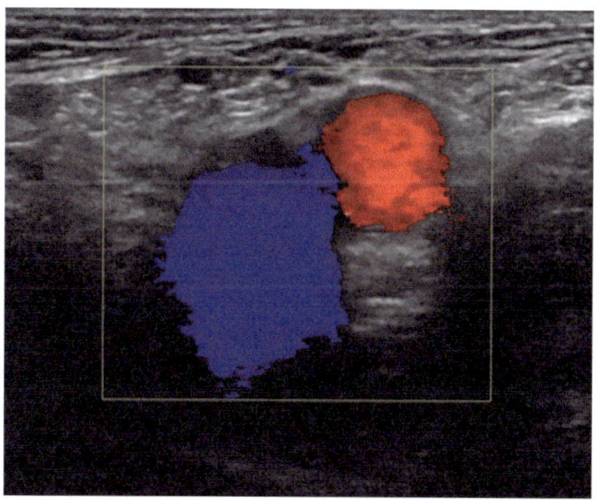

Fig. 15.3 Color Doppler image of left common femoral artery (red) and common femoral vein (blue)

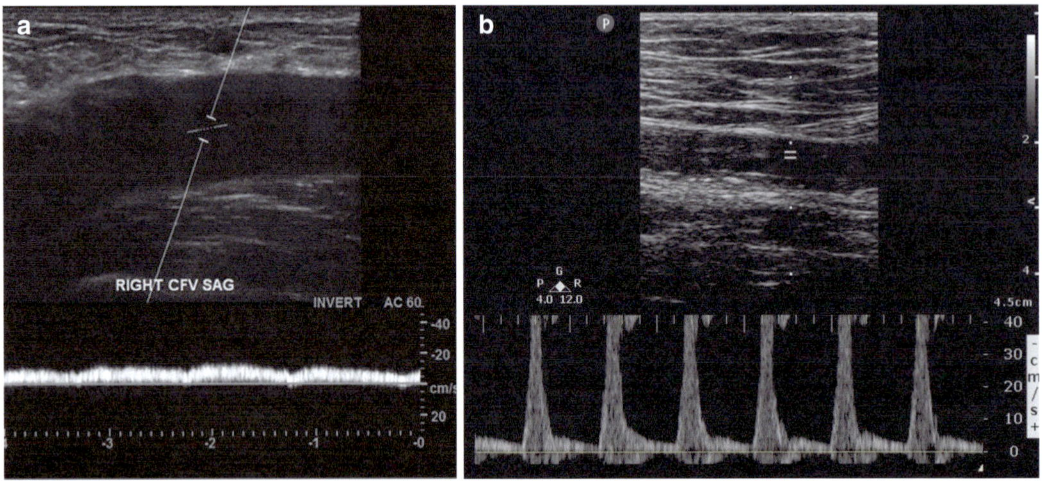

Fig. 15.4 (**a**) Common femoral vein – spectral Doppler waveform showing phasic flow. (**b**) Common femoral artery – spectral Doppler waveform showing pulsatility

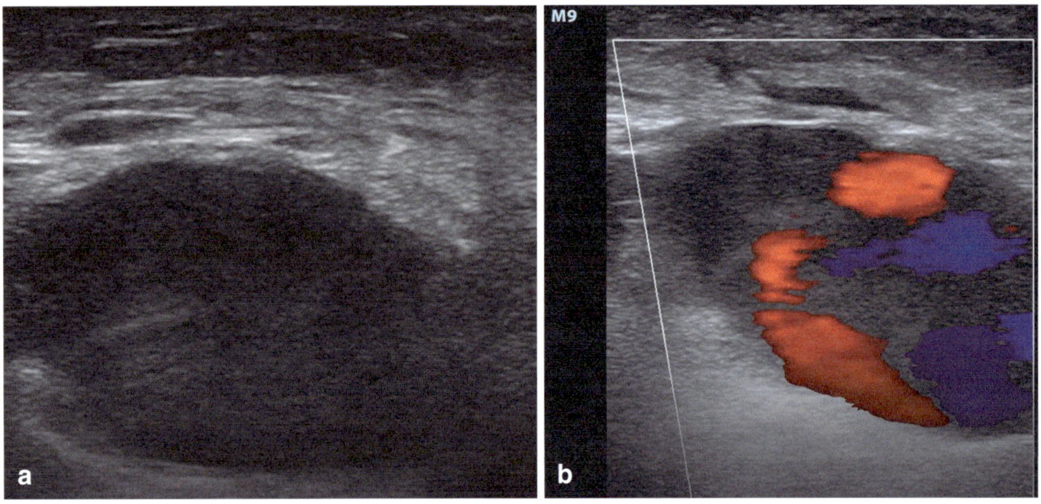

Fig. 15.5 Femoral artery pseudoaneurysm. (**a**) Gray-scale ultrasonography shows a well-defined anechoic mass. (**b**) Color Doppler shows swirling blood flow pattern within the mass

Contraindications

The contraindications to direct percutaneous thrombin injection therapy include:

1. Ruptured pseudoaneurysm
2. Coexisting arteriovenous fistulous component
3. Associated ipsilateral deep venous thrombosis
4. Prior treatment/exposure to bovine thrombin due to concern for allergic reactions
5. Increased risk of vessel thrombosis such as patients with hypercoagulable disorders
6. Infected pseudoaneurysms or overlying skin erosion/breakdown due to risk of infection
7. Inability to access the site for injection due to scarring

Equipment/Probe Selection

- An ultrasound system capable of adequate image quality and soft tissue penetration is essential. The ultrasound system should have a linear array transducer, although obese

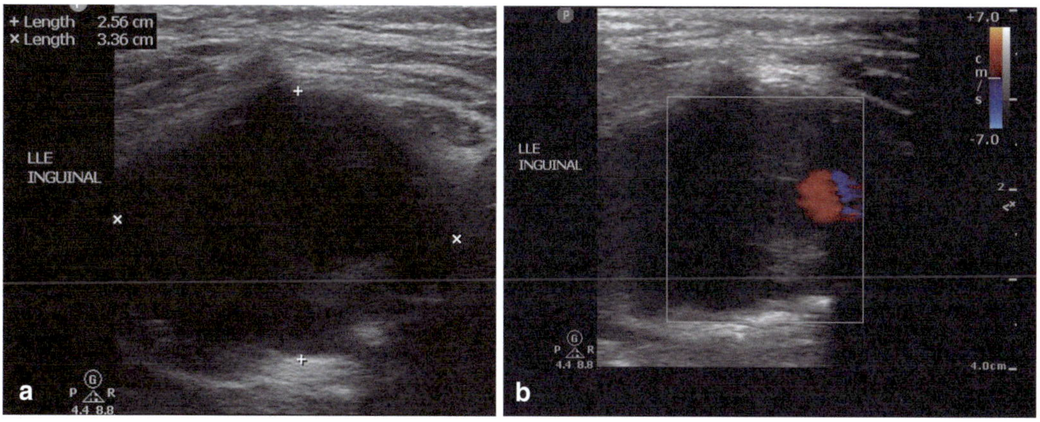

Fig. 15.6 Partially thrombosed femoral artery pseudoaneurysm (**a**) B-mode image. (**b**) Color Doppler image

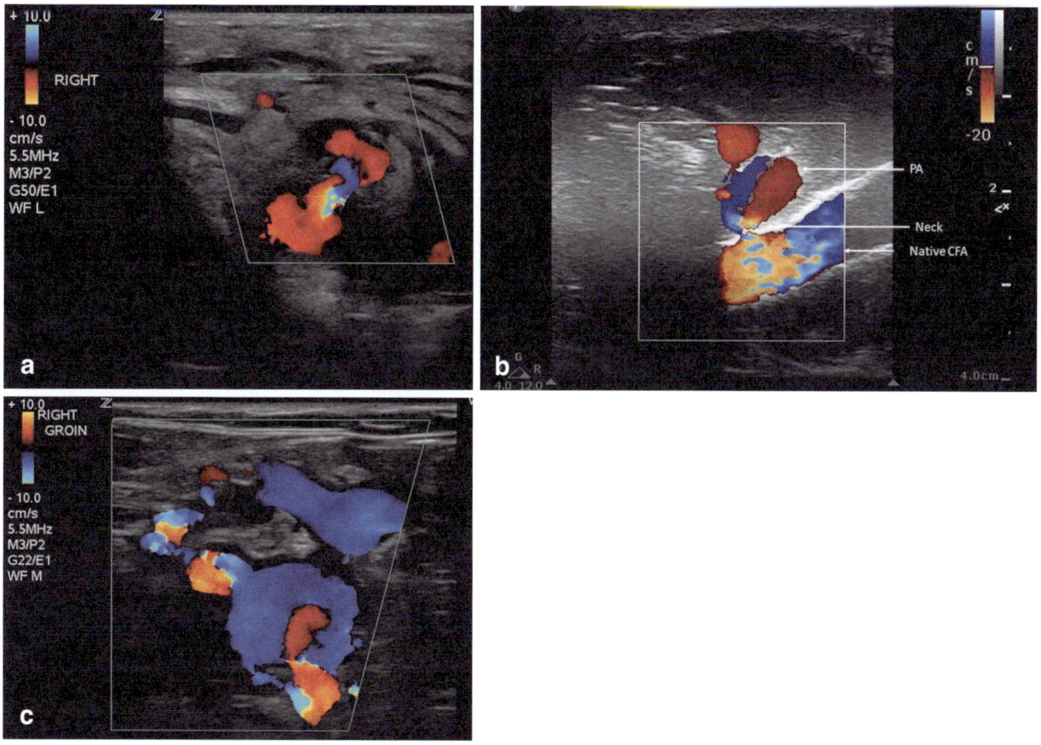

Fig. 15.7 Color Doppler images of three patients with femoral artery pseudoaneurysms demonstrating bidirectional swirling turbulent blood flow in the sac (**a**-**c**)

patients may require the use of a curvilinear probe. Color and pulsed-wave Doppler capability are important adjuncts.

- Recombinant or bovine thrombin (100–1000 units/ml).
- 20 G or 22 G needle with syringe.
- Local anesthetic (1% lidocaine).
- 25 G needle for anesthetic infiltration.
- Sterile drapes, gown, gloves, mask, and cap.
- Sterile ultrasound probe cover.
- Gauze.

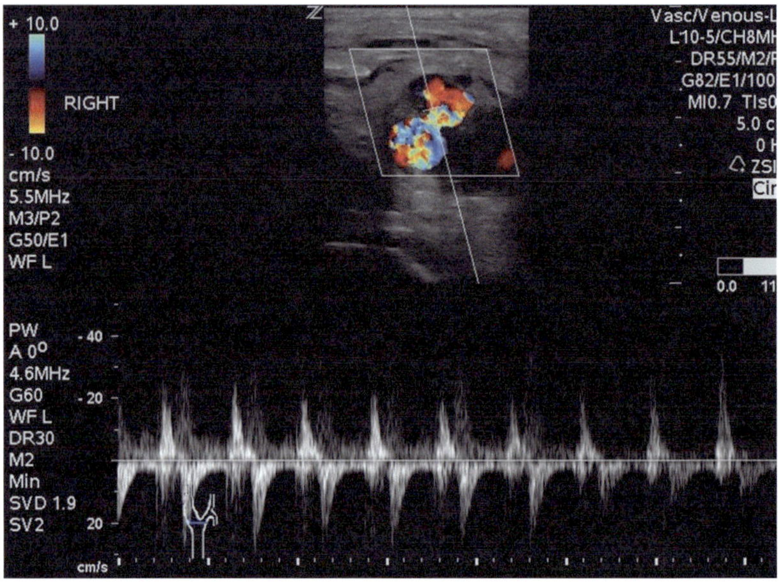

Fig. 15.8 Pulsed-wave Doppler showing a "To and Fro" Doppler pattern (blood entering the sac during systole and leaving during diastole) in the neck of pseudoaneurysm

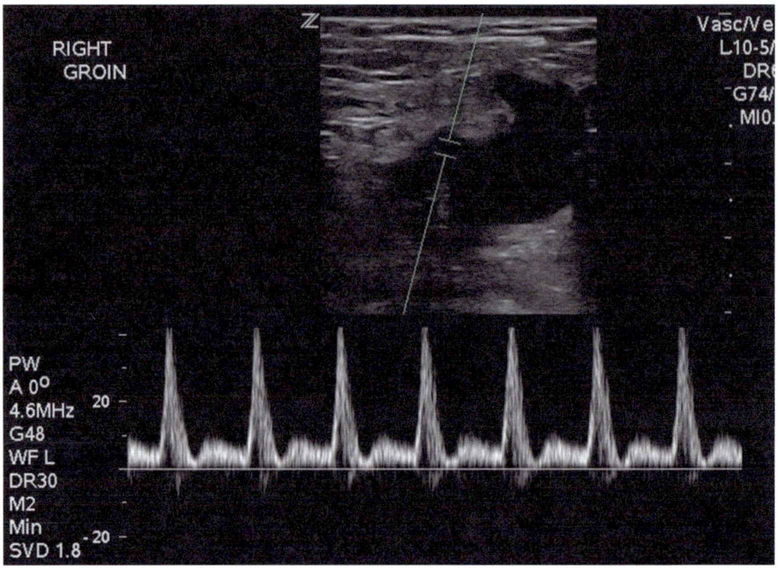

Fig. 15.9 Spectral Doppler demonstrating preserved native arterial flow distal to the neck of the pseudoaneurysm sac

Preparation/Pre-procedural Evaluation

Ultrasound assessment of the pseudoaneurysm involves scanning the suspected area in two orthogonal planes and documenting the following: site of origin of the aneurysm (common femoral vs. femoral/deep femoral artery), waveform pattern of outflow artery, size of the aneurysm, number of lobes and the dimensions of each lumen, and length and diameter of the neck of the aneurysm. After evaluating the extent of the pseudoaneurysm in two orthogonal planes, it is time to prepare for thrombin injection. The procedure should be performed under standard hospital sterile procedure guidelines similar to that of a central line placement. The ultrasound transducer should be disinfected and then sterilely dressed in an appropriate sterile ultrasound transducer sheath cover. Sterile gel should be utilized once the injection site has been prepped according to hospital sterile procedure guidelines. Prior to the procedure, it is important to check for vascular compromise distal to the location of the pseudoaneurysm, and in the case of the femoral artery pseudoaneurysm, the posterior tibial and dorsalis pedis pulses should be assessed with palpation or Doppler signals should be documented. In-plane needle visualization and guidance is likely to yield the best results in avoiding nearby structures and injection of thrombin into the injured artery. Local anesthetic administration under dynamic ultrasound guidance can be exceedingly helpful which allows depositing anesthetic throughout the path of the needle. A thin needle (20–22 G) can be utilized for thrombin injection. Using a 25 or 27 G needle will make it harder to visualize the needle on ultrasound. A small syringe can be used to draw thrombin (recombinant or bovine) for injection [19].

Procedure

The injection should be performed under real-time ultrasound guidance. Using B-mode imaging, the sterile needle should be placed to one side of the long axis of the linear array transducer directly in the middle of the transducer. The needle is slowly introduced through the skin under real-time ultrasound guidance. Once the needle tip and shaft are identified, after having been inserted several millimeters under the skin, the needle tip is directed into the sac of pseudoaneurysm. The operator should take extreme care to direct the needle tip to the periphery of the aneurysm away from the neck of pseudoaneurysm. This reduces the possibility of thrombin administration into the pseudoaneurysm neck and, possibly, into the arterial circulation. Under ultrasound guidance, the sac is injected with 0.1 mL aliquots of thrombin until the blood flow in the sac is successfully obliterated. Alternate color Doppler and B-mode assessments should be performed to assess for thrombosis and disappearance of color signal and confirm pseudoaneurysm closure. After successful thrombosis is accomplished, the distal arterial circulation is assessed and compared with pre-procedural findings. For patients in whom thrombin is not initially successful, repeat injection can be attempted. The patient must remain supine after the procedure and should be observed for 6 hours. Thereafter, the native common femoral artery should be assessed with Doppler ultrasound to confirm patency. An ultrasound should ideally be performed the following day to confirm hemostasis (Figs. 15.10, 15.11, and 15.12) [19, 20].

Complications

The most serious complications following thrombin injection are arterial thrombosis or distal embolization, which are extremely rare (<1%). Other potential complications include allergic reactions related to bovine thrombin, infection, pseudoaneurysm rupture, and inadvertent injection of the thrombin into adjacent structures instead of pseudoaneurysm [19, 20].

Pearls/Pitfalls

A thorough assessment of pseudoaneursym should be performed prior to the procedure to determine the risk and benefit of the procedure. Thrombin injection is effective in patients who are already receiving anticoagulation with heparin or warfarin. A second injection can be performed if initial injection is not successful. Bovine thrombin is a foreign substance and, as such, may cause an allergic reaction after repeated exposures. Although downstream embolization is extremely rare, it may well be that some thrombin does in fact leave the pseudoaneurysm sac and travel into the native artery and systemic circulation. Pitfalls largely include the general mistakes providers make with ultrasound-guided procedures: advancing the needle without visualization and injury of nearby structures.

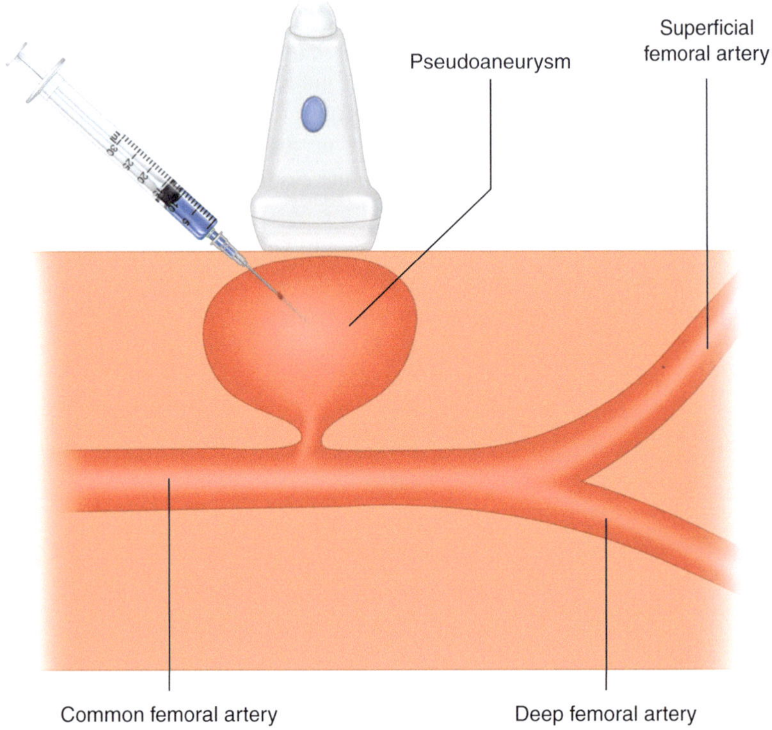

Fig. 15.10 Ultrasound-guided thrombin injection

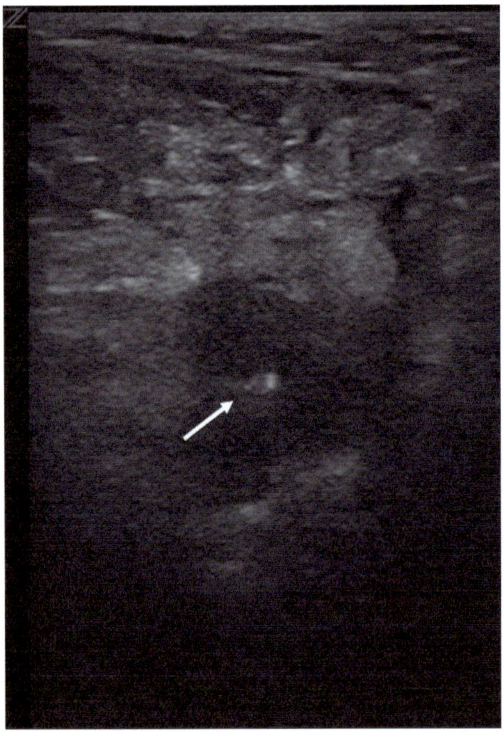

Fig. 15.11 Echogenic needle tip (arrow) is visualized in B-mode in the pseudoaneurysm sac

Integration into Clinical Practice

Femoral artery pseudoaneurysm after cardiac catheterization is not common but a well-recognized complication. Patients with femoral artery pseudoaneurysm are often initially evaluated in the emergency department. Providers with ultrasound skills can rapidly evaluate these patients for the presence of pseudoaneurysm. Depending on the practice setting and availability of resources, same providers can perform the thrombin injection in conjunction with cardiology consultation.

Evidence

Compelling evidence exists regarding the effectiveness of thrombin injection for pseudoaneurysm treatment. A recent study by Ehieli et al. looked at 326 patients who underwent thrombin injection for femoral artery pseudoaneurysm formation. The procedure was successfully completed in 98.2% of cases. Complete thrombosis

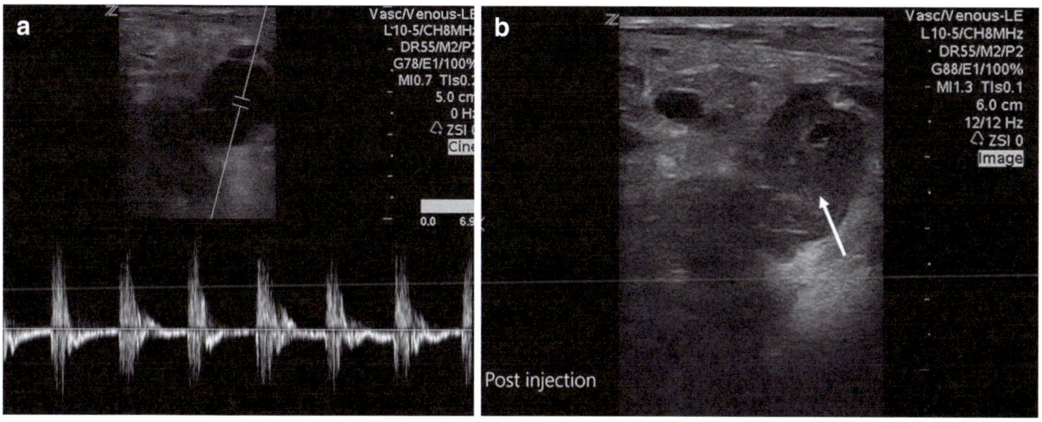

Fig. 15.12 (**a**) Pseudoaneursym sac prior to thrombin injection. (**b**) Post thrombin injection, successful thrombosis (arrow) is accomplished

of the psuedoaneurysm was achieved in 74.5% of patients within the first 24 hours. Those patients who required a second injection had a 97% success rate [14]. In a study done by Paulson et al., percutaneous ultrasound-guided thrombin injection had a high success rate of 96%, in comparison to the 74% success rate of ultrasound-guided compression [21]. In another prospective non-randomized study of femoral artery pseudoaneurysms treated with thrombin injection, the overall success rate was 97% and was not adversely affected by anticoagulation use [19].

- Do not inject a pseudoaneurysm with a sac size <1 cm because of risk of arterial thrombosis.
- Use the minimal amount of thrombin required to occlude the pseudoaneurysm, and always perform post-procedural assessment, including Doppler and color flow imaging of the native femoral artery.
- Anticoagulated patients are less likely to have complete thrombosis.

Key Points

- Use in-plane needle visualization and guidance for best results.
- Follow sterile precautions as with other similar procedures like central venous access.
- Alternate between B-mode and color Doppler assessments during thrombin injection to detect for thrombosis and disappearance of color signal.
- Maintain the needle tip in the periphery of the aneurysm sac and direct the needle away from the neck of the sac.
- Use a curvilinear probe to assess the aneurysm sac in obese patients.

Peripherally Inserted Central Catheter (PICC) Placement

Peripherally inserted central catheters (PICCs) are useful in patients with limited peripheral venous access or in those who require intermediate-term access. Ultrasound guidance has been shown to have a significant impact on the overall clinical performance of PICCs. With ultrasound guidance, the practice of placing PICCs in the antecubital veins has been completely abandoned. By placing the PICCs in the deeper veins in the upper arm, ultrasound guidance has been associated with a 95–99% success rate and a considerable reduction in early and late complications [22]. Ultrasound guidance helps reduce complications such as inadvertent puncture of the brachial artery and median nerve. Ultrasound is a valuable tool for selecting the most appropriate vein prior to the procedure and for the navigation of the catheter. Typically, access is through the cephalic, basilic, or brachial veins of the upper arm. The paired brachial veins follow the brachial artery, but the cephalic and basilic veins have no accompanying artery. Due to their variable location, smaller size, and lower patency rates, blind procedures can be challenging. The use of ultrasound guidance for PICC placement has been shown to increase overall success rates while decreasing risk of phlebitis and thrombosis [23, 24].

Anatomy

PICC lines are often placed in the superficial veins proximal to the antecubital fossa (usually in the basilic, brachial, or cephalic veins) (Fig. 15.13).

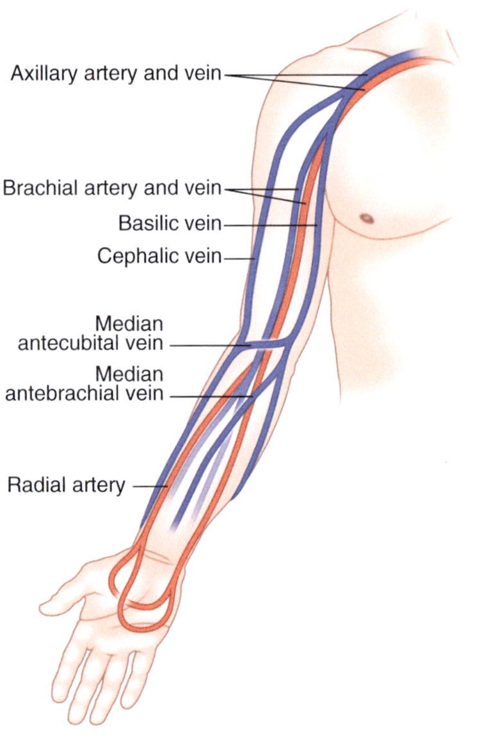

Fig. 15.13 Venous anatomy of the lower extremity

Sonographic anatomy of peripheral veins is discussed in Chap. 12. Briefly, many of the vessels targeted for cannulation occur as paired artery and vein, and they must be distinguished from each other. While both are tubular and have an anechoic lumen, the artery has a thicker wall and may demonstrate visible pulsations. Veins are more readily compressible than arteries, are often larger than their arterial counterpart, and contain valves (Fig. 15.14). Although usually not necessary, color and spectral Doppler can be used to distinguish arteries from veins by virtue of flow direction and pulsatility.

Indications

- Difficult intravenous access
- Limited peripheral venous access
- Duration of intravenous therapy expected to continue more than a week (e.g., antibiotics, antifungals, etc.)
- Ambulatory chemotherapy
- Frequent restarts of peripheral intravenous lines
- Serial transfusions of blood products
- Infusion of hyperosmolar solutions or substances with extreme pH (total parenteral nutrition)
- Serial lab draws/serial radiographic studies
- Thrombocytopenia or coagulopathy which prevents placement of a permanent infusion device
- Infusion of vesicant/irritant/painful intravenous medications
- Patient choice

Contraindications

- Burns, trauma, skin infections, radiation, vascular surgery, and history of venous thrombosis at the site of insertion
- Active bacteremia or septicemia
- Chronic renal failure and end-stage renal disease (vasculature should be preserved for potential dialysis catheter placement or AV fistula)

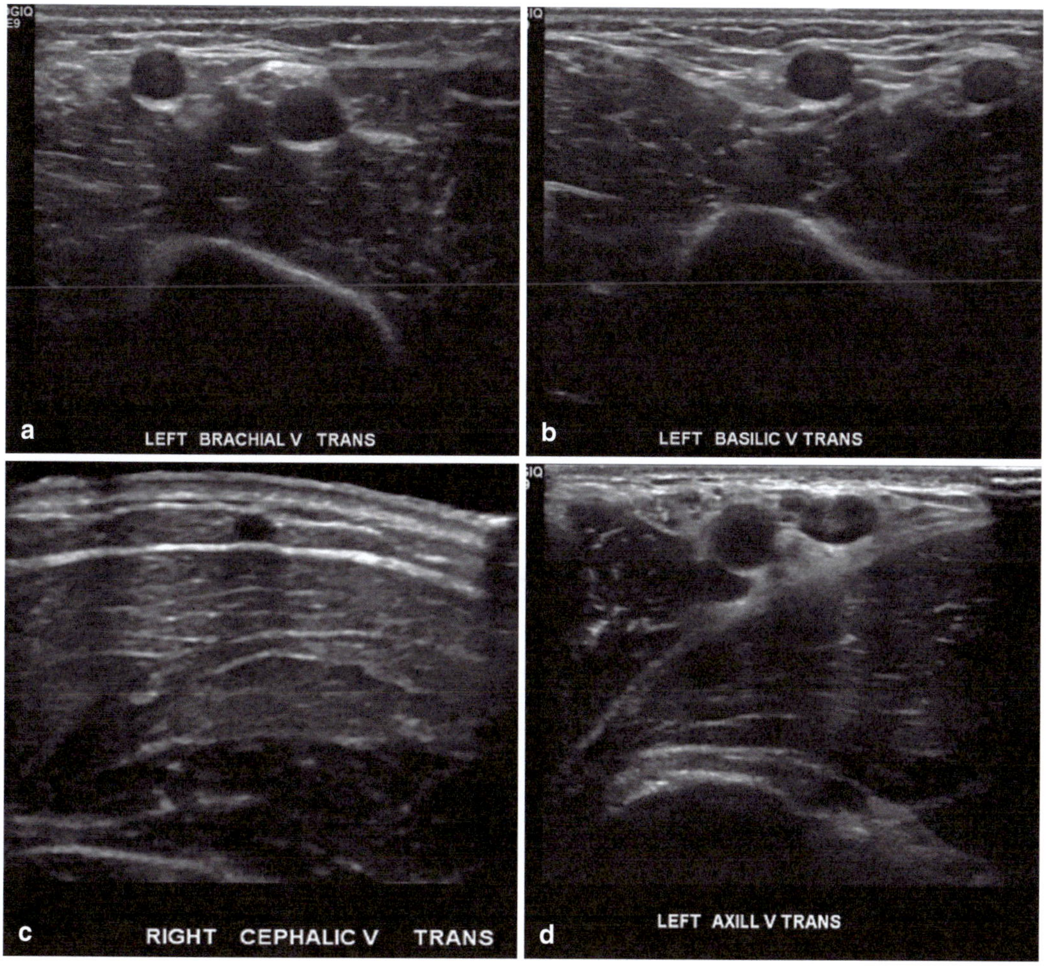

Fig. 15.14 B-mode image of (**a**) brachial veins, (**b**) basilic vein, (**c**) cephalic vein, (**d**) axillary vein

- Small diameter of arm veins (<3–4 mm)
- Prior mastectomy and lymph node dissection (since lymph system is compromised and unable to drain)
- Crutch walking and other upper body activities which can cause migration of the catheter tip
- Persistent cough and vomiting (increased intrathoracic pressure can lead to catheter migration, malposition, or erosion)
- Allergy to PICC components
- Physical or mental health conditions affecting care and maintenance of PICC line
- Conditions that prevent the ability to secure the catheter
- Severe edema in the affected limb
- Extremity contractures
- Sensory or motor deficits of the arm, which might delay recognition of complications.

Equipment/Probe Selection

- Ultrasound system with a linear array probe
- Sterile probe sheath cover for ultrasound probe
- Ultrasound gel
- Sterile gloves and gown, mask with face shield, and hat
- Sterile drape and towels
- Skin disinfectants (chlorhexidine/alcohol)
- Sterile saline flushes

- PICC catheter (Fig. 15.15)
- Needles of varying gauges
- 10 mL syringes
- Guidewire
- Dilator
- Introducer
- Small blade
- Local anesthetic (usually lidocaine)
- Suture material
- Sterile dressing kit (transparent and semi-permeable)
- BioPatch

Preparation/Pre-procedural Evaluation

PICCs are typically inserted at the bedside under ultrasound guidance. As with any procedure, preparation is key and ensuring that all essential equipment and materials are present is critical for successful outcomes (Fig. 15.16). Patient consent should be obtained. The patient's arm circumference should be measured which will serve as a reference if any edema occurs due to complications from PICC placement. Sterile technique is crucial for this procedure to reduce the risk of catheter-related bloodstream infections. Before inserting the PICC, ultrasound should be used to differentiate arteries from veins and select the optimal vein for PICC placement. The choice of vein should take into consideration factors such as size of the vein, depth from surface, course of the vein, adjacent structures, proximity to the axilla and antecubital fossa, and adjacent pathology (such as overlying cellulitis or abscess). The vein should be evaluated for patency and presence of valves, which can interfere with catheter passage and if damaged lead to worse venous function. It is crucial to select a vein away from arteries and nerves if possible. The basilic vein is ideal for PICC placement since it has the largest diameter of all upper extremity vessels and offers a non-tortuous entry into the subclavian vein and not in proximity with arteries and nerves.

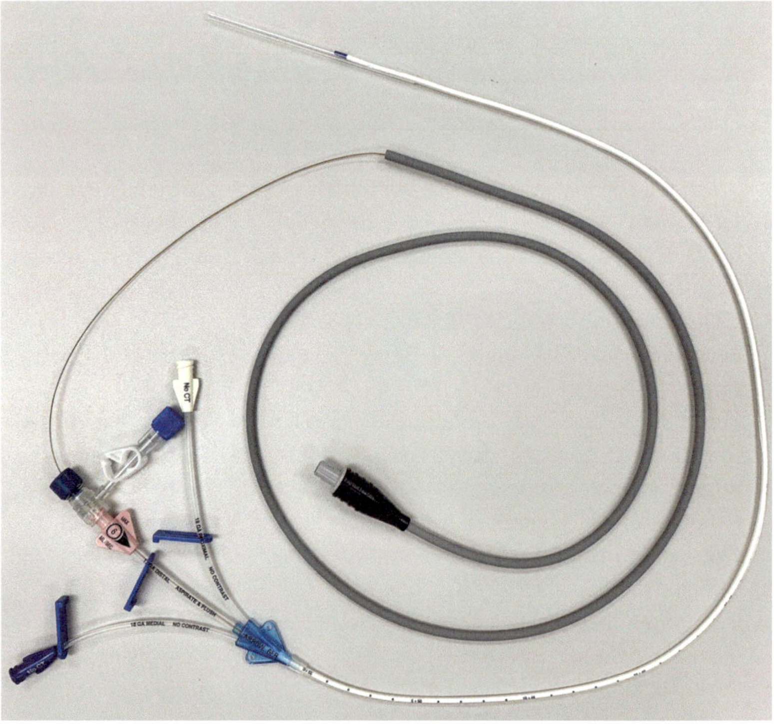

Fig. 15.15 Peripherally inserted central catheter

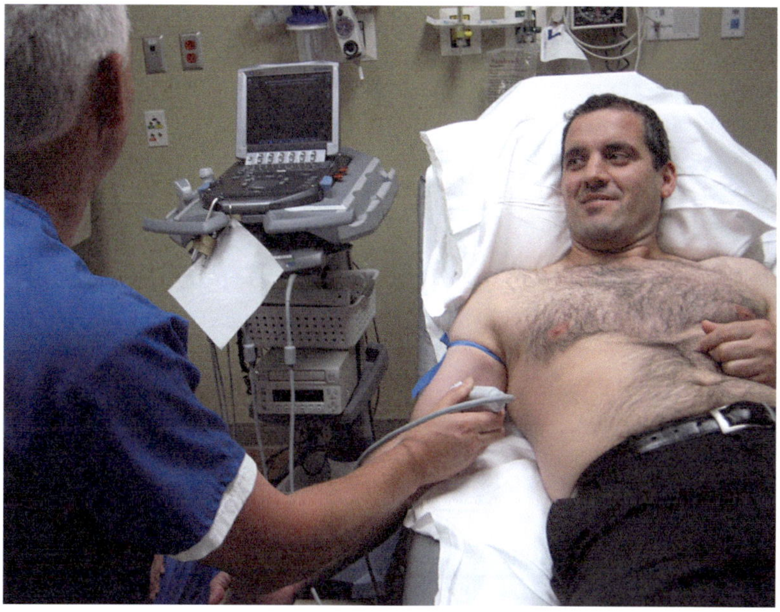

Fig. 15.16 Patient and ultrasound machine positioning

Procedure

The Seldinger technique is the most commonly used method for placing PICCs. A tourniquet should be applied proximal to the site of insertion. Use of a tourniquet is helpful to distend the vein lumen. The distance the catheter needs to be advanced to reach the SVC/right atrial junction should be measured (from the site of insertion to the mid-right mid-clavicular line and down to the third intercostal space). The upper arm should be prepped with chlorhexidine. A sterile field should be created by placing sterile towels and drape. The ultrasound probe must be covered with a sterile probe cover (discussed in Chap. 6). The skin should be anesthetized and the target vein should be re-identified using ultrasound. The vein should be accessed under real-time guidance using in-line approach technique (discussed in Chap. 12). Once the needle is inserted in the vein, the guidewire should be advanced through the needle. Then the needle should be removed, and guidewire placement in the vein should be confirmed using ultrasound. Then a small nick should be made with a scalpel at the insertion site alongside the guidewire to accommodate the dilator. The dilator and introducer should be inserted over the guidewire. Then the guidewire and dilator should be removed, leaving only the introducer in place. This should be followed by insertion of the catheter through the introducer to the predetermined length, and the introducer should be removed. The tourniquet should be removed. The proper placement of the catheter in atriocaval junction should be confirmed using the flush test (discussed in Chap. 6). Additionally, a chest radiograph should be ordered to determine the location of the tip of the PICC line. Once inserted, the catheter should be secured to sterile skin and the insertion site and hub are then covered with occlusive dressing (Figs. 15.17 and 15.18) [25].

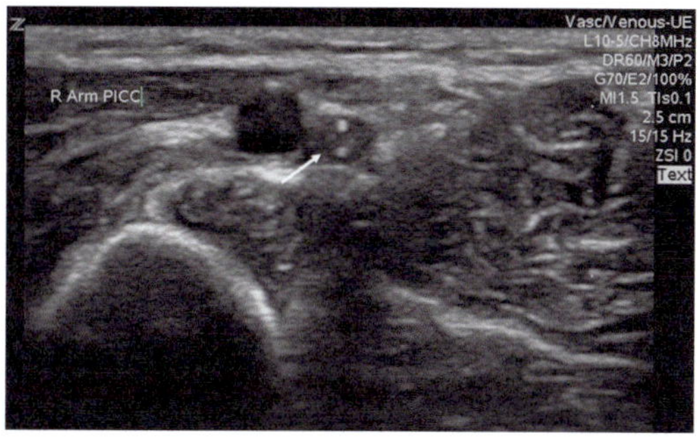

Fig. 15.17 Peripherally inserted central catheter (arrow) seen in the basilic vein in transverse plane

Complications

The complications of PICCs include infection, catheter malposition, migration of the catheter, mechanical malfunction, air embolism, phlebitis, thrombosis, infiltration, catheter occlusion (thrombotic and non-thrombotic causes), arrhythmias, line fracture/embolization, and accidental withdrawal [25].

Pearls/Pitfalls

Use of out-of-plane approach for venous access can lead to posterior wall penetration and inadvertent puncture of adjacent strictures. Malposition of the PICC line in the jugular vein can be assessed using linear array transducer (Fig. 15.19). Infection rates are higher for PICC lines inserted in the antecubital fossa compared to lines placed in the upper arm veins. Post-procedural routine PICC line care and patient education are critical to prevent infection.

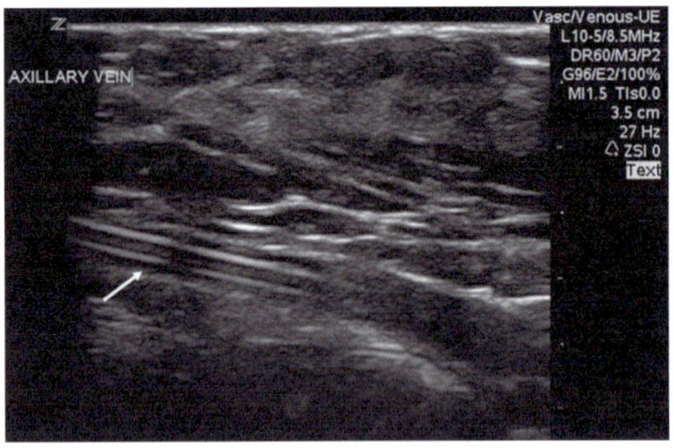

Fig. 15.18 Peripherally inserted central catheter (arrow) seen in the axillary vein in long axis

Integration into Clinical Practice

PICC lines are very effective for long-term intravenous use and are used in a variety of clinical settings. PICCs are particularly appropriate for patients who need regular outpatient-based therapy. PICCs have several advantages over central venous catheters. They provide medium-term access for several weeks up to 6 months, and they have been shown to be more cost-effective and have lower complication rates than central venous catheters. It is crucial to understand the fundamentals of needle guidance under ultrasound to successfully perform PICC line placement. With widespread availability of portable ultrasound and rapid proliferation of training programs, ultrasound-guided PICC line placement can make a significant impact on patient care in a wide variety of clinical settings.

Evidence

The use of ultrasound guidance for PICC line placement is a well-established technique with a success rate of approximately 95%. PICC lines are associated with decreased incidence of complications such as mechanical phlebitis and

Fig. 15.19 Peripherally inserted central catheter (PICC) line tip seen in the internal jugular vein (IJV)

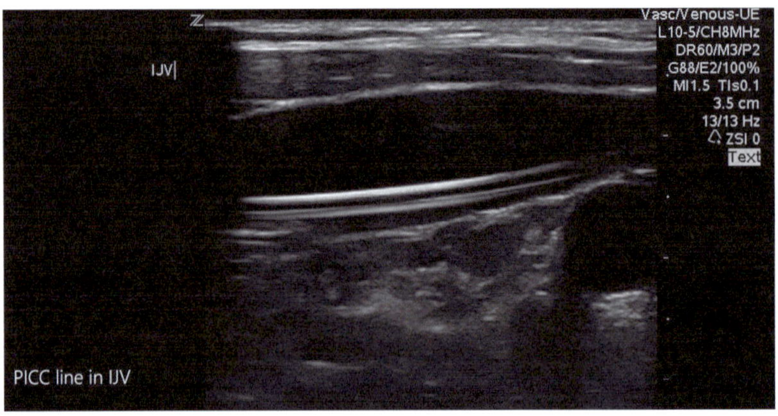

thrombosis [26]. One systematic review found a low infection rate of 2.1 per 1000 catheter days in hospitalized patients with PICC lines [27]. When performed by neonatologists with ultrasound expertise, real-time ultrasound-guided insertion of PICCs was found to be a more efficient method than standard line placement [23, 28–30].

Key Points

- Follow sterile precautions while placing PICC lines under ultrasound guidance, which includes covering the ultrasound probe with sterile probe cover.
- Differentiate veins from arteries using B-mode and Doppler imaging.
- Pulsed-wave Doppler is the only reliable method for differentiating the artery from vein, regardless of how low the blood pressure is, as low flow states can create confusing results on color Doppler interrogation.
- Choose the appropriate vein based on the size of the vein, depth from surface, course of the vein, adjacent structures, proximity to the axilla and antecubital fossa, and adjacent pathology (such as overlying cellulitis or abscess).
- Always assess the vein for patency and presence of valves.
- The basilic vein is ideal for PICC placement since it is not close to nerves or arteries.
- Use in-plane approach to insert the needle in the vein.
- Confirm the guidewire placement using ultrasound.
- Proper placement of the catheter can be confirmed using the flush technique.

Ultrasound-Guided Placement of a Midline Catheter

A midline catheter is an 8–12 cm catheter inserted in the upper arm with the tip of the catheter positioned just below the axilla. A midline catheter does not pass through central veins and is considered a useful alternative for peripheral venous access. The usual dwell time is approximately 14 days, but this catheter can last up to a month. The pre-procedural evaluation and the ultrasound technique for insertion are similar to PICC line placement, which is discussed above. Ultrasound should be used to select the largest vein, away from arteries and nerves. The optimal vein for insertion is generally the basilic vein. Similar to PICC lines, the basilic and brachial veins are preferred over the cephalic vein for midline catheter placement due to lower complication rates from higher flow. Ideally, midline catheter should be inserted above the elbow (distal enough from the axilla to ensure an 8–12 cm midline catheter will not cross the axilla), and avoid the antecubital fossa since catheters inserted at this location are associated with higher infection and thrombosis rates. The midline catheter should be placed using sterile barrier precautions. We recommend using an ultrasound-guided in-line approach to obtain venous access using 20 G catheter over the needle after anesthetizing the skin with lidocaine. After cannulating the vein, a guidewire should be placed through the cannula using the modified Seldinger technique similar to PICC placement. Then the cannula should be removed leaving the wire in situ. Then the midline catheter should be advanced over the wire, and the wire should be removed (Figs. 15.20, 15.21, and 15.22). Once the catheter is in the vein, its patency should be confirmed (discussed in the Chap. 12) [31, 32].

Ultrasound-Guided Arterial Catheterization

Arterial catheters are used for diagnostic and therapeutic procedures, as well as for physiologic monitoring purposes. Sites for access may include the femoral, radial, axillary, and brachial arteries. Arterial access is usually guided by palpating the arterial pulse, but ultrasound-guided access is superior over landmark technique, especially in patients with altered anatomy, obesity, states of low cardiac output, and severe atherosclerotic disease.

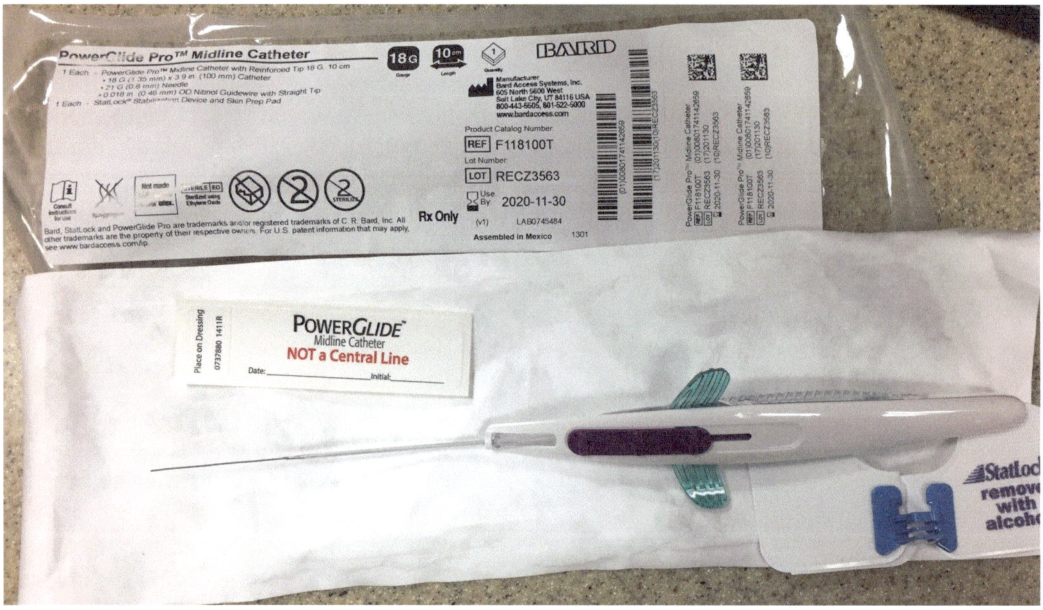

Fig. 15.20 Midline catheter

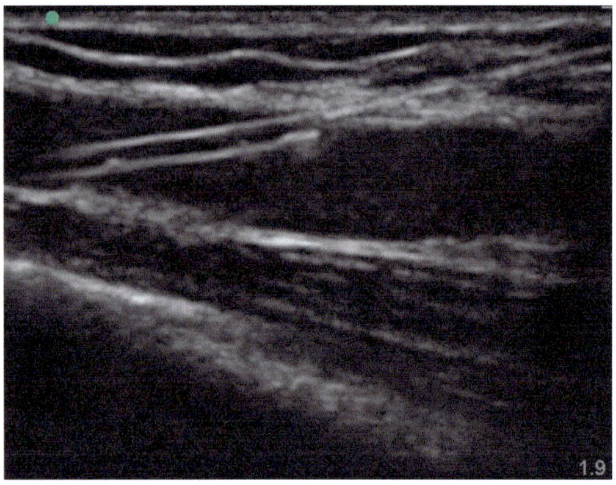

Fig. 15.21 B-mode image of midline catheter cannula seen in long axis

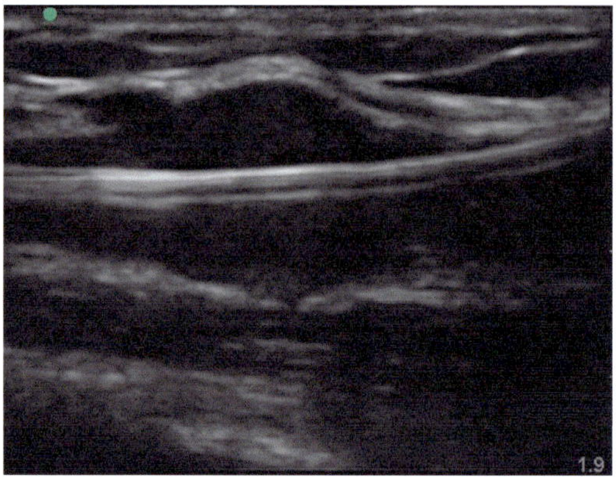

Fig. 15.22 Midline catheter seen in the basilic vein in long axis

Anatomy

The two most common locations used for arterial line placement are the radial and femoral arteries. The radial artery is most often selected because of its superficial location. In a majority of patients, the radial artery originates from the brachial artery just distal to the elbow. The radial artery descends laterally in the forearm until it reaches the wrist. In the proximal forearm, the artery runs underneath the supinator longus muscle. In the mid-forearm, down to the wrist, it lies in between the supinator longus and the flexor carpi radialis tendons. It is superficial in the thenar area of the wrist where the radius articulates with the metacarpal bones. The radial artery is smaller in caliber than the ulnar artery at their origins, but it is equal or larger than the ulnar artery at the level of the wrist (Fig. 15.13).

The common femoral artery is the continuation of the external iliac artery and lies lateral to the common femoral vein below the inguinal ligament. It is found just medial to the midpoint of the inguinal ligament, approximately halfway between the anterior superior iliac spine and pubic tubercle. The femoral nerve lies lateral to the common femoral artery but outside the femoral sheath. The common femoral artery bifurcates into the superficial femoral artery and profunda femoris artery in the proximal thigh.

On B-mode imaging, the arteries look round, with anechoic lumen, thicker wall, and visible pulsations. Arteries are not easily compressible when compared to veins. Color and spectral Doppler can be used to distinguish arteries from veins by virtue of flow direction and pulsatility (Fig. 15.23).

Indications

- Continuous blood pressure monitoring in critically ill patients including those who are in shock, patients on vasopressors, hypertensive emergency, stroke, etc.
- Patients who need frequent blood draws
- Patients on mechanical ventilation needing ABGs
- Cardiac function monitoring in conjunction with other technologies
- Cardiac catheterization and radiological interventional procedures, manual or automated exchange transfusions, plasmapheresis, and extracorporeal membrane oxygenation

Contraindications

- Infection at the site of insertion
- Impaired collateral circulation
- Severe peripheral vascular disease
- Severe coagulopathy
- Raynaud syndrome
- Full-thickness burns

Equipment/Probe Selection

- Ultrasound system with linear array probe
- Sterile ultrasound probe cover
- Sterile ultrasound gel
- Transducer kit with all IV lines, transducer cables, and appropriate monitor setup.
- Chlorhexidine or other disinfectant solution
- Sterile towels or drapes
- Insertion needle with a guidewire
- Lidocaine with syringe/needle
- Suture material (silk or other nonabsorbable suture)
- Needle driver or sutures on a straight needle
- 11 Gauze
- Tegaderm
- BioPatch

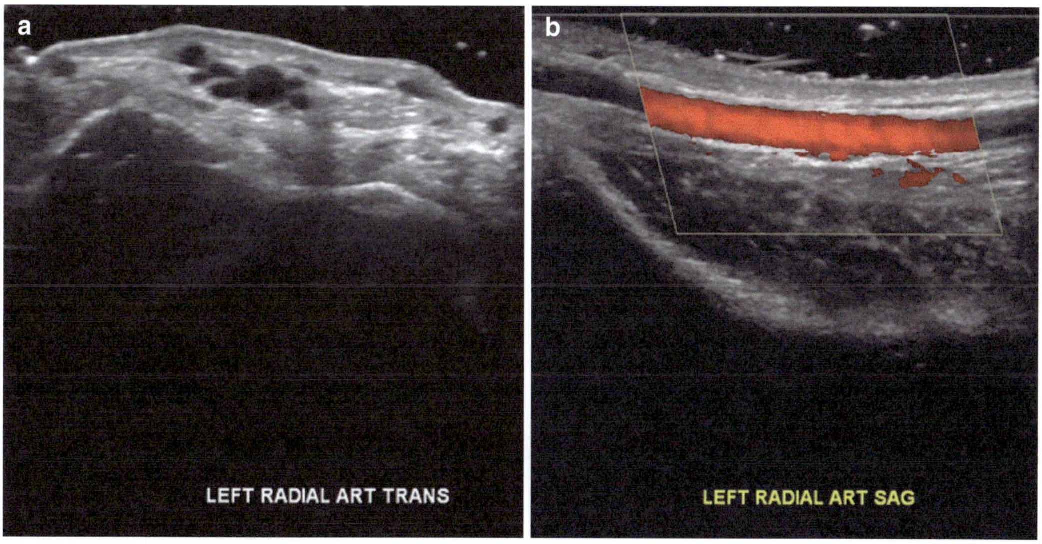

Fig. 15.23 B-mode and color Doppler images of the radial artery (**a**) short axis, (**b**) long axis

Preparation/Pre-procedural Evaluation

The anatomy of the selected insertion site should be assessed. Allen test should be performed prior to radial artery cauterization. The ultrasound machine should be positioned across the operator to allow real-time visualization of the needle. The patient's wrist should be secured to an arm board using tape after dorsiflexion of the wrist to approximately 60° over a small towel roll or Kerlix gauze roll.

On B-mode imaging, the radial artery is identified using a linear array transducer. The artery will be seen as an anechoic structure with visible pulsations of the vessel. Compression of the artery may make the pulsation of the artery easier to detect, although excessive pressure may collapse the artery in patients with shock. Poor perfusion may make it difficult to distinguish artery from vein. Doppler mode can be used to identify the artery if it is challenging on B-mode imaging. Visualization can be improved by adjusting the depth and gain on the ultrasound system.

The insertion site should be cleaned with chlorhexidine, and a sterile field needs to be created by draping sterile towels around the insertion site. A sterile probe cover should be placed over the ultrasound probe. Sterile field should be maintained throughout the procedure.

Procedure

An in-line approach where the probe is oriented parallel to the vessel and where the vessel appears as a tubular structure darkened area on the screen should be used. The skin is punctured parallel to the probe and the needle will be seen on the monitor from either the left or right, depending on the probe's orientation. The needle tip should be followed into the artery using ultrasound. In some cases, the needle may lie outside the vessel parallel to the artery but may appear to have penetrated the artery on ultrasound, but no blood return will be seen in the catheter chamber. In this case, the needle should be withdrawn and the probe should be recentered on the long axis of the artery, followed by reinsertion of the needle.

After successfully cannulating the vessel, the black tab on the catheter should be slid toward the needle which will advance the wire into the artery. Then the needle should be stabilized and the catheter should be advanced over the wire and into the artery. The catheter should then be connected to the pressure tubing, quickly flushed, and the adequacy of the arterial trace should be determined for optimal damping. The catheter should be sutured in place (Figs. 15.24 and 15.25) [33, 34].

Complications

- Bleeding
- Infection
- Thrombosis

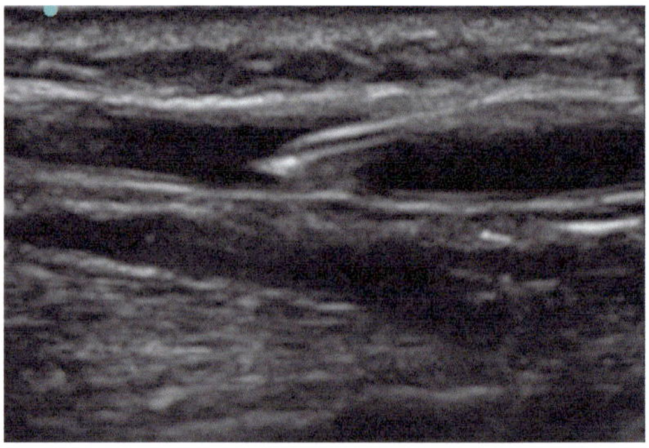

Fig. 15.24 B-mode of the radial artery (note intimal layer) with needle puncturing the artery in in-plane approach

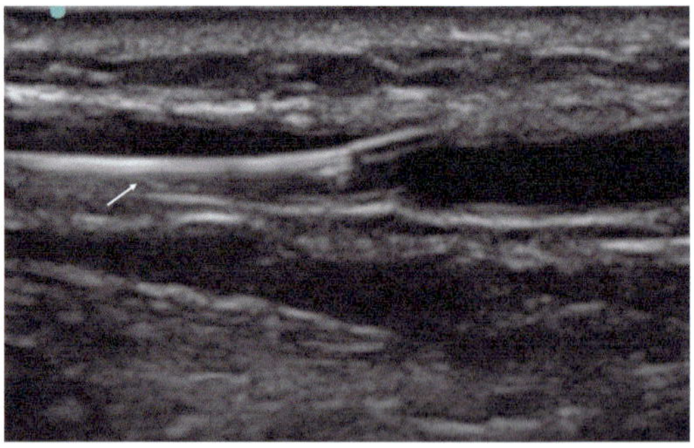

Fig. 15.25 Guidewire (arrow) being advanced into the radial artery

- Pain
- Embolization
- Ischemia
- Arteriovenous fistula

Pearls/Pitfalls

The main challenge when performing ultrasound-guided catheterization is visualization of the needle tip since radial artery is a very superficial structure. The unseen needle tip could be inserted more deeply than the operator is aware and can cause injury to deeper structures. For this reason, continuous visualization of the needle tip is critical during angiocatheter insertion. Another challenge encountered in patients with shock is vasospasm, which may prevent the operator from advancing the catheter into the arterial lumen. If this happens, ultrasound guidance should be used to find a more proximal location for insertion.

Integration into Clinical Practice

Radial artery catheterization is a common procedure in the care and management of critically ill patients in acute care settings. Arterial lines play a vital role in the management of critically ill requiring vasoactive medications, stroke patients where blood pressure titration is needed, and patients in the intensive care units requiring frequent blood draws for ABGs. Radial line cannulation is relatively simple procedure that has become even easier with the increasing use of ultrasound. All emergency physicians, intensivists, or anesthesiologists should be competent in using ultrasound for radial artery cannulation. Knowledge of sonographic anatomy and attention to the location of the needle tip during the procedure are essential aspects of the technique.

Evidence

A clinical trial comparing fluoroscopic and sonographic guidance for femoral artery catheterization demonstrated a significant advantage for ultrasound in the 30% of patients with a high femoral artery bifurcation. Several studies have shown the benefit of increased success rate of radial artery catheterization using ultrasound guidance in the emergency setting [35–37]. A recent meta-analysis of randomized controlled trials demonstrated that radial artery cannulation under ultrasound guidance increases the first-attempt success rate [38]. Improved success rates using ultrasound for arterial cannulation in pediatric patients have also been documented in the literature. Most recent Cochrane Systematic Review suggested that ultrasound guidance for radial artery cannulation improves first- and second-attempt success rates and decreases the rate of complications when compared with palpation or Doppler auditory assistance [39]. Ultrasound guidance can also decrease catheter-related infections due to reduction in insertion attempts and increased first-attempt success rates [40].

Key Points

- Ultrasound-guided arterial catheterizations have been associated with reduction in complications, improved first-attempt success rates, and decrease in infection rates.
- Aseptic precautions should be followed while placing arterial catheters.
- Use in-plane technique and follow the needle tip continuously after skin puncture.
- Excessive pressure may collapse the artery in patients with shock.
- Poor perfusion may make it difficult to distinguish artery from vein.

References

1. Moore CL, Copel J. Point-of-care ultrasonography. N Engl J Med. 2011;364:749–57.
2. Keenan SP. Use of ultrasound to place central lines. J Crit Care. 2002;17:126–37.
3. Maecken T, Grau T. Ultrasound imaging in vascular access. Crit Care Med. 2007;35:S178–85.

4. Leung J, Duffy M, Finckh A. Real-time ultrasonographically-guided internal jugular vein catheterization in the emergency department increases success rates and reduces complications: a randomized, prospective study. Ann Emerg Med. 2006;48:540–7.
5. Paul-Andrè C, Kendall J. Ultrasound guidance for vascular access. Emerg Med Clin N Am. 2004;22:749–73.
6. Augoustides J, Horak J, Ochroch A. A randomized controlled clinical trial of real-time needle-guided ultrasound for internal jugular venous cannulation in a large university anesthesia department. J Cardiothorac Vasc Anesth. 2005;19:310–5.
7. Mallory D, McGee W, Shawker T, Brennen M, Bailey K, Evans R, et al. Ultrasound guidance improves the success rate of internal jugular vein cannulation. A prospective, randomized trial. Chest. 1990;98:157–60.
8. Lamperti M, Caldiroli D, Cortellazzi P, Vailati D, Pedicelli A, Tosi F, et al. Safety and efficacy of ultrasound assistance during internal jugular vein cannulation in neurosurgical infants. Intensive Care Med. 2008;34:2100–5.
9. Serafimidis K, Sakorafas G, Konstantoudakis G, Petropoulou K, Giannopoulos G, Danias N, et al. Ultrasound-guided catheterization of the internal jugular vein in oncologic patients; comparison with the classical anatomic landmark technique: a prospective study. Int J Surg. 2009;7:526–8.
10. Troianos C, Jobes D, Ellison N. Ultrasound-guided cannulation of the internal jugular vein. A prospective, randomized study. Anesth Analg. 1991;72:823–6.
11. Karakitsos K, Labropoulos N, DeGroot E, Patrianakos AP, Kouraklis G, Poularas J. Real-time ultrasound-guided catheterisation of the internal jugular vein: a prospective comparison with the landmark technique in critical care patients. Crit Care. 2006;10:R162.
12. Denys B, Uretsky B, Reddy P. Ultrasound-assisted cannulation of the internal jugular vein: a prospective comparison to the external landmark-guided technique. Circulation. 1993;87:1557–62.
13. Etemad-Rezai R, Peck DJ. Ultrasound-guided thrombin injection of femoral artery pseudoaneurysms. Can Assoc Radiol J. 2003;54:118–20.
14. Ehieli WL, Bozdogan E, Janas G, Jaffe TA, Miller CM, Bashir MR, Allen BC. Imaging-guided percutaneous thrombin injection for the treatment of iatrogenic femoral artery pseudoaneurysms. Abdom Radiol (NY). 2019;44(3):1120–6.
15. Kacila M, Vranic H, Hadzimehmedagic A, Sehovic S, Granov N. The frequency of complications of pseudoaneurysms after cardiac interventional diagnostic and therapeutic interventions. Med Arh. 2011;65(2):78–81.
16. Hashemi Fard O. Iatrogenic femoral artery pseudoaneurysm (review of treatment options). ARYA Atheroscler. 2010;6(2):74–7.
17. Kronzon I. Diagnosis and treatment of iatrogenic femoral artery pseudoaneurysm: a review. J Am Soc Echocardiogr. 1997;10(3):236–45.
18. Chun E. Ultrasonographic evaluation of complications related to transfemoral arterial procedures. Ultrasonography. 2018;37(2):164–73.
19. Stone P, Campbell J, AbuRahma A. Femoral pseudoaneurysms after percutaneous access. J Vasc Surg. 2014;60:1359–66.
20. Bydawell G. Percutaneous thrombin injection for pseudoaneurysm treatment. S Afr J Radiol. 2013;17(1):41–2.
21. Paulson EK, Sheafor DH, Kliewer MA, Nelson RC, Eisenberg LB, Sebastian MW, et al. Treatment of iatrogenic femoral arterial pseudoaneurysms: comparison of US-guided thrombin injection with compression repair. Radiology. 2000;215:403–8.
22. Parás-Bravo P, Paz-Zulueta M, Sarabia-Lavin R, et al. Complications of peripherally inserted central venous catheters: a retrospective cohort study. PLoS One. 2016;11(9):e0162479.
23. Nichols I, Humphrey JP. The efficacy of upper arm placement of peripherally inserted central catheters using bedside ultrasound and microintroducer technique. J Infus Nurs. 2008;31:165–76.
24. Schweickert WD, Herlitz J, Pohlman AS, Gehlbach BK, Hall JB, Kress JP. A randomized, controlled trial evaluating postinsertion neck ultrasound in peripherally inserted central catheter procedures. Crit Care Med. 2009;37:1217–21.
25. Gonzalez R, Cassaro S. Percutaneous Central Catheter (PICC) [Updated 2019 Feb 11]. In: StatPearls [Internet]. Treasure Island: StatPearls Publishing; 2019. Available from: https://www.ncbi.nlm.nih.gov/books/NBK459338/.
26. Stokowski G, Steele D, Wilson D. The use of ultrasound to improve practice and reduce complication rates in PICC insertions. Art Sci Infus Nurs. 2009;32:145–55.
27. Pratt RJ, Pellowe CM, Wilson JA, et al. epic2: national evidence-based guidelines for preventing healthcare-associated infections in NHS hospitals in England. J Hosp Infect. 2007;65(Suppl 1):S1–64.
28. Katheria AC, Fleming SE, Kim JH. A randomized controlled trial of ultrasound-guided peripherally inserted central catheters compared with standard radiograph in neonates. J Perinatol. 2013;33:791–4.
29. Parkinson R, Gandhi M, Harper J, Archibald C. Establishing an ultrasound guided peripherally inserted central catheter (PICC) insertion service. Clin Radiol. 1998;53:33–6.
30. Sofocleous CT, Schur I, Cooper SG, et al. Sonographically guided placement of peripherally inserted central venous catheters: review of 355 procedures. AJR Am J Roentgenol. 1998;170:1613.
31. Yokota T, Tokumine J, Lefor AK, Hasegawa A, Yorozu T, Asao T. Ultrasound-guided placement of a midline catheter in a patient with extensive postburn contractures: a case report. Medicine. 2019;98(3):e14208.
32. Adams DZ, Little A, Vinsant C, Khandelwal S. The midline catheter: a clinical review. J Emerg Med. 2016;51(3):252–8.

33. Pierre L, Keenaghan M. Arterial lines. [Updated 2018 Dec 13]. In: StatPearls [Internet]. Treasure Island: StatPearls Publishing; 2019. Available from: https://www.ncbi.nlm.nih.gov/books/NBK499989/.
34. Ailon J, Mourad O, Chien V, Saun T, Dev SP. Videos in clinical medicine. Ultrasound-guided insertion of a radial arterial catheter. N Engl J Med. 2014;371(15):e21.
35. Shiver S, Blaivas M, Lyon M. A prospective comparison of ultrasound-guided and blindly placed radial arterial catheters. Acad Emerg Med. 2006;13:1275–9.
36. Seto AH, Abu-Fadel MS, Sparling JM, Zacharias SJ, Daly TS, Harrison AT, et al. Real-time ultrasound guidance facilitates femoral arterial access and reduces vascular complications: FAUST (Femoral Arterial Access With Ultrasound Trial). JACC Cardiovasc Interv. 2010;3:751–8.
37. Pachikara R, Gallagher P, Watcha M. Evaluation of ultrasound-guided radial artery cannulation in children. Pediatr Crit Care Med. 2009;10:45–8.
38. Bhattacharjee S, Maitra S, Baidya DK. Comparison between ultrasound guided technique and digital palpation technique for radial artery cannulation in adult patients: an updated meta-analysis of randomized controlled trials. J Clin Anesth. 2018;47:54–9.
39. Aouad-Maroun M, Raphael CK, Sayyid SK, Farah F, Akl EA. Ultrasound-guided arterial cannulation for paediatrics. Cochrane Database Syst Rev. 2016;(9):CD011364.
40. Miller AG, Bardin AJ. Review of ultrasound-guided radial artery catheter placement. Respir Care. 2016;61(3):383–8.

Index

S. Adhikari, M. Blaivas (eds.), *The Ultimate Guide to Point-of-Care Ultrasound-Guided Procedures*, https://doi.org/10.1007/978-3-030-28267-7

V

MIX
Papier aus verantwortungsvollen Quellen
Paper from responsible sources
FSC® C105338

If you have any concerns about our products,
you can contact us on
ProductSafety@springernature.com

In case Publisher is established outside the EU,
the EU authorized representative is:
Springer Nature Customer Service Center GmbH
Europaplatz 3, 69115 Heidelberg, Germany

Printed by Libri Plureos GmbH
in Hamburg, Germany